Asian American Mental Health
Assessment Theories and Methods

International and Cultural Psychology Series

Series Editor: **Anthony Marsella**, *University of Hawaii, Honolulu, Hawaii*

ASIAN AMERICAN MENTAL HEALTH
Assessment Theories and Methods
Edited by Karen S. Kurasaki, Sumie Okazaki, and Stanley Sue

Asian American Mental Health
Assessment Theories and Methods

Edited by

Karen S. Kurasaki
The California Endowment Funds
Sacramento, California

Sumie Okazaki
University of Illinois at Urbana-Champaign
Champaign, Illinois

Stanley Sue
University of California
Davis, California

Springer Science+Business Media, LLC

Library of Congress Cataloging-in-Publication Data

Asian American mental health: assessment theories and methods/edited by Karen S. Kurasaki, Sumie Okazaki, Stanley Sue.
    p.   cm. — (international and cultural psychology)
   Includes bibliographical references and index.
   ISBN 978-1-4613-5216-7   ISBN 978-1-4615-0735-2 (eBook)
   DOI 10.1007/978-1-4615-0735-2
    1. Asian Americans—Mental health. 2. Asian Americans—Mental health services. I. Title: Asian American mental health. II. Kurasaki, Karen S. III. Okazaki, Sumie. IV. Sue, Stanley. V. Series.

RC451.5.A75 A83 2001
362.2'089'95073—dc21

2002025685

ISBN 978-1-4613-5216-7

©2002 Springer Science+Business Media New York
Originally published by Kluwer / Plenum Publishers, New York in 2002
Softcover reprint of the hardcover 1st edition 2002

10 9 8 7 6 5 4 3 2 1

A C.I.P. record for this book is available from the Library of Congress

All rights reserved

No part of this book may be reproduced, stored in a retrieval system, or transmitted
in any form or by any means, electronic, mechanical, photocopying, microfilming, recording,
or otherwise, without written permission from the Publisher, with the exception of any material
supplied specifically for the purpose of being entered and executed on a computer system,
for exclusive use by the purchaser of the work.

ABOUT THE AUTHORS

Doris F. Chang, Ph.D., earned her doctorate in clinical psychology from the University of California, Los Angeles. She is currently a NIMH postdoctoral fellow at the Department of Social Medicine, Harvard Medical School. Her interests include cross-cultural psychiatric diagnosis and treatment, domestic violence, and community mental health initiatives in Asian communities in the U.S. and China.

Yulia Chentsova-Dutton, is currently a graduate student in the Department of Psychology at Stanford University. She received her B.A. at Williams College and her master's degree in Clinical Science and Psychopathology at the University of Minnesota. Her research interests include cultural influences on emotional processes in healthy, depressed, and socially anxious individuals.

Fanny M. Cheung, Ph.D., is chairperson and professor of the Department of Psychology at The Chinese University of Hong Kong. She is principal investigator of the Chinese Personality Assessment Inventory project, published the Chinese Minnesota Multiphasic Personality Inventories, and was founding chairperson of the Equal Opportunities Commission of Hong Kong from 1996-1999. Her research interests are personality assessment, psychopathology, and gender studies.

Jean Lau Chin, Ed.D./ABPP, is president of CEO Services, providing clinical, educational, and organizational development services, and on the faculty of Center of Minority Training in Psychology, Boston Medical Center. Her professional interests include cultural competence, women's issues, community-based services, racial/ethnicity, integrating health and mental health, and systems outcomes.

Rita Chi-Ying Chung, Ph.D., is associate professor in the Counseling and Development Program, Graduate School of Education, George Mason University. Her research focuses on psychosocial adjustment of refugees and immigrants, interethnic group relations and racial stereotypes, coping strategies in dealing with racism and its impact on psychological well-being, and multicultural issues in mental health, achievement motivation and aspirations.

Richard H. Dana, Ph.D., is research professor (honorary) at Regional Research Institute, Portland State University. His interests are in multicultural assessment-intervention process model application to California public mental health services utilizing research findings on matching, acculturation, and cultural competency measures; textbook for assessment courses and book on exemplar instrument, TEMAS (with Giuseppe Costantino).

Adam J. Darnell is a doctoral student in community psychology in the Department of Psychology at Georgia State University. His research interest is in the assessment and promotion of cultural competence at the organizational level in mental health agencies.

ABOUT THE AUTHORS

Nancy Farwell, Ph.D., is assistant professor of social work, University of Washington. She has extensive practice experience with refugee families, and conducts community-based research with multiethnic youth in public housing. Her research interests in community mental health, psychosocial issues of war-affected children, and post-conflict recovery have taken her to Asia and Africa.

Marjorie Kagawa-Singer, Ph.D., R.N, M.N., is associate professor of Public Health and Asian American Studies Center, University of California, Los Angeles. Her research focuses on the disparities in physical and mental health care outcomes of ethnic minority populations, primarily Asian Americans/Pacific Islanders, with chronic illnesses. Presently, her research focuses on developing standards of cultural competence in health care.

Ellen S. Kim is a doctoral student in Counseling Psychology at New York University. She is currently an intern at Mt. Sinai School of Medicine, Rehabilitation Psychology and Clinical Neuropsychology Service. Her research interests are in the areas of emotional intelligence and cultural aspects of cognitive abilities.

Su Yeong Kim is a doctoral candidate in the Human Development Graduate Program, housed in the Department of Human and Community Development at the University of California, Davis. Her research examines how cultural and family factors influence the social, emotional, and academic adjustment of ethnic minority adolescents and children of immigrants.

Alan K. Koike, M.D., MSHS, is assistant clinical professor in the Department of Psychiatry, University of California Davis Medical School. His research interests include Asian American mental health and health services.

Karen S. Kurasaki, Ph.D., is program officer at The California Endowment in Sacramento, California. Her research interests include ethnic and racial identity development, children's mental health systems of care, and community-based prevention interventions to strengthen youth and families.

Richard M. Lee, Ph.D., is assistant professor in the Department of Psychology at University of Minnesota, Twin Cities. His research focuses on cultural socialization processes within Asian American families, including acculturation, ethnic identity, and parent-child relationships. He also conducts research on social and cultural influences on social connectedness.

Frederick T. L. Leong, Ph.D., is professor of psychology at Ohio State University. He obtained his Ph.D. from the University of Maryland with a double specialty in Counseling and Industrial/Organizational Psychology. His major research interests are in vocational psychology (career development of ethnic minorities), cross-cultural psychology (particularly culture and mental health and cross-cultural psychotherapy), and organizational behavior.

ABOUT THE AUTHORS

Keh-Ming Lin, M.D., MPH, is professor of psychiatry, University of California in Los Angeles, and Director of NIMH/Harbor-UCLA Research Center on the Psychobiology of Ethnicity. He is the founder of two major Asian mental health centers in Los Angeles and has made significant contributions on cross-ethnic psychopharmacology, pharmacogenetics, psychiatric nosology, epidemiology and refugee mental health.

Margaret T. Lin, M.D., is currently a 4th year resident in the Department of Psychiatry at Harbor UCLA Medical Center. As an APA/CMHS Minority Fellowship fellow (2001-2002), she has been working with Dr. Keh-Ming Lin on a number of projects related to issues of culture in psychiatry. Her special area of interest is in help-seeking behavior and compliance of psychiatric treatment in elderly Asian women.

Michael Lynch Maestas, Ph.D., is on the staff of the Counseling Center at the University of Missouri-Columbia. His professional interests include American ethnic minority issues, acculturation, ethnic identity development and retention, multicultural counseling and assessment competencies, training in professional psychology, and psychological evaluation and assessment.

Tamiko Mogami is a doctoral student in Counseling Psychology at New York University. She has just completed a psychology research fellowship at the Tibly Foundation affiliated with Montefiore Hospital, Albert Einstein College of Medicine. Her research and professional interests are in the areas of psychopathology, cognitive functioning, and schizophrenia.

Sumie Okazaki, Ph.D., is assistant professor in the Clinical Community Division in the Department of Psychology at the University of Illinois at Urbana-Champaign. Her research interests include Asian American mental health, the roles of culture and ethnicity in emotion and psychopathology, and cultural validity of assessment instruments.

Gargi Roysircar, Ph.D., is professor and director of the Multicultural Center for Research and Practice (www.multiculturalcenter.org) in the Department of Clinical Psychology, Antioch New England Graduate School of Antioch University. She conducts research on the interface of acculturation and ethnic identity with the mental health of immigrants and ethnic minorities, worldview differences between and within cultural groups, multicultural competencies and training in professional psychology, and multicultural assessment and instrumentation.

Jonathan Sandoval, Ph.D., is professor of education at the University of California, Davis, and is former President of APA's Division of School Psychology. His research interests include issues in applied measurement, the prevention of school failure, the training of education professionals, and the promotion of mental health in schools.

ABOUT THE AUTHORS

Michael Smukler, Ph.D., is a management consultant specializing in behavioral outcomes management and quality assessment/improvement in publicly funded mental health systems. His research and publications have focused on the development of culturally-competent level-of-care schemes for community mental health systems, and equity and access in public mental health programs.

Stanley Sue, Ph.D., is professor of psychology, psychiatry, and Asian American Studies at the University of California, Davis. He received a B.S. from the University of Oregon and Ph.D. in psychology from University of California, Los Angeles. His research interests include ethnicity and cultural competency, Asian American mental health, treatment, and community psychology.

Lisa A. Suzuki, Ph.D., is an associate professor in the Department of Applied Psychology at New York University. Her main research interests have been in the areas of multicultural assessment, training, and qualitative research methods. She is the coeditor of the *Handbook of Multicultural Assessment* and the *Handbook of Multicultural Counseling*.

Mei Tang, Ph.D., is an assistant professor in the Counseling Program at the University of Cincinnati, has done research and teaching in career development of minority group members, cross-cultural counseling, counseling in schools, and research and assessment in counseling. She is also editorial board member for *Career Development Quarterly* and *Journal of College Counseling*.

Jeanne L. Tsai, Ph.D., is currently an assistant professor in the Department of Psychology at Stanford University. She received her Ph.D. in Clinical Psychology at UC Berkeley. Her research focuses on three main topics: (1) cultural identity and orientation, (2) cultural influences on emotional processes, and (3) minority mental health.

Edwina S. Uehara, Ph.D., is an associate professor of social work, University of Washington. She has extensive ethnographic research experience, particularly with ethnic minority communities and populations. Her interests include multicultural mental health practice, critical theory and critical pedagogy, and the integration of ethnography and clinical practice.

Vivian Y. Wong is a doctoral student in the Development of Human and Community Development at the University of California, Davis. She is interested in the socio-emotional development of children and adolescents. Her research interests include cross-cultural research with Asians and Asian Americans and the interactions between parents and children.

Greg Yamashiro is a doctoral student at the University of Washington, School of Social Work. His interests include the conceptualization of culture and its use in social work research and practice, mental health, gerontology, cross-generational

ABOUT THE AUTHORS

issues among cultural minority groups, and use of temporality in theoretical and research models.

Joyce Wu Yeh, Ph.D., has been in private practice in the Los Angeles area since 1988. She was psychologist and coordinator of the Children's Program at Coastal Asian Pacific Mental Health Services, Los Angeles County, from 1984 to 1998. She has been actively serving the community as a speaker on cross-cultural and parenting issues since 1984.

May Yeh, Ph.D., is assistant professor of psychology at San Diego State University; research scientist, Child and Adolescent Services Research Center, San Diego Children's Hospital and Health Center; adjunct assistant professor of psychiatry, University of California in San Diego; and a licensed clinical psychologist. Her primary interests are cultural issues in mental health service delivery to children.

Yu-Wen Ying, Ph.D., is professor at the School of Social Welfare, University of California, Berkeley. Her major research interests include immigrant and refugee adaptation, acculturation and ethnic identity formation, family relationships in migrant families, cross-cultural conception of depression, and culturally competent mental health prevention and treatment interventions, with a special focus on Asian American populations.

Nolan W. S. Zane, Ph.D., is director of the National Research Center on Asian American Mental Health and associate professor of psychology and Asian American studies at the University of California, Davis. His research interests include outcomes of culturally oriented treatments for ethnic minority clients, change mechanisms in mental health interventions, evaluation of behavior change programs, and cultural determinants of addictive behaviors among Asians.

ACKNOWLEDGEMENTS

This book is a result of a truly collective effort. We would like to thank Dr. Jennifer Lee, Su Yeong Kim, Kim Schimmel, Arnold Ho, Soojin Myoung, and Billie Gabriel of the National Research Center on Asian American Mental Health for their capable administrative and editorial assistance, and Dr. Richard Dana for his sage editorial advice. Our thanks to Dr. Anthony Marsella, the Series Editor, for his encouragement and support of this book project, and Joyce F. Liu for her excellent assistance with the final editorial procedures. Special thanks are also due to Christiane Roll, our publishing editor at Kluwer Academic Press, for her support, patience, and guidance in bringing this book to fruition. This project was supported in part by the grants from the NIMH (1R01-MH44331 & 1R01-MH59616) and the University of California Humanities Research Institute. And finally, we would like to express our gratitude to all the contributors to this volume for their patience with the arduous editorial process and for their collective wisdom that makes this book a valuable source book for the field of Asian American psychology.

Karen Kurasaki
Sumie Okazaki
Stanley Sue

TABLE OF CONTENTS

1. **Introduction**   1
   Karen S. Kurasaki
   Sumie Okazaki

SECTION I: CULTURAL RELEVANCE OF DIAGNOSTIC CATEGORIES: A CONCEPTUAL DISCUSSION

2. **Understanding the Rates and Distribution of Mental Disorders**   9
   Doris F. Chang

3. **Examining the Usefulness of DSM-IV**   29
   Richard H. Dana

4. **Toward a New Paradigm: A Cultural Systems Approach**   47
   Marjorie Kagawa-Singer
   Rita Chi-Ying Chung

5. **Challenging the Myth of a Culture Free Nosological System**   67
   Keh-Ming Lin
   Margaret Lin

SECTION II: THEORIES OF RELEVANT SOCIOCULTURAL VARIABLES

6. **Assessing Acculturation and Cultural Variables**   77
   Gargi Roysircar
   Michael Lynch Maestas

7. **Models of Cultural Orientation: Differences Between American-born and Overseas-born Asians**   95
   Jeanne L. Tsai
   Yulia Chentsova-Dutton

8. **Cultural Variations in Self-Construal as a Mediator of Distress and Well-being**   107
   Sumie Okazaki

CONTENTS

9. **The Use of Culturally-Based Variables in Assessment: Studies on Loss of Face** 123
Nolan Zane
May Yeh

SECTION III: ISSUES OF PSYCHOMETRIC EQUIVALENCE ACROSS CULTURES

10. **Universal and Indigenous Dimensions of Chinese Personality** 141
Fanny M. Cheung

11. **Interpreting Cultural Variations in Cognitive Profiles** 159
Lisa A. Suzuki
Tamiko Mogami
Ellen S. Kim

12. **The Conception of Depression in Chinese Americans** 173
Yu-Wen Ying

13. **Assessing Asian and Asian American Parenting: A Review of the Literature** 185
Su Yeong Kim
Vivian Y. Wong

SECTION IV: CULTURALLY INFORMED ASSESSMENT, RESEARCH, AND PRACTICE

14. **Assessing Psychiatric Prevalence Rates Among Asian Americans** 205
Karen S. Kurasaki
Alan K. Koike

15. **The Place of Ethnographic Understanding in the Assessment of Asian American Mental Health** 219
Edwina S. Uehara
Nancy Farwell
Greg Yamashiro
Michael Smukler

16. **The Clinical Assessment of Asian American Children** 233
May Yeh
Joyce Wu Yeh

CONTENTS xv

17. **Examining the Role of Culture in Educational Assessment** 251
Jonathan Sandoval

18. **A Cultural Accommodation Approach to Career Assessment**
with Asian Americans 265
Frederick T. L. Leong
Mei Tang

19. **Theory and Method of Multicultural Counseling Competency**
Assessment 283
Richard M. Lee
Adam J. Darnell

20. **Assessment of Cultural Competence in Mental Health Systems of** 301
Care for Asian Americans
Jean Lau Chin

SECTION V: CONCLUSIONS

21. **Advances in the Scientific Study of Asian Americans** 317
Stanley Sue

SUBJECT INDEX 323

AUTHOR INDEX 331

KAREN S. KURASAKI AND SUMIE OKAZAKI

CHAPTER 1

INTRODUCTION

1. BOOK DEVELOPMENT AND PURPOSE

Ethnicity and culture profoundly influence people's beliefs about mental illness, their experiences of psychiatric distress, and communication of distress. Conducting culturally valid assessments of Asian Americans' cognitive, emotional, psychological, and social functioning is a major challenge that confronts both research and practice today. Mental health assessments with Asian Americans raise a number of intriguing questions. For example, how universal are the Big Five personality characteristics? Is the Diagnostic and Statistical Manual (DSM) system universally useful with members of various ethnic groups? Which diagnostic categories are relevant to Asian Americans, and what measurement instruments are available? How do we measure acculturation and ethnic identity of Asian Americans, and are such constructs best conceptualized as a unidimensional or multidimensional process? How do we develop linguistically appropriate measurement instruments?

In 1998, the National Research Center on Asian American Mental Health, with funding from the University of California Humanities Research Institute and the National Institute of Mental Health, convened a two-day conference to discuss the current state of knowledge as well as the challenges facing Asian American mental health assessment. Scholars in the fields of anthropology, Asian American studies, counseling, education, history, psychiatry, psychology, and sociology gathered to examine the conceptual and methodological issues related to conducting culturally valid mental health assessments of Asian Americans. This book is the culmination of the works presented at the 1998 conference, with additional contributions from experts on a wide range of topics that are essential to practice and research.

The nature of assessing mental health and illness across diverse ethnic and cultural groups is complex and fascinating. Current assessment methods generally entail administration of Western designed instruments and application of Western criteria across cultural groups. Rarely are instruments translated into all (or even the most) common Asian languages or norms properly established for different Asian American cultural and linguistic populations. By using the available assessment instruments and norms on Asian Americans, we assume equivalent diagnostic concepts across cultures and ethnicity; a questionable assumption given how meanings related to health and illness are socially constructed. For example, culturally laden meanings of health and illness are evident in the linguistic differences we find in describing human emotions. Individuals from Western cultures commonly describe emotions using color imagery – someone in distress feels *blue*, whereas individuals from Eastern cultures may express feelings using physiological metaphors—something pressing on the heart or chest (Kleinman, 1982). There is an ongoing debate as to whether physiological conceptualizations of health and illness, such as those documented more commonly among individuals of Asian heritage, may lead one to manifest distress primarily through physical or bodily symptoms. New evidence also raises questions as to whether thresholds for what is seen as pathological or not may be culture based and vary across groups. This book addresses such central questions in diagnosing and conceptualizing mental disorders.

There is danger in not responding to individuals within our diverse society with assessment techniques that are sensitive to cultural variations in symptom presentation. Assessments that are not culturally informed can result in missed diagnoses of real and treatable psychological problems, as well as over-pathologizing culturally normal thoughts and behaviors. How then do we distinguish between psychopathology and culturally appropriate thoughts and behaviors? This book seeks to provide some insights into this and similar questions.

Another important challenge in conducting assessments with Asian Americans is that the population, whose members we seek to assess, is a moving target of a sort. The sheer demographic heterogeneity within this population group with respect to national origin, language, religion, immigration history, socioeconomic status, generational status, community contexts, and other dimensions is reflected in the diverse psychological experiences of individuals of Asian heritage residing in the United States today. Adding complexity to this population heterogeneity is the ever-shifting backdrop of immigration patterns, the changing nature of the Asian diaspora across the world, and fluid movements of persons of Asian heritage and their families across continents, nations, and cultures. Looking to the future, what appears certain is that Asian American population in the U.S. will continue to grow in size and complexity. From 1970 to 1990, the Asian American population doubled in size every decade. It is projected that by the year 2020, the Asian American population will be approximately 20.2 million, or about 8 percent of the total U.S. population. Such rapid projected population growth of Asian Americans beseeches us to seriously examine issues related to culturally valid mental health assessment among this population. This book examines some of the central issues in characterizing the diversity within the population.

Indeed, in order to conduct culturally valid assessments with Asian Americans, state-of-the-art resources are needed to: 1) guide researchers on methodological and conceptual issues in conducting culturally valid assessment of psychological experiences with Asian American; 2) provide practical guidelines for researchers and clinicians on techniques and approaches specific to conducting culturally valid assessment with Asian Americans; and 3) educate students in mental health fields regarding specific cultural considerations for assessing the psychological status of

INTRODUCTION

Asian Americans. This book was compiled to respond to the gap in the available literature with cutting-edge guidelines and thorough analyses of the critical issues related to assessing Asian American mental health. While recognizing their within-group diversity, there are also common psychosocial experiences that broadly affect Asian American individuals' well-being and distress due to shared cultural values, shared immigrant experience, or shared ethnic minority experience. For these reasons, the issues concerning Asian American mental health assessment are addressed in here in a single volume. To the extent that it is possible, given the current state of knowledge, ethnic- and culture-specific conceptual, research, and practice issues are addressed as well.

2. BOOK ORGANIZATION

This book is organized in five sections that cover conceptual, theoretical, methodological, and practice issues related to Asian American mental health assessment. **Section I** includes four chapters that provide a conceptual discussion of the cultural relevance of Western diagnostic categories. In Chapter 2, Doris Chang critically examines the methodological procedures used in psychiatric epidemiological research here and abroad. D. Chang also provides valuable guidelines for interpreting the rates and distribution of mental disorders among ethnic minorities, and particularly Asian Americans, that have been obtained from these studies. In the third chapter, Richard Dana discusses the goodness-of-fit between standard assessment instruments, which rely on the DSM-IV categories, and use with multicultural populations, particularly Asian Americans. In Chapter 4, Marjorie Kagawa-Singer and Rita Chung provide a conceptual overview of how meanings of health and illness are socially constructed and how assessment strategies that decontextualize human behavior from their cultural context can lead to findings that are merely artifacts of the methodology itself. Their chapter thoroughly addresses the theoretical assumptions and methodological fallacies that underlie the search for universals rather than the cultural specificity of mental illness. Finally in Chapter 5, Keh-Ming Lin and Margaret Lin argue that the term *culture bound syndrome*, while often used to highlight the power of culture in shaping the experience and expression of distress, also implicitly endorses the deep-rooted bias that the current nosological system (i.e., DSM-IV) is *culture free*.

Section II is comprised of four chapters that examine relevant sociocultural theories and variables used to characterize individual differences within the Asian American population. In Chapter 6, Gargi Roysicar and Michael Maestas present a thorough discussion of the research covering the domains of acculturation, acculturative stress, and ethnic identity. In the seventh chapter, Jeanne Tsai and Yulia Chentsova-Dutton summarize the current state-of-the-art in the conception and assessment of cultural orientation in Asian Americans and present innovative research findings that support the use of different models for assessing cultural orientation in immigrant versus U.S.-born Asian Americans. In Chapter 8, Sumie Okazaki critically examines the assessment of independent and interdependent self-construals and the complex relationship between self-construals and psychological distress in Asian Americans. In Chapter 9, Nolan Zane and May Yeh examine how incorporating interpersonally-based variables such as loss of face into the treatment process may be the key to improving access and care to Asian American clients. Together, these chapters provide much needed clarity to the definitions of cultural variables that are critical to understanding the pathogenesis and treatment of mental illness among Asian Americans.

Section III contains four chapters that examine issues of psychometric equivalence across cultures. In Chapter 10, Fanny Cheung presents research findings from a comparison between Hong Kong and U.S. Chinese norms on the Big Five personality factors. In Chapter 11, Lisa Suzuki, Tamiko Mogami, and Ellen Kim discuss the psychometric properties of tests of intelligence, abilities, and achievement and their appropriateness for use with Asian Americans. In Chapter 12, Yu-Wen Ying examines research evidence that suggests that the meaning of depression is inextricably linked with the culturally defined sense of self. In Chapter 13, Su Yeong Kim and Vivian Wong provide an overview of the parenting literature from both the quantitative and qualitative research paradigms. Their review of parenting concepts, goals, and values provides a foundation for developing more culturally relevant measures to assess Asian American parenting.

Section IV presents applied models for conducting culturally informed assessment research and practice. In Chapter 14, Karen Kurasaki and Alan Koike provide recommendations for conducting culturally valid research to estimate psychiatric prevalence rates among Asian Americans. In the next chapter, Edwina Uehara, Nancy Farwell, Greg Yamashiro, and Michael Smukler provide a model for incorporating qualitative research methods into the mental health assessment of Asian Americans in both research and practice settings. In Chapter 16, May Yeh and Joyce Yeh survey the available research on behavior checklists and projective tests that are widely used in assessing children, and how such measures have faired in clinical evaluations of Asian American children. Yeh and Yeh also provide practical strategies for interpreting findings from clinical evaluations of Asian American children from a cultural framework. In Chapter 17, Jonathan Sandoval provides a conceptual discussion of and practice strategies for a culturally informed approach to evaluating the education performance of Asian American children, with particular attention to children whose primary language is not English. In Chapter 18, Frederick Leong and Mei Tang review the literature on career development assessment with Asian Americans, including a brief discussion of the problems of psychometric equivalence across cultures in both personality and career development assessment. Leong and Tang also provide a thorough presentation of research findings supporting the innovation of a more integrative model to improve the validity of career development assessment with Asian Americans. In Chapter 19, Richard Lee and Adam Darnell survey the models used to assess practitioner cultural competency among those providing services to Asian American clients. Finally in the last chapter of this section, Jean Lau Chin provides a history of how measurement tools for assessing cultural competence in mental health care systems have been developed, and presents quality of care guidelines at both the system and client levels that promote culturally valid assessments of service delivery outcomes with Asian Americans.

INTRODUCTION

Section V, the final chapter of this book by Stanley Sue, synthesizes and extends the ideas and issues put forth in this compendium volume. Our goal for this book is to move the field forward by focusing attention on some of the most important questions about the cultural nature of diagnostic and assessment processes facing the mental health community. In editing this volume, we were delighted to see the progress being made on conceptual, methodological, and practical fronts, yet humbled by the many challenges that still remain in conducting culturally valid assessment research and practice with Asian Americans. It is our hope that this volume will be a valuable resource to students and professionals who engage in psychological research and practice that involve Asian American groups and individuals.

SECTION I: CULTURAL RELEVANCE OF DIAGNOSTIC CATEGORIES: A CONCEPTUAL DISCUSSION

2. **Understanding the Rates and Distribution of Mental Disorders**
Doris F. Chang

3. **Examining the Usefulness of DSM-IV**
Richard H. Dana

4. **Toward a New Paradigm: A Cultural Systems Approach**
Marjorie Kagawa-Singer
Rita Chi-Ying Chung

5. **Challenging the Myth of a Culture Free Nosological System**
Keh-Ming Lin
Margaret Lin

DORIS F. CHANG

CHAPTER 2

UNDERSTANDING THE RATES AND DISTRIBUTION
OF MENTAL DISORDERS

1. INTRODUCTION

The increasing diversity of the American public has challenged mental health professionals to expand their knowledge base to include issues of race, culture, and ethnicity. A fundamental issue is whether or not the rates and distribution of mental disorder in the community vary by ethnic group. Unfortunately, this deceptively simple question has not been satisfactorily answered despite the growing number of studies examining mental illness among European Americans, African Americans, Latinos, and more recently American Indians and Asian Americans. Critical methodological and conceptual problems have complicated our understanding and assessment of ethnic differences and highlight the need for improvements in research methods and assessment practices. This chapter will review the available community prevalence data for Asian Americans compared to other groups and discuss the conceptual and methodological issues that have influenced the state of the field. In addition, within-group variables that influence the prevalence of mental disorders will be discussed.

For over three decades, significant controversy has surrounded the assessment of mental disorders in Asian Americans. Two opposing hypotheses have been advanced in predictions about the prevalence of psychiatric problems among Asian Americans. The first suggests that rates will be low because Asian Americans are seen as an extremely well-adjusted group, as exemplified in the "model minority" stereotype. Low rates of psychiatric disorders may also be related to the tendency by persons of Asian heritage to manifest their psychic distress as physical ailments. The second hypothesis suggests that rates of psychiatric problems will be high in this group due to the stress associated with immigration and acculturation. In fact, data from a variety of domestic and international studies have provided partial support for both hypotheses, suggesting that prevalence estimates for Asian Americans must be interpreted against the conceptual and methodological framework of each particular study. In particular, how each study grapples with issues such as sampling, demographic diversity, language, variations in symptom expression, and case identification may have important implications for the validity and generalizability of the findings. This chapter will begin with a review of findings from psychiatric epidemiological surveys conducted in the United States and in overseas Asian communities, followed by a discussion of important conceptual and methodological issues that influence the assessment of Asian American mental health. Although a number of early studies on Asian Americans examined their use of treatment services (e.g., S. Sue & McKinney, 1975; Kitano, 1969), this chapter will not include estimates of treated prevalence due to space limitations. Moreover, because data suggest that Asian Americans are less likely than the general population to use services, prevalence estimates of psychopathology based solely on clinical samples are likely to paint a biased picture (S. Sue, D. W. Sue, L. Sue, & Takeuchi, 1995).

2. ETHNIC DIFFERENCES IN EPIDEMIOLOGICAL SURVEYS

The following review of epidemiological surveys of mental disorders includes studies conducted in the United States as well those conducted in overseas Asian communities. Specifically, only those studies that administered structured diagnostic research interviews capable of generating reliable psychiatric diagnoses by trained lay persons in the general populations were included in this review. A summary of lifetime prevalence rates of selected disorders is presented for each study in Tables 1 and 2. Missing data in the table results from differences in the number of disorders assessed for each study, as well as differences in the level of analysis (i.e., "any phobia" versus agoraphobia, simple phobia, and social phobia).

The earliest psychiatric epidemiological study conducted using a structured interview schedule in a community setting was the Epidemiological Catchment Area (ECA) study. Conducted in conjunction with five major universities, the ECA study examined the prevalence and incidence of mental disorders in five community catchment areas: New Haven, Connecticut (Yale University); Baltimore, Maryland (John Hopkins University); St. Louis, Missouri (Washington University); Durham, North Carolina (Duke University); and Los Angeles, California (University of California, Los Angeles). Over 20,000 respondents aged 18 years or older were interviewed, with each site sampling more than 3,000 community residents and 500 institutional residents. The National Institute of Mental Health (NIMH) Diagnostic Interview Schedule (DIS), a structured interview designed for administration by nonprofessional interviewers, was used to generate Diagnostic and Statistical Manual of Mental Disorders (Third Edition) (DSM-III) diagnoses. Results indicated that nearly 20% of the U.S. population were currently experiencing at least one of 17 DSM-III mental disorders, or had experienced one within the past six months (Robins & Reiger, 1991). Table 1 summarizes key ECA study results for the total sample (N = 19,640). The most common lifetime psychiatric diagnosis was phobia (14.3%), followed by alcohol abuse/dependence (13.8%), generalized anxiety disorder (8.5%), major depressive episode (6.3%) and dysthymia (3.2%).

UNDERSTANDING THE RATES AND DISTRIBUTION OF MENTAL DISORDERS 11

Table 1. Lifetime Prevalence Rates of Mental Disorders by Study: DIS or DSM-III for the United States

Mental Disorder	ECA[a] (N=19,640)	United States ECA Asians[b] (n=242)	ECA-LA Asians[b] (n=161)
Mood Disorders			
Major depressive episode	6.3	3.4	3.2
Dysthymia	3.2	3.0	3.3
Manic episode	0.8	0.0	0.0
Anxiety Disorders/ Somatization			
Generalized anxiety disorder	8.5†	—	—
Panic disorder	1.6		
Any phobia	14.3	6.6	5.6
Agoraphobia	5.6	—	—
Simple phobia	11.3	—	—
Social phobia	2.7	—	—
Obsessive-compulsive disorder	2.6	1.0	0.2
Somatization	0.1		
Substance Use Disorders			
Alcohol abuse/dependence	13.8	7.1	7.1
Drug abuse/ dependence	6.2	2.3	2.1
Other Disorders			
Schizophrenia/ schizophreniform	1.5	0.2	
Antisocial personality	2.6	0.2	0.2

Note: Not all disorders assessed for each study. Empty cells indicate zero cases found.
† Assessed in only 3 of 5 sites.
[a] Robins & Regier (1991).
[b] A. Y. Zhang & Snowden (1999).

Table 2. Lifetime Prevalence Rates of Mental Disorders by Study: DIS or DSM-III, International Rates

Mental Disorder	Taipei, Taiwan[a] (N=5,005)	Shanghai, China[b] (N=3,098)	Shatin, Hong Kong[c] (N=7,229)	Seoul, Korea[d] (N=3,134)
Mood Disorders				
Major depressive episode	0.9	0.2	1.9	3.3
Dysthymia	0.9	0.3	2.0	2.4
Manic episode	0.2	0.0	0.2	0.4
Anxiety Disorders/ Somatization				
Generalized anxiety disorder	3.7	—	9.5	3.6
Panic disorder	0.2	0.1	0.3	1.1
Any phobia	4.2	1.5	2.1	5.9
Agoraphobia	1.1	—	—	2.1
Simple phobia	0.6	—	—	5.4
Social phobia	3.6	—	—	0.5
Obsessive-compulsive disorder	0.9	0.1	1.1	2.3
Somatization	0.0	0.0	0.2	0.0
Substance Use Disorders				
Alcohol abuse/dependence	5.2	0.5	4.5	21.7
Drug abuse/ dependence	0.1	—	0.2	0.9
Other Disorders				
Schizophrenia/ schizophreniform	0.3	0.2	0.1	0.3
Antisocial personality	0.1	—	1.6	2.1

Note: Not all disorders assessed for each study. Empty cells indicate zero cases found.

[a] Hwu et al. (1989).

[b] C. H. Wang et al. (1992).

[c] Chen et al. (1993).

[d] C. K. Lee et al. (1990).

UNDERSTANDING THE RATES AND DISTRIBUTION OF MENTAL DISORDERS

Mental Disorder	NCS[a] (N=8,098)	CAPES[b] (N=1,701)
Mood Disorders		
Major depressive episode	17.1	6.9
Dysthymia	6.4	5.2
Manic episode	1.6	0.1
Anxiety Disorders/ Somatization		
Generalized anxiety disorder	5.1	1.7
Panic disorder	3.5	0.4
Any phobia	—	—
Agoraphobia	5.3	1.6
Simple phobia	11.3	1.1
Social phobia	13.3	1.2
Obsessive-compulsive disorder	—	—
Somatization	—	—
Substance Use Disorders		
Alcohol abuse/dependence	23.5	—
Drug abuse/ dependence	11.9	—
Other Disorders		
Schizophrenia/ schizophreniform	—	—
Antisocial personality	3.5	—

Note: Not all disorders assessed for each study. Empty cells indicate zero cases found.

[a] Kessler et al. (1994).
[b] Takeuchi et al. (1998), Y.-P. Zheng et al. (1997).

What did the ECA study reveal with regard to the mental health of Asian Americans, in particular? Although the majority of ECA study reports have excluded Asian Americans in their ethnic comparisons (e.g., Holzer, Swanson, & Shea, 1995; Weissman, Bruce, Leaf, Florio, & Holzer, 1991), one exception is a recent report by Zhang and Snowden (1999). Zhang and Snowden examined the ECA study's community sample to determine the prevalence of 16 DSM-III mental disorders among European American, African American, Latino, and Asian American respondents (N=18,152). The 420 community residents who did not fall into one of these four ethnic categories were omitted from the analyses. In addition, the Los Angeles site (n=2,939) was selected for separate analysis because the majority of Latinos and Asian Americans (91% and 67%, respectively) were sampled from that site.

Although Asian Americans had lower overall rates of mental disorders, the pattern of lifetime prevalence rates was similar to that found in the total sample (see Table 1). Excluding generalized anxiety disorder, which was not included in their study, the most common psychiatric disorder for Asian Americans across all 5 sites was alcohol use/dependence (7.1%), followed by phobia (6.6%), major depressive episode (3.4%), and dysthymia (3.0%). After controlling for demographic characteristics, ethnic differences were still notable. For the total sample, Asian Americans exhibited a significantly lower rate of schizophreniform disorder, manic episode, bipolar disorders, panic disorder, somatization disorder, drug and alcohol abuse or dependence, and antisocial personality than European Americans (p<.01). Asian Americans were not statistically different from European Americans in their rates of schizophrenia, major depressive episode, major depression, dysthymia, atypical bipolar disorder, obsessive-compulsive disorder, phobia, and anorexia nervosa. The majority of these ethnic patterns were replicated in the analysis of the Los Angeles site data with the exceptions that Asian Americans had significantly lower rates of schizophrenia, atypical bipolar disorder, and obsessive-compulsive disorder compared to European Americans. There were no disorders found to be more prevalent for Asian Americans than for European Americans.

Zhang and Snowden (1999) reported that compared to European Americans, ethnic minorities as a whole had an **equal** or **lower** lifetime prevalence rate for most disorders including substance use disorders, when demographic characteristics were controlled. The only exceptions to this general finding were that African Americans were significantly **more** likely to have a history of phobia or somatization disorder than European Americans (19.9% versus 11.5% and 0.5% versus 0.1%, respectively). Despite the general trend of lower prevalence of mental disorders among ethnic minority respondents, the pattern of difference frequently varied across groups. For example, compared to European Americans, African Americans had a similar rate of manic disorders, but a lower rate of depressive disorders (data not included in Table 1). In contrast, Asian Americans had a similar rate of depressive disorders, but a lower rate of manic disorders compared to European Americans.

These findings challenge previous assumptions that rates of depression among Asian Americans are exceptionally low in contrast to other groups. Also counter to previous assumptions, Asian Americans were found to be significantly **less** likely than European Americans to meet criteria for somatization disorder (0.0% versus 0.1%). Although the ECA study did not assess for other, less severe somatoform disorders, these results suggest that it may be erroneous to assume that Asian Americans as a whole do not experience depression to the extent that other groups

UNDERSTANDING THE RATES AND DISTRIBUTION OF MENTAL DISORDERS   15

do, or that somatization is the predominant presentation style among persons of Asian heritage.

3. INTERNATIONAL STUDIES IN ASIAN COMMUNITIES

In the 1980s following the success of the ECA study, four major surveys were conducted in Taiwan, China, Hong Kong, and Korea using modified, translated versions of the DIS to generate DSM-III diagnoses. The application of the DIS/DSM-III criteria for case definition provides an opportunity for a cross-national comparison of rates of mental disorder. The following review focuses on urban samples, which may be more socioeconomically and culturally similar to Asian Americans. However, unlike the ECA study, these international studies did not include patients or subjects in institutional settings. In addition, because the number of disorders surveyed varied across studies, the lifetime prevalence of having any disorder are not strictly comparable.

The Taiwan Psychiatric Epidemiological Project (TPEP), conducted from 1982 to 1986, used a Mandarin Chinese version of the DIS (DIS-CM) that incorporated several additional disorders considered to be important in the Taiwan-Chinese patient population (i.e., generalized anxiety, and psychophysiological and paranoid disorders) (Hwu, Yeh, & Chang, 1989). After psychometric investigations found the DIS-CM to be a reliable case-identification tool, multistage random sampling was used to obtain a representative Taiwanese sample of adults aged 18 and over living in metropolitan Taipei (n=5,005), two small towns (n=3004), and six rural villages (n=2995). Comparing the Taipei sample to the ECA study sample, which used a similar community sampling design, prevalence rates of all mental disorders were much lower among the Taiwan Chinese although the pattern of results was similar (see Table 2). The lifetime prevalence for having any of 25 psychiatric disorders (excluding tobacco dependency) was 16.3% for residents of Taipei. Among DSM-III disorders only, the lifetime prevalence rate was highest for alcohol use/abuse (5.2%), followed by phobic disorders (4.2) and generalized anxiety disorder (3.7%). Rates of major depression and dysthymia were substantially lower compared to the ECA study findings at 0.9% each.

Around the same time that the TPEP was being conducted, another Mandarin Chinese version of the DIS was independently developed by the Shanghai Psychiatric Hospital and the Pacific/Asian American Mental Health Research Center at the University of Illinois at Chicago (Yu, Zhang, Xia, & Liu, 1987). In 1983, this Mandarin version was adopted as the case-finding tool for a psychiatric epidemiological survey of the Xuhui District of Shanghai (Wang et al., 1992). A random cluster sampling design was employed to obtain a sample of 3,098 respondents between 18 and 64 years of age. Again, the data indicated that the specific rates of DSM-III mental disorders were low, compared to those reported by the ECA study (Table 1). The lifetime prevalence of having any of 10 core DSM-III diagnoses included in the study was 2.6%; the rate dropped to 2.1% when alcohol abuse/dependence was excluded. Unlike the ECA study and the TPEP, the prevalence of phobic disorders ranks first (1.5%) among the disorders covered by the Shanghai study, followed by alcohol abuse/dependence (0.5%), dysthymia (0.3%) and major depression (0.2%).

Between December 1984 and October 1986, Chen et al. (1993) conducted a large-scale community survey in Shatin, Hong Kong, using a Cantonese translation of the DIS. A random cluster sampling design was used to identify 7,229 respondents between 18 and 64 years of age. The study used a two-phase design of data collection. The Self-Reporting Questionnaire (SRQ) was used for case screening in the first phase, and the DIS was used for case identification in the second phase. Twenty-five percent of the original random sample was subsampled and "flagged" for administration of both the SRQ and the DIS. For the remaining sample, only respondents with SRQ-positive responses were administered the DIS. The number of false-negative cases in the nonflagged subsample was estimated from the false-negative rate of the flagged subsample. As shown in Table 2, the most common DIS/DSM-III disorder was generalized anxiety disorder (9.5%), followed by alcohol abuse/dependence (4.5%), phobia (2.1%), dysthymia (2.0%), and major depression (1.9%).

Lee et al. (1990) conducted an epidemiological survey to estimate the prevalence of mental disorders in Korea. Two-stage cluster sampling was used to identify a final sample of 3,134 respondents aged 18 to 65 living in Seoul and 1,966 living in rural areas. The DIS was translated into Korean and a series of field trials indicated that it was a reliable case finding tool. Results indicated that 39.8% of the Seoul sample reported a lifetime history of at least one of the 17 disorders covered by the Korean DIS. When substance use disorders were excluded, this rate dropped to 13.4%. The most common lifetime DSM-III disorders were alcohol abuse/dependence (21.7%), followed by phobic disorders (5.9%), generalized anxiety disorder (3.6%), and major depression (3.3%).

Taken together, these studies reveal a number of interesting insights regarding the mental health of Asian Americans compared to Asians in Asia. First, the lifetime prevalence of DIS/DSM-III mental disorders was generally lower in overseas Asian communities compared to the ECA study's total sample. Second, while the ECA study's Asian American sample had significantly **lower** rates of most disorders compared to European Americans, their rates were generally **higher** than their overseas Asian counterparts for mood disorders, phobic disorder, and substance use/abuse disorders, in particular. Third, lifetime prevalence rates of obsessive-compulsive disorder, somatization disorder, and schizophrenia across the four Asian studies were generally comparable to those reported for the ECA study's Asian American sample. This finding may suggest that the presentation of these latter three disorders may be less influenced by the acculturation process. Finally, the variability in prevalence rates across the Taiwanese, Chinese, Hong Kong, and Korean studies suggests that while overseas Asians may have lower overall rates of mental disorder compared to American populations, the heterogeneity of Asian cultures may yield important within-group differences as well (e.g., high rates of alcohol use/abuse disorders in the Seoul sample compared to the Shanghai sample).

4. NATIONAL COMORBIDITY STUDY

Further developments in psychiatric epidemiology led to the National Comorbidity Study (NCS) in the early 1990s. Improving upon the methodology used by the ECA study researchers, the NCS was lauded as the first psychiatric epidemiologic study to be conducted on a representative national sample. Selected using stratified, multistage area probability sampling, a total of 8,098 noninstitutionalized respondents aged 15 to 54 years of age participated in the survey. A modified version of the Composite International Diagnostic Interview (UM-CIDI), which was based on the DIS, was used to estimate the prevalence of 14 Diagnostic and Statistical Manual of Mental Disorders (Third Edition-Revised) (DSM-III-R) diagnoses. The NCS results indicated that psychiatric disorders were more prevalent than the ECA and other studies had estimated. Nearly 50% of those interviewed reported at least one UM-CIDI/DSM-III-R disorder, and nearly 30% met criteria for at least one disorder within the past year (Kessler et al., 1994). As summarized in Table 3, the most common lifetime diagnosis was alcohol use/abuse (23.5%), followed by major depression (17.1%), social phobia (13.3%), drug use/dependence (11.9%), and simple phobia (11.3%).

Kessler et al. (1994) attributed the higher prevalence rates of some disorders to secular trends as well as a number of methodological factors that distinguished the NCS from previous studies. For example, the NCS is based on a national sample, concentrates on a younger age range, uses a correction weight to adjust for nonresponse bias, and applies the DSM-III-R as a diagnostic standard rather than the DSM-III. In addition, although the UM-CIDI is very similar to the DIS, variations exist with regard to word choice, depth of probing, and refinements to aid recall of lifetime episodes, all of which may have resulted in higher prevalence estimates.

While the NCS represents the most comprehensive and rigorous prevalence study of psychiatric disorders in the United States, there have been no studies to date that have reported NCS prevalence statistics for the Asian American respondents. Because of their small sample size, Asian American respondents were aggregated and placed in an "Other" category, which comprised 3.3% of the total sample and were not included in the ethnic comparisons conducted by Kessler et al. (1994).

5. CHINESE AMERICAN PSYCHIATRIC EPIDEMIOLOGICAL STUDY

The Chinese American Psychiatric Epidemiological Study (CAPES) is the largest, most rigorous, and carefully conducted survey of mental health on any Asian American group. It was designed to address many of the methodological and sampling problems that have impeded earlier efforts to estimate the prevalence of mental disorder in Asian Americans. Focusing on only one ethnic group, Chinese Americans living in Los Angeles County, CAPES used a multistage sampling procedure, and included respondents that speak either English or one of the two most common Chinese dialects, Mandarin or Cantonese. The final sample consisted of adult respondents (18 years and older) from 1,747 Chinese American households.

As in the NCS, the UM-CIDI was used as the major diagnostic instrument to obtain prevalence estimates for selected DSM-III-R mental disorders.

Although different sample weights and procedures make it difficult to compare across studies, results from this survey indicated that Chinese Americans living in Los Angeles had relatively lower rates of mental disorders than have been found in national surveys (S. Sue et al.,1995; Takeuchi et al., 1998). Compared to the NCS, the Chinese Americans in CAPES had a much lower prevalence of major depression and anxiety disorders. Specifically, the lifetime prevalence of major depressive disorder was 6.9%, compared to 17.1% in the NCS total sample (12-month prevalence was 3.4% and 10.3%, respectively). However, the lifetime prevalence of dysthymia was more comparable, with 5.2% of the CAPES and 6.4% of the NCS sample meeting DSM-III-R criteria (12-month prevalence was 0.9% and 2.5%, respectively). Compared to the NCS sample, the CAPES respondents had a substantially lower lifetime prevalence of generalized anxiety (1.7% versus 5.1%), panic disorder (0.4% versus 3.5%), agoraphobia (1.6% versus 5.3%), simple phobia (1.1% versus 11.3%), and social phobia (1.2% versus 13.3%).

Recognizing the cultural loading of the DSM-III-R, the CAPES also obtained a 12-month prevalence rate for neurasthenia (Zheng et al., 1997), a disorder commonly diagnosed and widely recognized in countries such as China, Hong Kong, and Taiwan but one that is no longer included in the DSM system. According to the International Classification of Diseases (ICD-10), neurasthenia is characterized by either physical or mental fatigue or weakness and is accompanied by a host of somatic, affective, and cognitive difficulties including muscular aches and pains, gastrointestinal problems, sleep disturbances, dizziness, irritability, and excitability (World Health Organization, 1992). The 12-month prevalence rate for "pure" neurasthenia (i.e., not comorbid with other current or lifetime DSM-III-R diagnoses) among Chinese Americans in Los Angeles was 3.6%, which was comparable to the 12-month rate for major depression (3.4%), but higher than phobia (1.7%), dysthymia (0.9%), generalized anxiety disorder (1.0%), and panic disorder (0.2%) (Zheng et al., 1997).

6. METHODOLOGICAL AND CONCEPTUAL CONSIDERATIONS

Attempts to understand the mental health of Asian Americans have been challenged by the group's heterogeneity and small sample size, in addition to the many difficulties associated with cross-ethnic assessment procedures. More than 50 distinct ethnic groups (including Pacific Islander Americans), speaking as many as 30 different languages, are included in the category of Asian American (S. Sue et al., 1995). Of these, some such as the Hmongs from Laos come from preliterate societies, while others, such as the Japanese and Hong Kong Chinese, come from very industrialized, modern societies (Fugita, 1990). Significant variations in socioeconomic status and educational attainment exist, with 90% of Indonesian Americans graduating from high school, compared to 22% of Hmong Americans. There are also pronounced differences in immigration history and generational status. For instance, Japanese immigration to the United States may be traced back to the late 19th century, while the majority of Hmong and other Southeast Asian refugees arrived after 1970.

The considerable cultural, generational, socioeconomic, and linguistic heterogeneity found among Asian Americans suggests the need for specific studies of these groups, rather than aggregate research (S. Sue et al., 1995). For example, the CAPES provides important discrete information about the mental health of one group, Chinese Americans, living in a large, ethnically-diverse urban setting. Unfortunately, small sample sizes and language needs result in a host of sampling difficulties and associated costs that have proven prohibitive for most researchers. As a result, many Asian American groups such as Asian Indians are simply overlooked in research (Durvasula & Mylvaganam, 1994), and findings from one Asian American group are often generalized to the entire population.

For example, although Zhang and Snowden (1999) make an important contribution to our understanding of the prevalence of mental disorders among Asian Americans, the sample itself is highly unique and should not be viewed as representative of Asian Americans as a whole. Only English-speaking respondents were included, therefore excluding the nearly 25% of Asian and Pacific Islanders Americans between 18 and 64 years of age who cannot communicate in English (Yoon & Chien, 1995). In addition, two-thirds of the Asian American respondents resided in Los Angeles, a large and ethnically diverse metropolitan city. Numerous Asian American groups were aggregated into a single category in order to retain statistical power; however, the study failed to report the ethnic breakdown of the aggregate category (e.g., Chinese Americans, Japanese Americans, Korean Americans). Thus, while Zhang and Snowden (1999) provide the only available estimate of mental disorders among the Asian American population as a whole, the cultural and socioeconomic heterogeneity of Asian Americans renders these results potentially misleading. While some Asian American groups may indeed be better adjusted, others such as Southeast Asian refugees and Asian American veterans have extremely high levels of depression and other disorders (Chun, Eastman, Wang, & S. Sue, 1998).

Another concern in assessing the rates of mental disorders is the validity of Western diagnostic concepts, such as those embodied in the DSM and upon which instruments like the DIS and UM-CIDI are based. Although the studies previously discussed have indicated that prevalence rates of mental disorder are lower among ethnic minority groups (Takeuchi et al., 1998; Zhang and Snowden, 1999; Zheng et al., 1997), Hinton and Kleinman (1993) and others have argued that the neo-Kraepelinian paradigm of the DSM system is culture-bound and fails to satisfactorily recognize the ethnic and cultural variations in illness expression and illness experience. For example, a large number of studies have found ethnic differences in symptom reporting style, idioms of distress, pain tolerance, psychiatric stigma, and explanatory models of illness (e.g., Cheung, Lee, & Chan, 1983; Kleinman, 1980, 1988; Luk & Bond, 1992). Although structured diagnostic interviews have made it possible for large-scale epidemiological studies to be conducted, the structure and content of these interviews rarely address these cultural components that may affect the diagnostic process. Yet, the reliability and validity of these interviews depend on three key assumptions.

First, it is assumed that questions posed by the interviewer have been appropriately interpreted and honestly answered, and that responses are successfully communicated to and understood by the interviewer. Clearly, successful communication is a basic requirement for reliable and valid diagnosis, which is one reason why non-English speakers were excluded in the ECA study and NCS. However, even for Asian Americans who have acquired English as a second language, response biases and communication problems may still emerge, particularly when discussing sensitive, embarrassing, or painful experiences such as past traumas, sexual difficulties, depressed or suicidal feelings. Good (1993) discussed the problem of narrative context to the extent that conversations between clients and clinicians (or lay interviewers) are heavily influenced by social context and cultural norms, which may have practical implications for the diagnostic task. For example, in a Chinese primary care study of somatization, Chang (2000) discovered that the Chinese physicians were extremely reluctant to probe for sexual dysfunction in unmarried individuals, claiming that to do so would imply that the patients had had pre-marital sex and cause them to lose face. Good (1993) argues that in certain cultural contexts, where questioning and revelation about the self may be restricted, structured interviews may have limited validity. In addition, variations in the cultural norms surrounding modes of communication may also affect the validity of diagnostic judgments (D. W. Sue & D. Sue, 1999). Interviewers unfamiliar with nonverbal communication patterns or "idioms of distress" may misinterpret respondents' symptoms, leading to diagnostic inaccuracies and biased estimates in epidemiological research.

A second assumption of epidemiological surveys is that the diagnostic categories and representative symptoms being assessed are universal. DSM categories are treated as the gold standard of diagnosis in the U.S., and structured diagnostic interviews are seen as reliable operationalizations of these reified categories. In fact, the research literature suggests that most major classes of disorders (i.e., affective disorders, psychotic disorders) have been identified across ethnic groups; however, cultural factors have been found to influence the presentation of these disorders in unique ways (e.g., Nakane et al., 1991; Katz et al., 1988). For example, there is considerable evidence that Chinese patients with depression tend to emphasize somatic aspects of their illness, underreporting the accompanying psychological distress (Cheung & Lau, 1982; Cheung, B. W. K. Lau, & Waldmann, 1980-81; Kleinman, 1982). Lee (1996) argued that the Diagnostic and Statistical Manual of Mental Disorders (Fourth Edition) (DSM-IV) symptom criteria for anorexia nervosa excludes some Hong Kong Chinese women whose self-starvation is motivated out of a desire to control their social environments, rather than an "intense fear of gaining weight or becoming fat" (American Psychiatric Association, 1994, p. 544). Thus, problems in diagnosis may arise not only from miscommunication between interviewer and respondent, but from differences in symptoms and cultural forms of particular disorders.

Related to this problem is a third assumption that the current taxonomy being applied is sufficient for categorizing the distress experiences of the sample. However, the research and training materials associated with the DSM-III and DSM-III-R, upon which the DIS and UM-CIDI were based, focus on a biological paradigm of psychopathology and do not directly address the role of ethnicity and culture in mental illness. Despite the early identification of culture-bound syndromes by psychiatrists and anthropologists (e.g., Simons & Hughes, 1985), the social context and indigenous clinical conditions found in non-White populations has traditionally been ignored or minimized (Guarnaccia & Rogler, 1999). Indeed, this bias is also reflected in most epidemiological surveys of mental disorder, with one exception.

The CAPES highlights in bold relief the importance of examining culture-bound syndromes such as neurasthenia as a means of capturing the illness experiences of specific cultural groups. Results indicate the salience of neurasthenia in the Chinese American community and highlight the need for systematic research to investigate the specificity of the disorder, compared to other DSM categories (see Guarnaccia & Rogler, 1999). Although neurasthenia has been artificially linked with undifferentiated somatoform disorder in the DSM-IV, Zheng et al. (1997) argue that the vague nature of this residual category does not do justice to the distinctiveness of neurasthenia as it appears in "pure" form. The majority of respondents with neurasthenia (77%) did not meet criteria for any other concurrent DSM-III-R diagnoses, and more than half (56.2%) did not meet criteria for any current or lifetime disorders. Other studies support the view that neurasthenia represents an important and specific form of psychiatric disorder that should be regularly included in psychiatric screenings of Chinese Americans and potentially, other Asian American groups (Zheng, Lin, Yamamoto, & D. Zheng, 1992). Moreover, the phenomenological overlap with chronic fatigue syndrome suggests that neurasthenia may also be quite prevalent in mainstream and other minority populations as well. These data argue for cross-cultural validation studies to demonstrate whether neurasthenia is best conceptualized as a culture-bound syndrome, a cultural variant of a standard psychiatric diagnosis, or a discrete entity that merits inclusion as a mental disorder in the DSM.

6.1 Within-Group Variables

What makes some groups of individuals more prone to mental disorder than others? While the CAPES indicates that Chinese Americans may have lower rates of some mental disorders than the general population, research has also identified other Asian American groups that are more vulnerable to psychological problems, including Southeast Asian refugees, the elderly, and Vietnam war veterans (Kinzie et al., 1990; Matsuoka & Hamada, 1991; Westermeyer, Neider, & Callies, 1989; Yee, Huang, & Lew, 1998). Historically, psychological investigations into the relationship between ethnicity and mental health have largely focused on minority status or social class as a means of differentiating between low- and high-risk groups. However, more recent efforts have sought to capture the factors that impact the ability of Asian Americans to cope with the stresses of migration and acculturation.

6.2 Social Class

Dohrenwend and Dohrenwend (1969) stated in their review of the literature that the association between mental disorder and socioeconomic status (SES) is one of the best substantiated findings of psychiatric research. However, empirical studies indicate that this relationship is neither stable nor linear across ethnic groups (Dohrenwend, 1990). Rather, SES has unique associations with discrete disorders, with the greatest increase in risk occurring primarily in the lowest SES category (Holzer et al., 1986; Kessler et al., 1994).

In a review of 20 international studies on the relationship between mental illness and SES, Neugebauer, Dohrenwend, and Dohrenwend (1980) reported that 17 showed higher overall rates of psychopathology in the lowest class. This general trend was upheld in the CAPES as well. For Chinese Americans in Los Angeles, the relationship between SES and rates of psychiatric disorder was most consistent for the lifetime prevalence of dysthymia (Takeuchi et al., 1998). Chinese Americans with less than a high school degree were twice as likely to report lifetime dysthymia than individuals with some college education. Those with annual household incomes below $25,000 were between four and six times more likely to report lifetime dysthymia than those with incomes higher than $25,000. Unemployment was also related to increased risk for lifetime and 12-month depressive episode, and for current dysthymia.

Because of the inverse relationship between SES and risk for some mental disorders, the majority of studies that examine ethnic differences in mental health statistically "control" for the effects of SES as a matter of course. However, SES alone was not sufficient to explain all of the ethnic differences found in the ECA study or the NCS (Holzer et al., 1995; Zhang & Snowden, 1999).

6.3 Immigration and Acculturative Stress

Although many recent immigrants of Asian heritage are in the lowest SES category, other factors such as the country of origin, reasons for immigration, age at immigration, number of years in the U.S., language ability, and available social networks have also been investigated for their relation to psychiatric disorder (Beiser, 1988; Kuo & Tsai, 1986; Tran, 1989). Empirical studies have demonstrated the high levels of distress and psychiatric illness among refugees, especially those from Southeast Asia, many of whom suffered enormous losses, massive trauma, and torture as the result of war (Gong-Guy, 1987; Lin, Tozuma, & Masuda, 1979). Estimates of the treated prevalence of post-traumatic stress disorder among these traumatized populations have ranged from 50-70%, with some groups such as the Mien showing an even higher risk (Kinzie et al, 1990). In general, research has demonstrated that undesired life changes, including being forced to leave one's homeland because of war or environmental catastrophe, are correlated with anxiety, depression, and physical symptoms (Sarason, Johnson, & Siegel, 1978).

In contrast, voluntary immigrants, including many from Taiwan, Hong Kong, Japan, India, and Korea, come to the U.S. for educational purposes or economic opportunities. These individuals may arrive with technical skills, personal resources, and extended social networks that provide them with a higher capacity for achieving social acceptance and stable employment. Moreover, immigrants who feel a sense of mastery or control over the events in their life and perceive change as an exciting opportunity for personal development are more likely to report positive adjustment experiences (Kuo & Tsai, 1986).

A number of studies have reported the relationship between adaptation difficulties and depression. Kuo and Tsai (1986) observed that although Korean, Chinese, Filipino, and Japanese immigrants varied in the level and type of adjustment difficulties reported, the intensity of life events, financial worries, and adjustment stress were positively related to respondents' depression score. Takeuchi et al. (1998) found that Chinese Americans who did not have a working knowledge of English were significantly more likely to have had a depressive episode or dysthymia in their lifetime, compared to those who spoke English as a primary language. Similarly, individuals who immigrated to the U.S. before the age of 21 were significantly less likely to report a lifetime episode of depression or dysthymia, possibly due to a higher adaptability with regard to language and culture. Compared to respondents without any psychiatric diagnoses, Chinese Americans with depression, anxiety, or neurasthenia also reported more negative life events, experienced significantly higher stress levels, and were less satisfied with their social support (Zheng et al., 1997).

Although factors such as locus of control, hardiness, and social support have been associated with cross-cultural adjustment (e.g., Dion, Dion, & Pak, 1992; Ying & Leise, 1994), continued research is needed to identify those factors that account for why some Asian American groups have a lower risk for psychological problems compared to other groups in the U.S. Moreover, epidemiological surveys of overseas Chinese communities using the updated UM-CIDI/DSM-III-R protocols are needed in order to generate hypotheses about cultural and environmental factors that may influence risk for mental disorder.

7. SUMMARY AND CONCLUSIONS

The vast ethnic, economic, and social diversity of persons of Asian heritage living in the United States poses many unique challenges to the assessment of mental disorder among this heterogeneous population. Not only are there considerable differences among the groups classified under the umbrella term Asian American, they also differ from mainstream European American society with regard to cultural values, ethnic history, and social status. These differences confound traditional diagnostic and assessment procedures and suggest the need for more inclusive procedures that recognize cultural forms of standard diagnostic categories as well as indigenous, or culture-bound syndromes. Unfortunately, small sample size and mainstream psychology's emphasis on internal rather than external validity has hindered the development of Asian American mental health research (S. Sue, 1999).

With these caveats in mind, only two large-scale epidemiological surveys, the Epidemiologic Catchment Area (ECA) study and the Chinese American Psychiatric

24 DORIS F. CHANG

Epidemiological Study (CAPES), have specifically examined Asian Americans. The findings reveal substantially **lower** rates of mental disorders compared to U.S. population estimates, but generally **higher** rates of mood disorders, substance use/abuse, and some anxiety disorders compared to international studies of Asian communities. These data suggest that the acculturative stress experienced by some Asian Americans increase their vulnerability to certain mental disorders; however, cultural or social factors continue to protect them to some degree from the even higher rates of psychological distress found in mainstream U.S. communities. Interestingly, research has revealed that recent immigrants (including those from other ethnic groups) have fewer psychiatric disorders in general than those who were born in the United States and more acculturated to the host society (Yamamoto, Rhee, & Chang, 1994; Karno et al., 1987).

Understanding the mental health of Asian Americans is a complex endeavor that requires specific assessments of such factors as ethnicity, immigration history, acculturative stress, social class, and culture-specific expressions of psychological distress. Examinations of Asian Americans along these dimensions reveal that some subgroups are at lower risk while others, such as Southeast Asian refugees, are at greater risk for mental disorder. While research on Asian Americans as an aggregate are useful and can have important policy implications, science will be more enhanced by research on specific groups, such as Asian Indians and other overlooked populations (S. Sue et al., 1995). Specific research may also help to identify the specific sociocultural traits that seem to protect certain Asian American groups from the psychological consequences of stress.

Lastly, as Guarnaccia and Rogler (1999) argue, culture-bound syndromes need to be investigated and understood on their own terms, as well as in relation to other psychiatric disorders. Particularly relevant for Asian Americans are the disorders *koro, latah, hwa-byung, shin-byung*, neurasthenia (*shenjing shuairuo*), *shenkui, shink-bu*, and *taijin kyofusho*, among others. Understanding the mental health of ethnic minority populations requires that we assess cultural variations of familiar disorders as well as specific culture-bound syndromes. Moreover, studies examining specific linkages between culture-bound syndromes and the standard psychiatric categories may offer significant insights into issues of psychiatric universality and cultural specificity.

8. REFERENCES

American Psychiatric Association (1994). Diagnostic and statistical manual of mental disorders (4th edition; DSM-IV). Washington, DC: Author.

Beiser, M. (1988). Influences of time, ethnicity, and attachment on depression in Southeast Asian refugees. *American Journal of Psychiatry, 145*, 46-51.

Chang, D. F. (2000). *The cultural validity of neurasthenia: Psychiatric diagnosis and illness beliefs in a Chinese primary care sample.* Unpublished doctoral dissertation, University of California, Los Angeles.

Chen, C.-N, Wong, J, Lee, N., Chan-Ho, M.-W., Lau, J. T.-F., & Fung, M. (1993). The Shatin community mental health survey in Hong Kong: II. Major findings. *Archives of General Psychiatry, 50*, 125-133.

Cheung, F. M., & Lau, B. W. K. (1982). Situational variations of help-seeking behavior among Chinese patients. *Comprehensive Psychiatry, 23*(3), 252-262.

UNDERSTANDING THE RATES AND DISTRIBUTION OF MENTAL DISORDERS 25

Cheung, F. M., Lau, B. W. K., & Waldmann, E. (1980-81). Somatization among Chinese depressive in general practice. *International Journal of Psychiatry in Medicine, 10*(4), 361-374.

Cheung, F. M., Lee, S. Y., & Chan, Y. Y. (1983). Variations in problem conceptualizations and intended solutions among Hong Kong students. *Culture, Medicine, and Psychiatry, 8,* 207-228.

Chun, K. M., Eastman, K. L., Wang, G. C. S. & Sue, S. (1998). Psychopathology. In L.C. Lee and N.W.S. Zane (Eds.), *Handbook of Asian American psychology* (pp. 457-484). Thousand Oaks, CA: Sage.

Dion, K. L, Dion, K. K., & Pak, A. W. P. (1992). Personality-based hardiness as a buffer for discrimination-related stress in members of Toronto's Chinese community. *Canadian Journal of Behavioural Science, 24,* 517-536.

Dohrenwend, B. P. (1990). Socioeconomic status (SES) and psychiatric disorders. *Social Psychiatry and Psychiatric Epidemiology, 25,* 41-47.

Dohrenwend, B. P., & Dohrenwend, B. S. (1969). *Social status and psychological disorder: A causal inquiry.* New York: Wiley.

Durvasula, R. S., & Mylvaganam, G. A. (1994). Mental health of Asian Indians: Relevant issues and community implications. *Journal of Community Psychology, 22,* 97-108.

Fugita, S. S. (1990). Asian/Pacific-American mental health: Some needed research in epidemiology and service utilization. In F. C. Serafica and A. I. Schwebel (Eds.), *Mental health of ethnic minorities* (pp. 66-84). New York: Praeger.

Gong-Guy, E. (1987). *The California Southeast Asian mental health needs assessment* (Contract No. 85-76282A-2). Sacramento: California State Department of Mental Health.

Good, B. J. (1993). Culture, diagnosis and comorbidity. *Culture, Medicine, and Psychiatry, 16,* 427-446.

Guarnaccia, P. J., & Rogler, L. H. (1999). Research on culture-bound syndromes: New directions. *American Journal of Psychiatry, 156*(9), 1322-1327.

Hinton, L. & Kleinman, A. M. (1993). Cultural issues and international psychiatric diagnosis. In J. A. Costa, E. Silva & C. Nadelson (Eds.), *International review of psychiatry, Volume 1* (pp. 111-129). Washington, DC: American Psychiatric Association Press.

Holzer, C. E., III, Shea, B. M., Swanson, J. W., Leaf, P. J., Myers, J. K., George, L. K., Weissman, M. M., & Bednarski, P. (1986). The increased risk for specific psychiatric disorders among persons of low socioeconomic status, evidence from the Epidemiologic Catchment Area Surveys. *American Journal of Social Psychiatry, 6,* 259-271.

Holzer, C. E., III, Swanson, J. W., & Shea, B. M. (1995). Ethnicity, social status, and psychiatric disorder in the Epidemiologic Catchment Area Survey. In R. K. Price, B. M. Shea, and H. N. Mookherjee (Eds.), *Social psychiatry across cultures.* New York: Plenum Press.

Hwu, H.-G, Yeh, E.-K., Chang, L. Y. (1989). Prevalence of psychiatric disorders in Taiwan defined by the Chinese Diagnostic Interview Schedule. *Acta Psychiatrica Scandinavica, 79,* 136-147.

Karno, M., Hough, R. L., Burnam, A., Escobar, J. I., Timbers, D. M., Santana, F., & Boyd, J. H. (1987). Lifetime prevalence of specific psychiatric disorders among Mexican Americans and non-Hispanic Whites in Los Angeles. *Archives of General Psychiatry, 44,* 695-701.

Katz, M. M., Marsella, A., Dube, K. C., Olatawura, M., Takahashi, R., Nakane, Y., Wynne, L. C., Gift, T., Brennan, J., Sartorius, N., & Jablensky, A. (1988). On the expression of psychosis in different cultures: Schizophrenia in an Indian and Nigerian community. *Culture, Medicine and Psychiatry, 12,* 331-355.

Kessler, R. C., McGonagle, K. A., Zhao, S., Nelson, C. B., Hughes, M., Eshleman, S., Wittchen, H.-U., & Kendler, K. S. (1994). Lifetime and 12-month prevalence of DSM-III-R psychiatric disorders in the United States. *Archives of General Psychiatry, 51,* 8-19.

Kinzie, J. D., Boehnlein, J. K., Leung, P. K., Moore, L. J., Riley, C., & Smith, D. (1990). The prevalence of posttraumatic stress disorder and its clinical significance among Southeast Asian refugees. *American Journal of Psychiatry, 147*(7), 913-917.

Kitano, H. H. (1969). Japanese-American mental illness. In S. Plog & R. Edgerton (Eds.), *Changing perspectives in mental illness* (pp. 256-284). New York: Holt, Rinehart Winston.

Kleinman, A. M. (1980). *Patients and healers in the context of culture: An exploration of the borderland between anthropology, medicine, and psychiatry.* Berkeley, CA: University of California Press.

Kleinman, A. M. (1982). Neurasthenia and depression: A study of somatization and culture in China. *Culture, Medicine, and Psychiatry, 6*(2), 77-190.

Kleinman, A. M. (1988). *Rethinking psychiatry: From cultural category to personal experience.* New York: The Free Press.

26 DORIS F. CHANG

Kuo, W. H., & Tsai, Y.-M. (1986). Social networking, hardiness and immigrant's mental health. *Journal of Health and Social Behavior, 27*, 133-149.

Lee, C. K., Kwak, Y. S., Yamamoto, J., Ree, H., Kim, Y. S., Han. J. H., Choi, J. O., & Lee, Y. H. (1990). Psychiatric epidemiology in Korea, Part I: Gender and age differences in Seoul. *Journal of Nervous and Mental Disease, 178*(4), 242-246.

Lee, S. (1996). Reconsidering the status of anorexia nervosa as a Western culture-bound syndrome. *Social Science and Medicine, 42*(1), 21-34.

Lin, K.-M., Tozuma, L., & Masuda, M. (1979). Adaptational problems of Vietnamese refugees. *Archives of General Psychiatry, 36,* 955-961.

Luk, C., & Bond, M. (1992). Chinese lay beliefs about the causes and cures of psychological problems. *Journal of Social and Clinical Psychology, 11*(2), 140-157.

Matsuoka, J., & Hamada, R. (1991). The wartime and postwar experiences of Asian-Pacific American veterans. *Journal of Applied Social Sciences, 16,* 23-36.

Nakane, Y., Ohta, Y., Radford, M., Yan, H., Wang, X., Lee, H. Y., Min, S. K., Michitsuji, S., & Ohtsuka, T., (1991). Comparative study of affective disorders in three Asian countries: II. Differences in prevalence rates and symptom presentation. *Acta Psychiatrica Scandinavica, 84,* 313-319.

Neugebauer, D. D., Dohrenwend, B. P., & Dohrenwend, B. S. (1980). The formulation of hypotheses about the true prevalence of functional psychiatric disorders among adults in the United States. In B. P. Dohrenwend, B. S. Dohrenwend, M. S. Goulde, B. Link, R. Neugebauer, & R. Wunsch-Hitzig (Eds.), *Mental illness in the United States.* New York: Praeger.

Robins, L. N., & Regier, D. A. (1991). *Psychiatric disorders in America: The Epidemiologic Catchment Area Study.* New York: The Free Press.

Sarason, I. G., Johnson, J. H., & Siegel, J. M. (1978). Assessing the impact of life changes: Development of the Life Experience Survey. *Journal of Consulting and Clinical Psychology, 46,* 932-946.

Simons, R. C., & Hughes, C. C. (1985). *The culture-bound syndromes: Folk illnesses of psychiatric and anthropological interest.* Dordrecht, The Netherlands: D. Reidel.

Sue, D. W., & Sue, D. (1999). *Counseling the culturally different: Theory and practice* (3rd Ed.). New York: John Wiley & Sons.

Sue, S. (1999). Science, ethnicity, and bias: Where have we gone wrong? *American Psychologist, 54*(12), 1070-1077.

Sue, S., & McKinney, H. (1975). *The mental health of Asian Americans.* San Francisco: Jossey-Bass.

Sue, S., Sue, D. W., Sue, L., & Takeuchi, D. (1995). Psychopathology among Asian Americans: A model minority? *Cultural Diversity and Mental Health, 1*(1), 39-51.

Takeuchi, D. T., Chung, R. C-Y., Lin, K.-M., Shen, H., Kurasaki, K., Chun, C-A., & Sue, S. (1998). Lifetime and twelve-month prevalence rates of major depressive episodes and dysthymia among Chinese Americans in Los Angeles. *American Journal of Psychiatry, 155*(10), 1407-1414.

Tran, T.V. (1989). Ethnic community supports and psychological well-being of Vietnamese refugees. *International Migration Review, 21,* 833-845.

Wang, C. H., Liu, W. T., Zhang, M. Y., Yu, E. S. H., Xia, Z. Y., Fernandez, M., Lung, C. T., Xu, C. L., & Qu, G. Y. (1992). Alcohol use, abuse, and dependency in Shanghai. In J. E. Helzer and G. J. Canino (Eds.), *Alcoholism in North America, Europe, and Asia* (pp. 264-286). New York: Oxford University Press.

Weissman, M. M., Bruce, M. L., Leaf, P. J., Florio, L. P., & Holzer, C. E., III (1991). Affective disorders. In L. N. Robins and D. A. Regier, *Psychiatric disorders in America: The Epidemiologic Catchment Area Study* (pp. 53-80). New York: The Free Press.

Westermeyer, J., Neider, J., & Callies, A. (1989). Psychosocial adjustment of Hmong refugees during their first decade in the United States: A longitudinal study. *Journal of Nervous and Mental Disease, 177*(3), 132-139.

World Health Organization (1992). *ICD-10: The ICD-10 classification of mental and behavioral disorders. Clinical descriptions and diagnostic guidelines.* Geneva, Switzerland: WHO.

Yamamoto, J., Rhee, S., & Chang, D.-S. (1994). Psychiatric disorders among elderly Koreans in the United States. *Community Mental Health Journal, 30*(1), 17-26.

Yee, B. W. K., Huang, L. N., & Lew, A. (1998). Families: Life-span socialization in a cultural context. In L. C. Lee and N. W. S. Zane (Eds.), *Handbook of Asian American psychology* (pp. 83-136). Thousand Oaks, CA: Sage.

Ying, Y., & Leise, L. H. (1994). Initial adjustment of Taiwanese students to the United States: The impact of postarrival variables. *Journal of Cross-Cultural Psychology, 25*(4), 466-477.

Yoon, E., & Chien, F. (1995). Asian American and Pacific Islander health: A paradigm for minority health. *Journal of American Medical Association, 275*(9), 736-737.

Yu, E., Zhang, M.-Y., Xia, Z.-Y, & Liu, W. T. (1987). Translation of instruments: Procedures, issues, and dilemmas. In W. T. Liu (Ed.), *The Pacific/Asian American Mental Health Research Center. A decade review of mental health research, training, and services. A report to the National Institute of Mental Health* (pp. 75-86). Chicago: P/AAMHRC.

Zhang, A. Y., & Snowden, L. R. (1999). Ethnic characteristics of mental disorders in five U.S. communities. *Cultural Diversity and Ethnic Minority Psychology, 5*(2), 134-146.

Zheng, Y.-P., Lin, K.-M., Takeuchi, D. Kurasaki, K., Wong, Y., & Cheung, F. (1997). An epidemiological study of neurasthenia in Chinese-Americans in Los Angeles. *Comprehensive Psychiatry, 38*(5), 249-259.

RICHARD H. DANA

CHAPTER 3

EXAMINING THE USEFULNESS OF DSM-IV

1. INTRODUCTION

The Diagnostic and Statistical Manual-IV (DSM-IV) (American Psychiatric Association, 1994) is an evolutionary product of a remedicalization of psychiatry that began in the 1970s to reintegrate psychiatry with medicine (Dana & May, 1986). DSM-IV provides the possibility for a reduction of the cultural bias present in earlier DSM versions by recognizing cultural diversity and improving the cultural boundaries for psychological disorders (Malgady, 2000). Nonetheless, this psychiatric awareness has resulted in a DSM vessel that is half-full or half-empty depending on an observer's perspective of the fairness and credibility of DSM diagnostic standards for multicultural populations in the United States.

Following a general historical description of DSM versions, this chapter will focus on reliability of the diagnostic process and validity of DSM-IV disorders for Asians and Asian Americans. The present status of psychopathology knowledge for this heterogeneous population will be described as a basis for a number of feasible interim and long-term DSM remediations designed to improve both the process and outcome of diagnosis. A more potable fulfillment of the promise in the DSM diagnostic vessel for all cultural/racial populations can provide directions for research and diagnostic assessment practice in professional psychology, psychiatry, and social work.

2. DSM: A EUROPEAN AMERICAN EMIC

The DSM was a major product of an identity crisis in psychiatry originating in a perception by other physicians of a deficient medical frame-of-reference. Psychiatry was believed to lack an empirical research basis for practice as a clinical science due to an over investment in psychoanalysis and community mental health between 1946 and 1975 (Dana & May, 1986). This crisis was ultimately resolved by a reaffirmation of biological factors in medical training for psychiatric specialization including a focus on pharmacological interventions for psychopathology and a paradigm shift reflected in the DSM. This shift was from a biopsychosocial model in DSM-I (American Psychiatric Association, 1952) to a disease-centered model in DSM-III (American Psychiatric Association, 1980) and DSM-IV (American Psychiatric Association, 1994). The DSM-IV has been described as the beginning of a new psychiatric paradigm in which cultural meaning systems, or emic categories of experience, are larger and more important than scientific paradigms (Castillo, 1996).

The transformation of the DSM from a formal process for collecting statistical information for census purposes into a European American emic system of psychopathology categories, ostensibly universal in application, has had untoward outcomes for cultural/racial populations in the United States. First, multicultural populations were subjected to invidious research comparisons with European American standards and psychopathology criteria. A substantial group difference literature emerged that was predicated on emic research methods and statistics. The overarching effect was support of ethnocentrism and the assumption in professional psychology that group differences were indeed minimal. These sources of bias have been addressed in reviews (Dana, 2000a; Okazaki & Sue, 1995) and by a recommendation to reverse the Null Hypothesis (Malgady, 1996, 2000). Malgady assumed that group differences in psychopathology were central rather than peripheral or distal and suggested the possible magnitude of Type I and Type II errors in our existing research-based knowledge of multicultural populations in the United States. My own efforts to develop an assessment-intervention model represent interim practice guidelines that follow Malgady's recommendations (Dana, 1997, 1998a, 1998b, 2000b). Second, as a consequence of these European American emics being used as etics, there has been DSM inattention to the meaning of group differences as exposed in symptomatology. These group differences also appear in the self, particularly in collectivist societies, as health-illness belief systems, and in the structure and contents of language used to describe emotional distress (Dana, 1993, 1998a, 1998c). Group differences have impacted directly on the perceived legitimacy or credibility and acceptability of European American clinicians, their methods and their service delivery style, or social etiquette, for multicultural populations. This chapter will emphasize the DSM-IV impact on Asian Americans, although it is recognized that the context for applications of DSM-IV includes assessment instruments and research methodology.

3. DSM-IV: ACKNOWLEDGING CULTURAL DIFFERENCES

DSM-IV has enhanced reliability and validity over earlier versions (Nathan, 1994; Nathan & Langenbucher, 1999). I concur with Malgady (2000) that this psychiatric recognition of cultural diversity is unprecedented, but continue to worry about the tokenism from a European American emic perspective that is portrayed by only 15 of 849 pages devoted to caveats regarding culture, age, and gender. DSM-IV cultural content may be likened to an exercise in politically-correct behavior used to create an appearance of cultural sensitivity without including all ingredients required for cultural competence in applications of this diagnostic system.

The heart of the difference between this DSM version and previous editions is the Appendix I Outline for Cultural Formulations that precedes a limited Glossary of Culture-Bound Syndromes. Cultural formulation provides an acceptable methodology for making use of cultural information in the diagnostic process that can result in more valid application of DSM-IV diagnostic criteria with multicultural clients. The location of the Outline and Glossary implies that cultural formulations are only to be used when culture-bound syndromes are suspected. However, the virtue of cultural formulations is that they can now be applied whenever cultural issues in a multicultural client are noteworthy in presenting problems and symptomatology. In fact, the Group on Culture and Diagnosis had recommended that the Outline appear at the beginning of DSM-IV and separately from the Glossary (Lewis-Fernandez, 1996). There are also problems with the sparse description of required content for a cultural formulation because psychologists, for example, have lacked sufficient training and cultural sensitivity to make use of the outline without intensive training. This sad fact was apparent in a national survey of professional psychologists who had considerable experience with multicultural faculty, diverse training cases, and their current clients (Allison, Echemendia, Crawford, & Robinson, 1996; Allison, Crawford, Echemendia, Robinson, & Knepp, 1994). A majority of these psychologists reported they were not competent to offer services to non-European Americans, with only 21% feeling competent with clients of Asian heritages.

To remedy this self-described inadequacy, the necessary training for preparation of cultural formulations should include careful attention to a volume describing what was omitted in DSM-IV. This volume was prepared by members of the Group on Culture and Diagnosis who collected and organized cultural information for each disorder (Mezzich, Kleinman, Fabrega, & Parron, 1996). In addition to this volume, it is necessary to have awareness of available general cultural information resources, specific readings on how to prepare cultural formulations, and familiarity with case examples from cultural/racial populations served by the diagnostician (Dana, 2001). Routine use of cultural formulations for some multicultural clients is now an ethical necessity (Dana, 1994), although this may not occur due to reluctance on the part of many diagnosticians to undertake an immensity of new learning within an already overcrowded agenda in their graduate education or professional practice. In workshops and classes, I have noted intellectual interest in the idea of cultural formulations but scant understanding of how much specific cultural knowledge is required for their preparation. I believe this lack of comprehension is due to the historic impact of ethnocentrism in this society that has resulted in a minimization among professional psychologists of group differences.

3.1 The Contents of a Cultural Formulation

At the onset, the outline for a cultural formulation requires delineating the client's cultural identity, the cultural orientation status or degree of acculturation, including language proficiency, use, and preference. Cultural explanations of illness include idioms, or symptoms used for communication of distress and need for social

32   RICHARD H. DANA

support. These explanations are always understood in terms of cultural reference group norms. Current factors in the psychosocial environment pertain to how stressors are interpreted and understood within a context of available social supports. Relationship to the clinician invokes similarities of social class, religion, culture, and language and how these characteristics relate to establishing a relationship and understanding normative versus pathological behaviors. Finally, the overall cultural considerations in the assessment are related to comprehensive diagnosis and care.

Each of these components of a cultural formulation requires some elaboration by the clinician based on cultural knowledge and assessment experience. First, cultural identity can be established for Asian Americans by using moderator variables for acculturation status. There are acculturation scales for Filipino Americans (Advincula & Ricco, 1998), Japanese Americans (Meredith, 1967), Southeast Asian Cambodians, Laotians, Vietnamese (Anderson et al., 1993), Taiwanese Americans (Yao, 1979), as well as a pan-Asian scale (Suinn, Rickard-Figueroa, Lew, & Vigil, 1987). There are also studies suggesting that items from acculturation scales can be used in interview format in settings eschewing instruments or with clients for whom testing is inappropriate (Tanaka-Matsumi, Hsia, & Fyffe, 1998; Zane, 1998).

Second, knowledge of health/illness beliefs provides the basis for cultural explanations. For example, traditional Chinese health/illness beliefs consider health as balance or harmony. Illness may be an outcome of imbalance in yin-yang, family relations, breathing/eating, bowel functions, sexual activities, or the result of any physiological excess. These imbalances occur at inner state, physical/psychological, and social levels. The outcomes of imbalance can be found in symptoms of numbness, anger, wildness, speech disturbances, and somatization, in culture-general disorders of depression and schizophrenia, and culture-bound disorders of neurasthenia, *shen-k'uei*, frigiphobia (fear of cold, regardless of actual temperature), or spirit possession (Dana, 1998b). These beliefs are often embodied in culture-bound syndromes in which the symptomatology evidences norms in the cultural reference group. For example, *Hwa-byung*, a Korean culture-bound syndrome, expresses the belief that suppressed anger is responsible for somatic illnesses and has been found among traditional Korean Americans (Pang, 1990).

Third, the psychosocial environment in collectivist societies stems from an extended self that incorporates family and social milieu as expanding influences on the individual by successive levels of intimate, operative, and wider society. *Jen,* or personage, has been described by levels of expressible conscious and intimate society/culture to provide a sociocentric human constant based on interpersonal transactions that conform to the standards of society (Hsu, 1971). Lewis-Fernandez and Kleinman (1994) offer the compelling examples of how face and favor interact to provide reciprocal relationships guided by moral norms. Face provides the ability to engage in these relationships using "favor based on human feelings and moral sensibility" (p. 69) as an emotional resource to be exchanged, owned, or gifted within social networks. Exchange of favor according to rules of reciprocity results in health for individuals and communities. Loss of face prohibits social power from being used constructively in daily living; one literally cannot look at others. As a consequence, loss of face is intimately connected to illness or personality development problems. Living in a collectivist society obliges a construction of social reality in which the forms of social conduct have little in common with social reality in non-collectivist societies. Similarly, levels of functioning are interpreted in social reciprocity idiom. The individual is expected to minimize distress using will power, symptom suppression, and avoidance of blatant affect. Unstinting emotional and physical support are provided by significant others to complete the equation and maintain harmony.

Finally, the relationship with the clinician is sustained by appropriate social etiquette during the delivery of services described by credibility and gift-giving (Sue & Zane, 1987). Credibility is found when a clinician behaves in socially expected and appropriate manner with a client. A relationship may be more readily established when the clinician has ascribed credibility, although any perceived lack of skills, or achieved status, may be responsible for premature termination (Sue, 1993). "A gesture of caring " to use Sue's words (p. 284) can include reduction of immediate depression or anxiety, clarification of issues for crisis management, and communication that their feelings, thoughts, and experiences are not unique. A clinician achieves credibility and has opportunity for gift-giving only when his/her social etiquette is appropriate and acceptable. However, social etiquette is culture-specific and embedded in linguistic forms and body language. For example, there is a ritual play in Chinese invitational discourse that emerges from and reinforces cultural identity simultaneously (Mao, 1992).

At the same time as culture-specific rules for professional engagement are invoked, behaviors during a clinical interview will be influenced more by relational cues than verbal contents for Koreans and other Asians (Ambady, Koo, Lee, & Rosenthal, 1996). Thus, the context of an interview can also determine what will be presented and discussed by a client. Within the interview context, however, subtle or muted expressions of affect and blandness must be understood as central to the definition and nature of the relationship with the clinician. The expression of symptoms varies with location and setting because the extent of self-disclosure is related to the identity and relationship of the person receiving the information, especially when the content concerns family members and intimate relationships. For this reason, a strong argument can be made for language and ethnicity matching of clients with clinicians to provide for an optimal relationship, particularly for Asian Americans who have underutilized mental health services historically.

3.2 Examples of Cultural Formulations

How difficult cultural formulations are to prepare is evidenced by the contents of the three published Asian-American cases (Barrett, 1997; Cheung & Lin, 1997; Lim & Lin, 1996). In this regard, the case of a Chinese-Vietnamese woman research participant (Cheung & Lin, 1997) merits comment. This cultural formulation could not have been prepared without knowledge of Chinese, the special circumstances of overseas Chinese communities, an understanding of refugee migration and relocation experiences as well as awareness of the magnitude of stress during the acculturation process in the United States. *Shenjing shuairuo*, or neurasthenia, was the patient's label for her distress as well as the label used by a Vietnamese

34 RICHARD H. DANA

psychiatrist. This psychiatrist and the authors of this article had knowledge concerning two classification systems not generally taught in the United States, the International Classification of diseases, Version 10 (ICD-10) and the Chinese Classification of Mental Disorders, version 2 (CCMD-2) as well as of DSM. These psychiatrists considered the relative acceptability to the patient of diagnoses from these different systems. Furthermore, the perception of severity of symptoms was related to cultural norms. This woman's family recognized adverse effects of stress on health but believed that her will power should have permitted her to ignore or suppress her symptoms. Her own explanation was somatic (i.e., running nose, sore throat, eye irritation) and social from the stressors due to overwork and pressure on the body stemming from cultural ideas concerning the necessity of moderation and balance for health. Her help-seeking was from Western-trained psychiatrists, although modern Western psychopharmacology provided her with only limited symptom relief. The intensity and immensity of stressors was apparent and these stressors occurred in a context of considerable social support including food, shelter, and emotional sustenance. Nonetheless, the degree of impairment was extreme. She was unable to work, had social and family relationship difficulties, and did not enjoy recreational activities. Even her ability to do routine household chores was impaired. Rapport and understanding of the complexity and nuances of her dilemmas were immensely facilitated by a clinician who spoke the same language and was from a similar culture and background. The final DSM-IV diagnoses here were Major Depression and Undifferentiated Somatoform Disorder and an Axis I, ICD-10 diagnosis of Neurasthenia.

4. PSYCHOPATHOLOGY

The DSM-IV relies heavily on the presence and expression of symptoms and the clustering of symptoms into disorders for diagnosis. Criteria validated in the United States are assumed to describe the presence and extent of disorders in other cultures with fidelity. The clusters of symptoms acceptable as DSM-IV diagnostic criteria represent expectations for European Americans in the United States. Symptoms are believed to be universal in spite of having different meanings in other cultures and differences in type, frequency, and duration. Different cultures also make different assumptions about symptoms that are subsequently used to interpret individual symptomatology. In non-Western societies, a family-group context for illness reduced the stigma of disease labels. Symptoms for a particular disorder may be expressed in somatic or psychological terms while clusters of symptoms can differ markedly for the same disorder.

A notable example is found in emotional words or symptoms for depression that were found to be clustered differently and with varied complexity or not amenable to clustering in eight countries (Brandt & Boucher, 1986). The requirements for a depression cluster were met in the United States, Sri Lanka, Japan, and Indonesia but not in Australia, Korea, Puerto Rico and Malaysia. These latter countries had depression-type words clustering into a sadness concept. In the United States, sadness was a primary ingredient of depression with anxiety, alienation, and shame-

EXAMINING THE USEFULNESS OF DSM-IV   35

guilt only marginally related. In Japan, however, anxiety, bored-lacking, misery, pain, regret-repent, and sadness were primary with 11 other secondary ingredients. This study suggested that the experience of depression may be conceptualized differently by using a variety of languages with specific vocabularies to structure the cultural meanings of the experience. Unfortunately, there has been no acceptable cross-cultural epidemiological research strategy to investigate depression, although Marsella (1987) suggested combining Western and indigenous definitions and sick roles, using similar case identification, sampling, and baselines for symptom frequencies, severity, and duration. Symptom patterns could be identified by multivariate analysis (Marsella, Sartorious, Jablensky, & Fenton, 1985).

In 1993, Sue reported that no large-scale prevalence studies on Asian Americans had been conducted. Nonetheless, he believed that prevalence rates had been underestimated in available research because this relatively small percentage of the population included many separate groups and samples of adequate size and representativeness had been difficult to assemble. In 1993-1994, the Chinese American Psychiatric Epidemiological Study (CAPES) was conducted and published research is now beginning to indicate the extent of underestimation (Takeuchi et al., 1998; Zheng et al., 1997). This section will examine studies of several major diagnostic categories including schizophrenia, depression, somatoform disorders, anxiety disorders, and culture-bound syndromes.

4.1 Schizophrenia

Schizophrenia occurs in almost all countries but prevalence rates differ markedly, symptom composition differs, and prognosis is much more favorable in developing countries than in the United States. The definition of schizophrenia also varies from a tight, narrow syndrome throughout much of the world (i.e., Western Europe, Asia, Latin America, Africa, Australia) to a broader, more inclusive syndrome in the Soviet Union and the United States (Westermeyer, 1985). Prevalence rates for DSM-IV schizophrenia in China and Japan are probably much lower than in the United States. Evidence for this assertion comes from differences in expression of symptoms, the use of different diagnostic systems in China and Japan, expectations for relatively good prognosis with home-care by families, and few hospitals for persons suffering from chronic mental illness (Cheung, 1991; Koizumi & Harris, 1992; Lin, 1953; Wilson & Young, 1988).

One study of the symptomatology of persons diagnosed with Schizophrenia in Japan and Taiwan will be used as an exemplar baseline for considering symptomatology displayed by traditional Asian Americans from these countries (Rin, Schooler, & Caudhill, 1973). The Japanese had clear symptom patterns with *shinkeishitsu* (depression/somatization), sleep disturbances, somatic/gastrointestinal complaints, inappropriate affect and hebephrenic-like acting-out, and apathy with rambling, distorted speech and restlessness. These authors described the Japanese symptoms as a turning against the self and problems with oneself. When compared with hospitalized, European Americans with a schizophrenia diagnosis in the United States, hospitalized Japanese patients were more physically assaultive, withdrawn,

36 RICHARD H. DANA

euphoric, emotionally labile, apathetic, had more sleep disturbances, fewer hallucinations, more bizarre ideas, and greater perplexity. Hospitalized Taiwanese patients had an outward focus with hostility, acting out, reality alterations, hypochondria, and headaches. These Taiwanese differed from mainland Chinese with a schizophrenia diagnosis, who exhibited a greater frequency of *shinkeishitsu* which was associated with relatively high social class status.

4.2 Depression

General medical practitioners are usually the first providers to see the majority of all persons with depression who generally present somatic and cognitive depressed symptoms (Lipowski, 1990). However, in many Asian American groups, somatic symptoms are the primary presenting complaints in psychiatric facilities. Thirty-five percent of refugees and immigrants to this country of Asian descent (i.e., Chinese, Filipino, Laotian, Mien, and Vietnamese) presented somatization complaints in primary care facilities with higher rates for refugees than immigrants (i.e., 43% vs. 27%) (Lin, Carter, & Kleinman, 1985). In fact, although the culturally determined array of presenting symptoms will often include somatization, the relative emphasis on these symptoms varies from culture to culture with more symptoms occurring among ethnic groups in which direct emotional expression is discouraged. More somatic symptoms have been associated with lower socioeconomic status, rural origins, and environmental stressors. Depression has been typically measured in Asian populations using translated measures without examination of translation adequacy or cross-cultural construct validity (Lin, 1989).

The Chinese may be the only group to have a clear depression pattern associated with somatic functioning (Marsella, Kinzie, & Gordon, 1973). However, the appearance of this pattern among Chinese in the United States may be associated with social class and age (unpublished study cited in Gaw, 1993). The prevalence of depression among Indochinese in the U.S. varies with the group and the length of time in the host country. In the U.S., Beiser (1988) reported fewer depressive symptoms over time among Laotians and Vietnamese except for unattached persons who had the highest symptom rates after 12 months. Beiser's sample of ethnic Chinese in the U.S. had low rates that continued to decrease over time with the presence of an established cultural community to provide support and affirm identity. A California study indicated that the highest rates for Khmer, with Khmer and Hmong having higher rates than Vietnamese or Chinese (Rumbaut, 1985). An Indochinese Refugee Program report described 28% of outpatients as having major depressive disorder (Kinzie & Manson, 1983).

A community survey using the Center for Epidemiologic Studies Depression Scale (CES-D) with Chinese American, Filipino American, Japanese American, and Korean American samples suggested a potential depression prevalence rate of about 19% (Kuo, 1984; Kuo & Tsai, 1986). Factor loading differences were examined for three CES-D factors among Chinese American, Korean American, and Japanese American and two factors for Filipino Americans. The pattern of similarities and differences among factor loadings for items was complex. The Chinese Americans

EXAMINING THE USEFULNESS OF DSM-IV   37

heavily somatized and had impaired interpersonal relations while the Japanese Americans somatized somewhat less frequently and had interpersonal relations characterized by greater fear and failure. Korean Americans emphasized loneliness, sadness, and less talk in their first factor while a second factor emphasized being happy and hopeful. Filipinos, however, presented very different factor loadings. These CES-D differences in depressive symptomatology among Asian Americans should be carefully examined by diagnosticians serving these groups. Comparisons should also be made with the 6.9% lifetime rates found in a very large sample in the Chinese American Epidemiological Study which used a version of the Composite International Diagnostic Interview (Takeuchi et al., 1998).

4.3 Somatoform Disorders

Somatization constitutes an attempt to communicate an experience of bodily symptoms and distress in response to psychosocial stressors often associated with depression and anxiety disorders, or worry and preoccupation with well-being (Lipowski, 1988). The most common somatic complaints are abdominal and chest pain, dyspepsia, headache, fatigue, cough, back pain, dizziness, and nervousness. Prevalence rates have been reported to be as high as 4% in the general population (Swartz, Blazer, George, & Landerman, 1986), although somatization accounted for 35% of illness visits in Southeast Asian primary care patients in this study (Lin, Carter, & Kleinman, 1985).

Much higher levels of somatic symptoms were also found among Hispanic psychiatric patients using diagnostic rating scales than were verifiable by DSM somatoform disorders criteria (Escobar, 1987). Escobar believed that the DSM system tends "to minimize cross-cultural differences in symptomatology and yield rather concordant syndromes stripped of their cultural character" (p. 178). As Fabrega (1991) has suggested in this context, the DSM flounders for multicultural populations because non-Western societies have not ordinarily provided unique disease labels due to belief in a multiplicity of causes while external validation for an illness is not required. Illness behaviors can reflect crises in relations with ancestors, social taboos, and political rivalries as well as family relations. Bodily language as expressed by somatic dialogue thus connects with, is responsible to, and reflects the self as well as social, natural, and supernatural phenomena.

4.4 Anxiety Disorders

Anxiety disorders are found in almost all cultures except among all aboriginal populations, although these individuals also experience anxiety and panic disorder in somatized form (Good & Kleinman, 1985). However, because culture-specific idioms are used to express anxiety complaints, anxiety, depression, and somatoform disorders (including neurasthenia, hypochondriasis and psychophysiological reactions) may overlap in symptomatologies and cannot readily be identified as separate clinical entities. The cultural context in which anxiety and fears occur may indicate whether or not the expression of these symptoms is pathological.

Pathological anxiety conditions can also be represented by culture-bound syndromes with various labels, prognosis, interventions, and outcomes. These culture-bound syndromes may be the equivalent of DSM panic disorders reported by 15% of respondents in a U.S. survey (Eaton, Kessler, Wittchen, & Magee, 1994). Sue (1993) suggested than anxiety symptoms are turned inward or internalized by Japanese Americans and later surface as physical complaints although more overt signs of conscious anxiety are largely absent. According to Sue (1993), Southeast Asians in the U.S. often experience fatigue, headaches, insomnia, memory loss, and impaired appetite because they focus more directly and immediately on somatic symptoms, or even specific organ dysfunctions.

The classification system for psychiatric diagnosis in China differs from either DSM in the United States or the ICD. When all three systems were applied to the same patients, the Chinese system identified the patients as suffering from neurotic disorders but the DSM and the ICD systems identified the same patients as suffering from depressive disorders (Nakane, Ohta, Uchino, & Takada, 1988). The diagnostic system used and the diagnostician's original culture largely determined the diagnostic label applied in cases of mental and physical fatigue coupled with decline of mental functions. The Chinese clinicians in China diagnosed the patients with neurasthenia, but clinicians in Japan and in the U.S. categorized the videotapes and brief, written case histories of patients as having adjustment reactions, anxiety disorders, and depression (Tseng, Xu, Ebata, Hsu, & Yuhua, 1986). Moreover, anxiety symptoms among Chinese in China were often represented by headaches, nausea, palpitations, and vertigo with references to emotions, as exemplified by angry liver, anxious heart and melancholy liver (Ots, 1990).

4.5 Culture-Bound Syndromes (CBS)

DSM-IV includes a selection of 25 CBSs in Glossary I. Described as folk conceptualization, or ethnopsychiatry, "the CBSs are commonly interpreted as patterned, pathologically exaggerated behavioral responses to culturally structured stress points, vulnerabilities, conflicts, or other sociocultural features (e.g., dominant social values) of a given person's environment" (Hughes & Wintrob, 1995, p. 567). The DSM-IV Glossary should be supplemented by use of the more complete 185 CBS version available in Simons and Hughes (1985, pp. 475-501).

CBSs probably occur with much greater frequency in immigrant, refugee, student, and sojourner populations in the United States than the DSM-IV Glossary location at the end of the volume would suggest. In fact, the CAPES of 1,747 Chinese American interviewees in Los Angeles county found that the neurasthenia (NT) prevalence rate without co-morbidity, as defined by the ICD-10, was 3.61% (Zheng at al., 1997). This high figure provided evidence that NT is probably a separate diagnostic category. As was also suggested in the CAPES, NT often occurs among Chinese Americans in a context with anxiety, depression, or fright (Lin, 1990). The CAPES report also contains the ICD-10 diagnostic criteria for NT, a resource useful for preparing cultural formulations in which fatigue is an important symptom. Moreover, this report suggested that NT may not even be properly

Examining the Usefulness of DSM-IV

identified as a CBS because a primary ICD-10 symptom is persistent and medically unexplained fatigue that has prevalence rates of 7% to 30% in Western communities. There are several other CBSs, including fright disorders, and the Sudden Unexpected Nocturnal Death Syndrome (SUNDS) manifested among Asians and Asian Americans that may have higher prevalence rates in the United States than hitherto suspected. Fright disorders are culture-specific expressions of intense and overwhelming anxiety (Good & Kleinman, 1985). For example, an altered trancelike state, *Latah*, occurs in Malaysia and Indonesia. In Korea, *shin-byung* appears with additional somatic complaints and possession by ancestral spirits and as *hwa-byung*, an anger syndrome with many physical symptoms, panic, and fear of death. Specific fears that the penis/vulva/nipples will shrink and recede into the body occur with *koro* in South China and among Chinese and Malaysian populations in Southeast Asia (Cheung, 1996). Sexual dysfunctions, or *shen-k'uei/shenkui* occurs in Chinese populations in contexts of extreme anxiety, or panic and somatic complains. In Japan, *shinkeishitsu*, a cluster of anxiety, fears of meeting people, inadequacy, and obsessive-compulsive symptoms, and *taijin kyofusho* consists of complaints that one's own bodily parts are offensive to others. Among Hmong men in the United States, SUNDS has been attributed to nocturnal spirit encounters (Adler, 1994). As with NT, these CBSs also occur in non-Asian cultures and may also have higher prevalence rates than hitherto suspected by European American psychiatrists.

The DSM-IV does disservice by ignoring cultural boundaries in extrapolation of diagnostic expectations for European Americans to Asian Americans. Asian Americans often express symptomatology using a somatic idiom, or with different symptom clusters for the same disorders. Moreover, psychopathology among Asian Americans contains a much larger representation of CBSs than was anticipated prior to CAPES. As a consequence, it behooves clinicians in the United States to be more aware of the disorders contained in diagnostic systems used in Asian countries and to use caution in applying the DSM-IV to Asian Americans without consideration of possible remediations to improve reliability.

5. DSM-IV REMEDIATIONS

Castillo (1996) suggested that the DSM-IV heralded the beginnings of a paradigm shift in psychiatry from a disease-entity conception to a holistic cultural-biopsychosocial model. This is occurring because the underlying disease-entity theory has not yielded unequivocal research documenting brain abnormalities as the causative factor in mental disorders. As a consequence, diagnosis and treatment should become "concerned with an individual who has thoughts, emotions, a social context, and a set of cultural schemas" (Castillo, p. 262). A new client-centered paradigm can synthesize knowledge from cultural, psychological, biological, and social factors. This model includes genetic sensitivity to culture-based and individually experienced stress/trauma. Individual culture-based feeling and thought responses to the environment serve to structure and alter neural networks in the brain. Biological and socio-cultural factors also influence duration of illness within clinical reality contexts that include "culture-bound syndromes, idioms of distress,

40   RICHARD H. DANA

professional diagnoses, and forms of deviant behavior structured in neural networks" (Castillo, p. 263). Within this model, culture-based treatments then provide culture-based psychological and neurological outcomes to demonstrate the permeable and changeable boundary between mental health and mental illness.

While I appreciate Castillo's integrated union of culture and biology, the importance of culture in the thinking and research of mental health scientists and practitioners falls far short of equivalence with biology in the present and immediate future. For this reason, I prefer approaches that affirm and strengthen cultural identity as the promised heart of psychological research, training, and practice (Dana, 1998b). From this perspective, more immediate and practical remediations include rendering DSM-IV more effective by using cultural formulations as described earlier in this chapter and by a more systematic diagnostic process. In addition, I believe that psychopathology can be re-conceptualized in etic-emic terms as a genuine cross-cultural psychology extension into the area of mental health.

5.1 A Systematic Diagnostic Process

Cultural formulations can increase DSM-IV reliability by transforming high inference assessment into low inference assessment (Dana, 2000a). High inference assessment can be transformed by an examination of reliability risk points in the diagnostic process (Wing, Nixon, Cranach & Strauss. 1980). These risk points occur in defining the symptoms, interviewing the patient, classifying the patient, including other clinical information and lab findings, reclassifying the symptoms, and considering presence-absence of etiological factors. Each of these risk points requires specific cultural competence skills as identified by Cuéllar and Gonzalez (2000, Table 25.2). It is recommended juxtaposing these risk points with DSM-IV cultural formulation components to increase reliability.

Cultural formulations, however, constitute only one of several important parts of the clinical process leading to a reliable DSM-IV diagnosis and subsequent treatment. My assessment-intervention model further delineates steps in the diagnostic process where relevant questions can be raised and cultural competency demonstrated by the helpfulness of cultural information resources for selecting and applying measuring instruments with a particular multicultural patient (Dana, 1997, 1998a, 2000b). These steps include evaluation of cultural orientation status for selection of assessment instruments, making decisions concerning the appropriateness of using existing European American emics, with or without modification, and/or use of available emic instruments. These instruments can provide further information for a cultural formulation whenever a clinical diagnosis is required and suggest whether a combined culture-general and culture-specific intervention will be beneficial (Dana, 1998b). When a diagnosis is not appropriate, an identity conceptualization that uses all available cultural information on personality and specific problems-in-living may be required for a culture-specific intervention.

This model also looks toward an eventual development of etic test derivatives from an etic-emic psychopathology theory analogous to what has been attempted in personality theory applied to the Thematic Apperception Test (DeVos & Vaughn, 1992). Such an enterprise is a natural development from the historic search in psychology for general laws of human behavior. Whenever etic or universal psychopathology constructs become available, these constructs may be combined with culture-specific or emic symptomatologies and syndromes using methodologies that are already available (e.g., Davidson, Jaccard, Triandis, Morales, & Diaz-Guerrero, 1976; Hui & Triandis, 1985).

5.2 Future DSM Versions

A cultural axis for the DSM could present an emic perspective from the standpoint of the patient and cultural reference group. Mezzich summarized the perspectives of proponents of a cultural axis: "the cultural meaning of a disorder has important influences on the reality of the illness, its accompanying social desirability, and its course. The authors recommend that the evaluator record in this axis the culture-specific illness category, explanatory model, illness idiom, predominant care-seeking patterns, and the perceived level of disability." (1996, p. 331). Mezzich believed that structure and codification of this proposal would be congruent with the consensual purposes and functions of DSM axes. Guarnaccia (1996) sees the utility of a cultural axis "for popular illness categories and for recording a patient's understanding of his or her disorder" (p. 336). He prefers a separate cultural axis to adding cultural syndromes to Axis I. Assessment of language abilities and acculturation is also considered germane to a cultural axis.

Byron Good (1996) has clearly identified the resistance within the psychiatric establishment to any emphasis on cultural contents in DSM-IV. There is clash between a belief in universal biological entities and the "forms of experience and cultural interpretations of that experience that occur in individuals and cultural groups" (Good, p. 349). The political correctness of the token cultural additions to DSM-IV are compelling evidences of underlying European American bias. The DSM-IV contains normative expectations for personhood, societal judgments concerning the major dimensions of aberrant behavior, basic categories to delineate these dimensions, and thought vs. affect and somatic vs. affective distinctions, among others, representative of a European American perspective on psychopathology. As a consequence, I do not believe that remediations in the form of a cultural axis will appear in subsequent DSM versions unless psychiatry can incorporate a commitment to human rights as complementary to its quest for a science of the human mind as Good has suggested is necessary.

5.3 Psychological Contributions

In the endeavor to protect human rights and avoid discrimination in the use of the DSM-IV, psychology can make a two-fold contribution. First, no other mental health area has the expertise to examine the European American methodology and statistics that undergird our research enterprise. Second, psychologists can share an advocacy role with other mental health professionals and social scientists in

42   RICHARD H. DANA

recognizing violations of human rights and implementing protections as a consequence of research that informs the entire mental health professional community.

Earlier in this chapter, the proposal to reverse the Null Hypothesis and implications for a cultural psychology were described as logical precursors to re-conceptualizing research process and methodology. There are available tools for competent cross-cultural and multicultural research (e.g., Allen & Walsh, 2000; van de Vijver, 2000). There is also a beginning of understanding that the cultural variance in clinical diagnostic instruments is of remarkably greater magnitude than was anticipated by a selective historic usage of methodology and statistics (e.g., Cuéllar, 2000; Nichols, Padilla, & Gomez-Macqueo, 2000). Moreover, there is now an investment in teaching clinical diagnostic assessment to professional psychologists on the basis of the entire available spectrum of relevant methodologies (e.g., López, 2000). This training can result in questioning the limits of usefulness of standard diagnostic instruments for multicultural populations and to researching new parameters for assessment practice in a multicultural society.

Finally, the protection of human rights and respect for the dignity and worth of individuals can be addressed by ethical codes that prioritize welfare of clients and patients (Payton, 1994) as well as by legitimizing advocacy in human science research (Wittig, 1985). Human science research can emphasize that knowledge of persons in social-cultural contexts is necessary using a systems approach and modified research methods in addition to tests. Our present ethical code in professional psychology (American Psychological Association, 1992) does not promote responsible clinical diagnostic assessment practice with multicultural populations (Dana, 1994, 1998b). Responsible assessment practice in a multicultural society is predicated on cultural competence. Cultural competence must be distinguished from professional competence per se; the requisite cultural knowledge cannot be acquired without awareness of professional competence boundaries. Responsibility for acquisition of this knowledge is a responsibility of the profession by specific training, practice, and experience. In the 1992 Ethics Code, the acquisition of such knowledge remained a responsibility of the individual psychologist. Similarly, the ethical code has not been supplemented by guidelines to include examples, vignettes and/or case materials, awareness of relevant assessment research, particularly concerning acculturation status, and a need for continuing self-examination by professional psychologists of their own cultural/racial identities (Dana, 1998b).

6. REFERENCES

Adler, S. R. (1994). Ethomedical pathogenesis and Hmong immigrants' sudden nocturnal deaths. *Culture, Medicine and Psychiatry, 18,* 23-59.

Advincula, A., & Ricco, R. (1998, August). *Development of the Filipino American Acculturation Scale.* Poster presented at the International Association for Cross-Cultural Psychology and Fourteenth International Silver Jubilee Congress, Bellingham, WA.

Allen, J., & Walsh, J. A. (2000). A construct-based approach to equivalence methodologies for cross-cultural/multicultural personality assessment research. In R. H. Dana (Ed.), *Handbook of cross-cultural and multicultural personality research* (pp. 63-85). Mahwah, NJ: Erlbaum.

EXAMINING THE USEFULNESS OF DSM-IV   43

Allison, K. W., Crawford, I., Echemendia, R., Robinson, L., & Knepp, D. (1994). Human diversity and professional competence: Training in clinical and counseling psychology. *American Psychologist, 49,* 792-796.

Allison,K. W., Echemendia, R., Crawford, I., & Robinson, L. (1996). Predicting cultural competence: Implications for practice and training. *Professional Psychology: Research and Practice, 27,* 386-393.

Ambady, N., Koo, J., Lee, F., & Rosenthal, R. (1996). More than words: Linguistic and nonlinguistic politeness in two cultures. *Journal of Personality and Social Psychology, 70,* 996-1011.

American Psychiatric Association (1952). *Diagnostic and statistical manual of mental disorders.* Washington, DC: Author.

American Psychiatric Association (1980). *Diagnostic and statistical manual of mental disorders* (3rd ed.). Washington, DC: Author.

American Psychiatric Association (1994). *Diagnostic and statistical manual of mental disorders* (4th ed.). Washington, DC: Author.

American Psychological Association (1992). Ethical principles of psychologists and code of conduct. *American Psychologist, 47,* 1597-1611.

Anderson, J., Moeschberger, M., Chen, M. S., Kunn, P., Wewers, M. E., & Guthrie, R. (1993). An acculturation scale for Southeast Asians. *Social Psycbiatry and Psychiatric Epidemiology, 28,* 131-141.

Barrett, R. J. (1997). Cultural formulation of psychiatric diagnosis. Death on a horse's back: Adjustment disorder with panic attacks. *Culture, Medicine and Psychiatry, 21,* 481-494.

Beiser, M. (1988). Influence of time, ethnicity, and attachment in Southeast Asian refugees. *American Journal of Psychiatry, 145,* 46-51.

Brandt, M. E., & Boucher, J. D. (1986). Concepts of depression in emotion lexicons of eight cultures. *International Journal of Intercultural Relations, 10,* 321-346.

Castillo, R. J. (1996). *Culture and mental illness: A client-centered approach.* Pacific Grove, CA: Brooks/Cole.

Cheung, F., & Lin, K.-M.. (1997). Neurasthenia, depression and somatoform disorder in a Chinese-Vietnamese woman migrant. *Culture, Medicine, and Psychiatry, 21,* 247-258.

Cheung, P. (1991). Adult psychiatric epidemiology in China in the 1980s. *Culture, Medicine and Psychiatry, 15,* 479-496.

Cheung, S. T. (1996). A critical review of Chinese Koro. *Culture, Medicine, and Psychiatry, 20,* 67-82.

Cuéllar, I. (2000). Acculturation as a moderator of personality and psychological assessment. In R. H. Dana (Ed.), *Handbook of cross-cultural and multicultural personality assessment* (pp. 113-129). Mahwah, NJ: Erlbaum.

Cuéllar, I., & Gonzalez, G. (2000). Cultural identity description and cultural formulation for Hispanics. In R. H. Dana (Ed.), *Handbook of cross-cultural and multicultural personality assessment* (pp. 605-621). Mahwah, NJ: Erlbaum.

Dana, R. H. (1993). *Multicultural assessment perspectives for professional psychology.* Boston: Allyn & Bacon.

Dana, R. H. (1994). Testing and assessment ethics for all persons: Beginning and agenda. *Professional Psychology: Research and Practice, 25,* 349-354.

Dana, R. H. (1997). Multicultural assessment and cultural identity: An assessment-intervention model. *World Psychology, 3(1-2),* 121-142.

Dana, R. H. (1998a). Multicultural assessment of personality and psychopathology in the United States: Still art, not yet science, and controversial. *European Journal of Psychological Assessment, 14,* 62-70.

Dana, R. H. (1998b). *Understanding cultural identity in intervention and assessment.* Thousand Oaks, CA: Sage.

Dana, R. H. (1998c). Personality and the cultural self: Emic and etic contexts as learning resources. In L. Handler & M. Hilsenroth (Eds.), *Teaching and learning personality assessment* (pp. 325-345). Mahwah, NJ: Erlbaum.

Dana, R. H. (2000a). Culture and methodology in personality assessment. In I. Cuéllar & F. A. Paniagua (Eds.), *Handbook of multicultural mental health: Assessment and treatment of diverse populations.* San Diego, CA: Academic Press.

Dana, R. H. (2000b). An assessment-intervention model for research and practice with multicultural populations. In R. H. Dana (Ed.), *Handbook of cross-cultural and multicultural personality assessment* (pp. 5-16). Mahwah, NJ: Erlbaum.

44   RICHARD H. DANA

Dana, R. H. (2001). Clinical diagnoses of multicultural populations in the United States. In L. A. Suzuki, J. Ponterotto, & P. Meller (Eds.), *The handbook of multicultural assessment* (2nd ed.) (pp. 101-131). San Francisco: Jossey-Bass.

Dana, R. H., & May, W. T. (1986). Health care megatrends and Health Psychology. *Professional Psychology: Research and Practice, 17,* 251-256.

Davidson, A. R., Jaccard, J. J., Triandis, H. C., Morales, M. L., & Diaz-Guerrero, R. (1976). Cross-cultural model testing of the etic-emic dilemma. *International Journal of Psychology, 11(1),* 1-13.

DeVos, G. A., & Vaughn, C. A. (1992). The interpersonal self: A level of psychocultural analysis. In L. B. Boyer & R. M. Boyer (Eds.), *The psychoanalytic study of society: Vol 17* (pp. 95-142). Hillsdale, NJ: Analytic Press.

Eaton, W. W., Kessler, R. C., Wittchen, H. U., & Magee, W. J. (1994). Panic and panic disorder in the United States. *American Journal of Psychiatry, 151,* 413-420.

Escobar, J. I. (1987). Cross-cultural aspects of the somatization trait. *Hospital and Community Psychiatry, 38,* 174-180.

Fabrega, H., Jr. (1991). Somatization in cultural and historical perspective. In L. J. Kirmayer, & J. M. Robbins (Eds.), *Current concepts of somatization: Research and clinical perspectives* (pp. 181-199). Washington, DC: American Psychiatric Press.

Gaw, A. C. (1993). Psychiatric care of Chinese Americans. In A. C. Gaw (Ed.), *Culture, ethnicity, and mental illness* (pp. 245-280). Washington, DC: American Psychiatric Press.

Good, B. J., (1996). Epilogue: Knowledge, power, and diagnosis. In J. E. Mezzich, A. Kleinman, H. Fabrega, Jr., & D. L. Parron (Eds.), *Culture and psychiatric diagnosis: A DSM-IV perspective* (pp. 347-351). Washington, DC: American Psychiatric Press.

Good, B. J., & Kleinman, A. M. (1985). Culture and anxiety: Cross-cultural evidence for the patterning of anxiety disorders. In A. H. Tuma & J. Maser (Eds.), *Anxiety and the anxiety disorders* (pp. 297-323).

Guarnaccia, P. J. (1996). Cultural comments on multiaxial issues. In J. E. Mezzich, A. Kleinman, H. Fabrega, Jr., & D. L. Parron (Eds.), *Culture and psychiatric diagnosis: A DSM-IV perspective* (pp. 335-338). Washington, DC: American Psychiatric Press.

Hughes, C. C., Wintrob, R. M. (1995). Culture-bound syndromes and the cultural context pf clinical psychiatry. In J. M. Oldham & M. B. Riba (Eds.), *Review of Psychiatry* (vol. 14, pp. 565-597). Washington, DC: American Psychiatric Press.

Hui, C. H., & Triandis, H. C. (1985). Measurement in cross-cultural psychology. *Journal of Cross-Cultural Psychology, 16,* 131-152.

Hsu, F. L. K. (1971). Psychosocial homeostasis and Jen: Tools for advancing psychological anthropology. *American Anthropologist, 73,* 24-44.

Kinzie, J. D., & Manson, S. (1983). Five years experience with Indochinese refugee psychiatric patients. *Journal of Operational Psychiatry, 14,* 105-111.

Koizumi, K., & Harris, P. (1992). Mental health care in Japan. *Hospital and Community Psychiatry, 43,* 1100-1103.

Kuo, W. H. (1984). Prevalence of depression among Asian-Americans. *Journal of Nervous and Mental Disease, 172,* 449-457.

Kuo, W, H., & Tsai, Y. (1986). Social networking, hardiness, and immigrants' mental health. *Journal of Health and Social Behavior, 37,* 133-149.

Lewis-Fernandez, R. (1996). Cultural formulation of psychiatric diagnosis. *Culture, Medicine and Psychiatry, 20,* 133-144.

Lewis-Fernandez, R., & Kleinman, A. M. (1994). Culture, personality, and psychopathology. *Journal of Abnormal Psychology, 103,* 67-71.

Lim, R. F., & Lin, K.-M. (1996). Cultural formulation of psychiatric diagnosis. Case No. 03. Psychosis following Qi-Gong in a Chinese immigrant. *Culture, Medicine and Psychiatry, 20,* 369-378.

Lin, E. H. B., Carter, W. B., & Kleinman, A. M. (1985). An exploration of somatization among Asian refugees and immigrants in primary care. *American Journal of Public Health, 75,* 1080-1084.

Lin, N. (1989). Measuring depressive symptomatology in China. *Journal of Nervous and Mental Disease, 177(3),* 121-131.

Lin, T. (1953). A study of the incidence of mental disorder in Chinese and other cultures. *Psychiatry, 16,* 313-336.

Lin, T. Y. (1990). Neurasthenia revisited: Its place in modern psychiatry? *Culture, Medicine, and Psychiatry, 14,* 105-129.

EXAMINING THE USEFULNESS OF DSM-IV

Lipowski, Z. J. (1988). Somatization: the concept and its clinical application. *American Journal of Psychiatry, 145,* 1358-1368.

Lipowski, Z. J. (1990). Somatization and depression. *Psychosomatics, 31,* 13-21.

López, S. R. (2000). Teaching culturally informed psychological assessment. In R. H. Dana (Ed.), *Handbook of cross-cultural and multicultural personality assessment* (pp. 669-687). Mahwah, NJ: Erlbaum.

Malgady, R. G. (1996). The question of cultural bias in assessment and diagnosis of ethnic minority clients: Let's reject the Null Hypothesis. *Professional Psychology: Research and Practice, 27,* 73-77.

Malgady, R. G. (2000). Myths about the Null Hypothesis and the path to reform. In R. H. Dana (Ed.), *Handbook of cross-cultural and multicultural personality assessment* (pp. 49-62). Mahwah, NJ: Erlbaum.

Mao, L. M. (1992). Invitational discourse and Chinese identity. *Journal of Asian Pacific Communication, 3,* 79-96.

Marsella, A. J. (1987). The measurement of depressive experience and disorder across cultures. In A. J. Marsella, R. M. A. Hirschfeld, & M. M. Katz (Eds.), *The measurement of depression* (pp. 376-397). New York: Guilford.

Marsella, A. J., Kinzie, D., & Gordon, P. (1973). Ethnic variations in the expression of depression. *Journal of Cross-Cultural Psychology, 4,* 435-459.

Marsella, A. J., Sartorius, N., Jablensky, A., & Fenton, F. R. (1985). Cross-cultural studies of depressive disorders: An overview. In A. Kleinman & B. Good (Eds.), *Culture and depression: Studies in the anthropology and anthropology of affect and disorder* (pp. 299-324). Berkeley, CA: University of California Press.

Meredith, G. M. (1967). Ethnic Identity Scale: A study in transgenerational communication patterns. *Pacific Speech Quarterly, 2,* 57-65.

Mezzich, J. E. (1996). Culture and multiaxial diagnosis. In J. E. Mezzich, A. M. Kleinman, H. Fabrega, Jr., & D. L. Parron (Eds.), *Culture and psychiatric diagnosis: A DSM-IV perspective* (pp. 327-334). Washington, DC: American Psychiatric Press.

Mezzich, J. E., Kleinman, A. M., Fabrega, H., Jr., & Parron, D. L. (1996) (Eds.). *Culture and psychiatric diagnosis: A DSM-IV perspective.* Washington, DC: American Psychiatric Press.

Nakane, Y., Ohta, Y., Uchino, J., & Takada, K. (1988). Comparative study of affective disorders on three Asian countries: Differences in diagnostic classification. *Acta Psychiatrica Scandinavica, 78,* 698-705.

Nathan, P. E. (1994). DSM-IV: Accessible, not yet ideal. *Journal of Clinical Psychology, 50,* 103-110.

Nathan, P. E., & Langenbucher, J. W. (1999). Psychopathology: Description and classification. *Annual Review of Psychology, 50,* 79-107.

Nichols, D. S., Padilla, J., & Gomez-Macqueo, E. L. (2000). Issues in the cross-cultural adaptation and use of the MMPI-2. In R. H. Dana (Ed.), *Handbook of cross-cultural and multicultural personality assessment* (pp. 247-266). Mahwah, NJ: Erlbaum.

Okazaki, S., & Sue, S. (1995). Methodological issues in assessment research with ethnic minorities. *Psychological Assessment, 7,* 367-375.

Ots, T. (1990). The angry liver, the anxious heart, and the melancholy spleen: The phenomenology of perception in Chinese culture. *Culture, Medicine and Psychiatry, 14,* 21-56.

Pang, K. Y. C. (1990). Hwabyung: The construction of a Korean popular illness among Korean elderly immigrant women in the United States. *Culture, Medicine, and Psychiatry, 14,* 495-512.

Payton, C. R. (1994). Implications of the1992 Ethics code for diverse groups. *Professional Psychology: Research and Practice, 25,* 317-320.

Rin, H., Schooler, C., & Caudhill, W. A. (1973). Culture, the social structure and psychopathology. *Journal of Nervous and Mental Disease, 157*(4), 296-312.

Rumbaut, R. (1985). Mental health and the refugee experience: A comparative study of Southeast Asian refugees. In T. C. Owan (Ed.), *Southeast Asian mental health: Treatment, prevention services, training, and research* (pp. 433-486). Bethesda, MD: NIMH.

Simons, R. C., & Hughes, C. C. (Eds.) (1985). *The culture-bound syndromes: Folk illnesses of psychiatric and anthropological interest.* Boston: Reidl.

Suinn, R. M., Rickard-Figueroa, K., Lew, S., & Vigil, P. (1987). The Suinn-Lew Asian Self-Identity Acculturation Scale: An initial report. *Educational and Psychological Measurement, 47,* 401-407.

Sue, S. (1993). Mental health. In N. Zane, D. T. Takeuchi, & K. Young (Eds.), *Confronting critical health issues of Asian and Pacific Islander Americans* (pp. 266-288). Thousand Oaks, CA: Sage.

Sue, S., & Zane, N. (1987). The role of culture and cultural techniques in psychotherapy: A critique and reformulation. *American Psychologist, 42,* 37-45.

Swartz, M., Blazer, D., George, L., & Landerman, R. (1986). Somatization disorder in a community population. *American Journal of Psychiatry, 143,* 1403-1408.

Takeuchi, D. T., Chung, R. C-Y., Lin, K.-M.., Shen, H., Kurasaki, K., Chun, C-A., & Sue, S. (1998). Lifetime and twelve-month prevalence rates of major depressive episodes and dysthymia among Chinese Americans in Los Angeles. *American Journal of Psychiatry, 155,* 1407-1414.

Tanaka-Matsumi, J., Hsia, C., & Fyffe, D. (1998, August). *Measurement of acculturation: An examination of psychometric properties.* Paper presented at the International Congress for Cross-Cultural Psychology 14th International and Silver Jubilee Congress, Bellingham, WA.

Tseng, W. S., Xu, D., Ebata, K., Hsu, J., & Yuhua, C. (1986). Diagnostic pattern for neurosis in China, Japan, and the United States. *American Journal of Psychiatry, 143,* 1010-1-14.

van de Vijver, F. (2000). The nature of bias. In R. H. Dana (Ed.), *Handbook of cross-cultural and multicultural personality assessment* (pp. 87-106). Mahwah, NJ: Erlbaum.

Westermeyer, J. (1985). Psychiatric diagnosis across cultural boundaries. *American Journal of Psychiatry, 142,* 798-805.

Wilson, L. G., & Young, D. (1988). Diagnosis of severely ill inpatients in China: A collaborative project using the Structured Clinical Interview for DSM-III (SCID). *Journal of Nervous and Mental Disease, 176,* 585-592.

Wing, J., Nixon, J., Cranach, M., & Straus, A. (1980). *Multivariate statistical methods used in the International Pilot Study of Schizophrenia* (DDDS Pub. No. ADM 80-630). Washington, DC: U.S. Government Printing Office.

Wittig, M. A. (1985). Metatheoretical dilemmas in the psychology of gender. *American Psychologist, 40,* 800-811.

Yao, E. L. (1979). The assimilation of contemporary Chinese immigrants. *Journal of Psychology, 101,*107-113.

Zane, N. W. S. (1998, December). *Major approaches to the measurement of acculturation: A conceptual analysis and empirical validation.* Paper presented at the International Conference on Acculturation: Advances in Theory, Measurement, and Applied Research, University of San Francisco, San Francisco, CA

Zheng, Y-P., Lin, K.-M., Takeuchi, D., Kurasaki, K., Wang, Y., & Cheung, F. (1997). An epidemiological study of neurasthenia in Chinese-Americans in Los Angeles. *Comprehensive Psychiatry, 38*(5), 249-259.

MARJORIE KAGAWA-SINGER AND RITA CHI-YING CHUNG[1]

CHAPTER 4

TOWARD A NEW PARADIGM: A CULTURAL SYSTEMS APPROACH

1. INTRODUCTION

Alice in Wonderland meets the Cheshire cat as she is traveling down a road and asks, "Would you tell me please which way I ought to go from here?" The Cheshire cat responds, "That depends on where you want to get to." She responds, "I don't much care where." To which he responds - " then it doesn't matter which way you go" (Carroll, 1946, p. 49).

Alice was unclear of her destination. Persons suffering from mental illness are often in the same state. However, even when the client is from an ethnic group different than that of the therapist, the therapist often presumes the European American clinical strategies are universally effective and therefore assumes the client wishes to travel down the same road and towards the same destination that the therapist has been trained to travel. Rarely does the therapist or researcher assess the appropriateness of the assumed destination or the means to get there beyond translating the existing road signs into the appropriate language.

2. TOWARD A NEW PARADIGM

The premise of this chapter is that culture is fundamental to the assessment of mental health status. An extensive body of literature in anthropology, sociology, and cross-cultural psychology clearly indicates that universal psychological needs of human beings, and the means to re-establish well-being are culturally defined (Angel & Thoits, 1987). Every culture has its own way of treating mental illness. Moreover, each culture establishes the parameters within which distress is defined—that is, what is normal versus abnormal behavior. In addition, each culture determines the etiology of and prescribes social responses to such distress such that treatment is congruent with culturally defined causative forces.

---

[1] We give special thanks to Thy Bich Nguyen and Regina Chinsio for their assistance with the preparation of this chapter.

The purpose of this chapter is to make explicit the influence of culture on the conceptualization and construction of mental illness. We first examine the theoretical assumptions and methodological fallacies that underlie the assumed universal patterns of expression of mental distress rather than cultural specificity of idioms of distress. Next, we demonstrate the need for extensive rethinking and restructuring of mental health theory for Asian Americans. We offer a different theoretical perspective for assessing the mental health of Asian American clients, and broadening the monocultural, European American paradigm to promote greater sensitivity in the assessment of cultural variations in emotional distress.

The theoretical framework presented in this chapter, Cultural Systems Approach, is based upon the following propositions.

- **Proposition 1:** The goal of human behavior is to fulfill the three universal human needs of safety and security, integrity, and a sense of belonging (Kagawa-Singer & Chung, 1994).
- **Proposition 2:** The construct of personhood or self and the means to fulfill these three universal needs for individuals are provided within a culturally informed social structure (Charmaz, 1991; Heelas & Lock, 1982; Kaufman & Cooper, 1999).
- **Proposition 3:** Psychological distress, both biologically and/or socially induced, is experienced in a socio-cultural context that can both potentiate and/or ameliorate the distress.
- **Proposition 4:** Psychological distress, as experienced in various cultures, may or may not have similar biological causes, but the expression of the distress or the psychopathology will primarily be communicated through the symbols provided within a particular cultural environment, and thus be culturally variant in construct and label, as well as meaning.

Following this line of logic, researchers and practitioners should interpret behavior according to its contextual meaning and accept the equal validity of various cultural constructions of the distress (Kagawa-Singer & Chung, 1994). Measures to capture these variations in constructs that would be cross-culturally valid and comparable would then be required to test universal and culture specific strategies for theory development, assessment accuracy, and intervention and treatment efficacy.

To understand the fundamental influence of culture on the expression and understanding of mental illness, we compare the Western basis of psychiatric diagnosis to potential variations in the different Asian American cultures. We begin with uniquely constructed indigenous concepts of the self or personhood (Averill, Opton, & Lazarus, 1969; Fabrega, 1974; Geertz, 1973; Kleinman, 1978; Paul, 1955; Rosenberg, 1979; Spiro, 1965; Tursky & Sternbach, 1967), and then proceed to a description of more specific Asian American concepts of health and mental health. We then present psychocultural frameworks from anthropology and sociology that form the basis of our proposed paradigm, the Cultural Systems Approach. We

TOWARD A NEW PARADIGM: A CULTURAL SYSTEMS APPROACH   49

proposed the Cultural Systems Approach as a cross-culturally based analytic framework for assessing psychological distress to guide future research with Asian Americans.

3. CULTURAL CONSTRUCTION OF THE SELF

The three basic human needs for psychological well-being are a sense of safety and security, integrity and meaning, and belonging (Kagawa-Singer, 1988). Behavior is directed to maintain these three needs through culturally prescribed behaviors that are sanctioned as appropriate. When these three needs are met within the socially sanctioned parameters, the culturally constructed sense of self or personhood is protected and promoted (Charmaz, 1991; Kaufman, 1986). Each culture, however, constructs the self with beliefs and values congruent with its own worldview. A worldview defines reality and consists of fundamental cognitive orientations by which people order their lives. It is historically conditioned, and therefore, culturally relative (Spiro, 1965). When the "self" is threatened, the psychological and social mechanisms evoked to protect the culturally constituted sense of self would vary as well as the prescribed modes of maintaining a positive self-image. The actual tools or skills available to protect one's sense of integrity, such as particular psychological defense mechanisms, may not differ so much across cultures as much as the pattern, emphasis, and occasion for their prescribed use. For example, only a few emotions are universal, such as pleasure, joy, anger, security, affection, grief and fear (Hinton, 1975). We are socialized to channel these basic emotions into nuanced and culturally prescribed ways of expressing feelings within social norms. Patterns of expression of emotional distress are, thus, culturally constituted constructs and are used within a social context to control thought and behavior. Each culture determines the parameters of acceptable social behavior and likewise, definitions of social deviance (Edgerton, 1985; Kutchins & Kirk, 1997). Crying appears to be a universal response to sadness, but how and when it is expressed is culturally determined. For example, the degree of keening and wailing at funerals of the Toraja of Indonesia (Wellenkamp, 1987) would not be the appropriate behavior at a Japanese Buddhist funeral or a Protestant funeral in the U.S. Hence, to display this degree and intensity of keening and wailing at the funerals in the latter two examples may be misinterpreted as needing psychological intervention.

3.1 European American Concepts of Self

In the dominant, middle-class, European American ethos, the individual is viewed as autonomous, egalitarian, rational, aggressive, self-assertive and self-aware (Lebra, 1976). Cultivation of the rational mind is of the essence, and healthy interpersonal relationships are characterized by open, verbal communication (Gudykunst & Ting-Toomey, 1988; Lazarus, 1983). In the European American ethos, individuals are believed to possess a sacred dignity and expected to control their destiny through rational means, and by verbally resolving those parts that are unsatisfying through interpersonal processes.

The present European American perspective has evolved from philosophical and cultural shifts expressed by writers of the Western Enlightenment period (Wellesz, 1973). During that period, the Cartesian duality of body and mind raised rationality above the emotional or animal nature of emotions, and evolved a belief in the self as unique, singular and exclusive, with the right to live and die with self-determined dignity. Dignity, however, is largely a New Testament and Christian contribution based on "the supreme value of the God-given soul" (Lukes, 1973, p. 46). Assuring one's dignity is a justifying moral argument in Western concepts (e.g., death with dignity) (Ersak, Kagawa-Singer; Blackhall, Barnes, & Koenig, 1998). Consequently, the goal in Western psychotherapy is to seek a clearer understanding of the dichotomy of the rational and emotional self. The objective is to mold one's self into the image of the "ideal" autonomous, self-reliant individual who strives to attain self-defined happiness.

These unstated values and assumptions about the universality of the individual direct much of psychological research. The transcultural applicability of these values and assumptions, although unsubstantiated, are not frequently questioned (Johnson, Marsella, & Johnson, 1974; Kleinman & Kleinman, 1991).

3.2 Concepts of the Self in Asian American Cultures

Concepts of the self or personhood in Asian American cultures may differ from that of the European American construct of the self. The pictograph of *person* in the Japanese and Chinese written languages (pronounced *jin* and *jen*, respectively) expresses the conceptualization of "self" in Asian culture. This character represents two human figures leaning against one another:

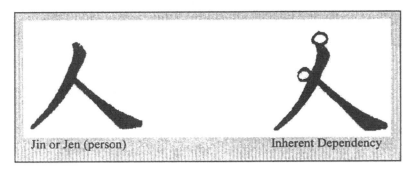

Figure 1. Pictograph of Person in Japanese and Chinese Written Language

Within the character for the individual person is the inherent concept of interdependency and support. The Japanese character for *human being—ningen—*is also a graphic expression of the interpersonal nature of human existence:

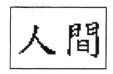

Figure 2. Graphical Expression of Interpersonal Nature of Human Existence

It literally translates: humanity is created between persons. Personal existence, reality, and the **rightness** or **wrongness** of a situation is defined in the space created between individuals. From this cultural perspective, neither reality nor the individual exists without participants (Lebra, 1976; Lock, 1982; Smith, 1983). These East Asian characters convey an interdependent conceptualization of the self, in contract to the Western concept of *I*, which is individuality. In the ideal Western ethos, individuals defend their individual boundaries against the intrusion of others (Bellah, Madsen, Sullivan, Swidler, & Tipton, 1985). Much time and effort is spent to declare clear ego boundaries between self and other. Indeed, this is the goal of most Western psychotherapy (Chang, 1988). In general, research that is based upon the Western concept of the self may have questionable validity when applied to Asian American individuals who adhere to more sociocentric concepts of the self than the Western-based concepts of individuality.

4. ANTHROPOLOGICAL AND SOCIOLOGICAL FRAMEWORKS FOR MENTAL HEALTH

Within the contexts of anthropology and sociology, mental health is primarily seen to be socially and culturally constructed. An acontextual definition of mental illness would be unusual. The context of illness, therefore, is not confined to the identified client. Rather, the "pathology" involves the entire community, for the social network is the group that provides the norms with which to label behavior as normal or abnormal, and importantly sanctions what is considered appropriate treatment. Furthermore, a treatment would be deemed appropriate if it corresponded with the socially sanctioned etiology of the disorder to which it is being applied. We use Fabrega's (1992) and Horwitz's (1999) categorizations to organize the various approaches that would inform an expanded, cross-culturally applicable framework for the study of Asian American mental health.

Fabrega (1992) organized the various approaches to the study of psychopathology into three types: radical, weak, and strong cultural relativism. Radical cultural relativism is the particularist view that states that all psychopathology is culture-bound and unique. In contrast, weak cultural relativism is the notion that culture shapes the particular presentation but not the underlying pathology (Lemelson, 1999). For example, paranoia is universal, but the content becomes culture specific: in the United States an individual may fear the CIA (Central Intelligence Agency), whereas in another culture an individual may fear witches or ghosts. Strong cultural relativism is a synthesis of radical and weak cultural relativism. That is, some characteristics of psychopathology may have a universal, neurophysiologic and pathophysiologic basis, but the existence and expression of these conditions is culturally and socially perceived and responded to by its members (Lemelson, 1999).

Horwitz (1999) grouped the prevalent approaches to the study of mental health in sociology into four categories within two dimensions (Table 1). The first dimension is comprised of the acontextual (universal) and the culturally dependent approaches. The second dimension consists of two categories that describe approaches that focus on either the *individual* exhibiting the symptoms or on the response of *members of the social network or society* to the individual exhibiting the symptoms. Only a brief description of each of these categories will be presented.

Table 1. Approaches to the study of mental health in sociology (adapted from Horowitz, 1999)

Object of Explanation	**Culturally Acontextual – Universal**	**Culturally dependent**
Individual	I. Etiological	III. Sociological Psychology
Responders	II.Social Response	IV.Social Constructionist

4.1 Acontextual or Universal Approaches

4.1.1 Etiological

The etiological approach focuses on how social systems are related to the development of mental illness (Aneshensel, 1992; Pearlin, 1989). Both mental and physical illnesses are viewed as clusters of symptoms that are independent of specific cultural context. The focus is on how chronic strains due to societal structure, such as poverty or discrimination, may be expressed as emotional symptoms of distress. The interest is why some people in a particular setting develop symptoms of mental illness while others do not.

4.1.2 Social response

The social response model seeks to explain not the emergence of psychiatric symptoms, but instead the responses that people make to these symptoms. For example, the World Health Organization (WHO) found that schizophrenia is found across cultures (Edgerton, 1967; Fabrega, 1992; Sartorius et al., 1976). However, schizophrenia found in developing countries appears to have a shorter course and is less debilitating. An interpretation of this is that compared to more economically developed societies, less developed societies place less stigma on the mentally

TOWARD A NEW PARADIGM: A CULTURAL SYSTEMS APPROACH

disordered, and allow greater latitude in behavior, and therefore have lower expectations for performance (Hopper, 1992; Waxler, 1974). Hence, social responses in different cultures may correlate with the prognosis of the disorder. One strength of this approach is its recognition that the biologic nature of psychiatric symptoms only partly determines how people react to psychiatric disorders. A variety of factors, including the relationship to the person who is ill, ethnicity, social class, age, gender, and social networks affect the definition, classification, and reaction to symptoms (Horowitz, 1982). These factors can either impede or enhance the optimal provision of mental health services (Mechanic, 1987).

4.2 Culturally Dependent Approaches

4.2.1 Sociological psychology

The socialological psychology approach is similar to Fabrega's (1992) radical cultural relativism in that cultural contexts fundamentally shape the types of mental disorder that *individuals* experience and display. Mental disorders are products of particular times and places including cultural contexts. The essential difference between sociologic models of etiology and sociologic psychology is that the former seeks social factors to explain universal symptoms of mental disorders and the latter perspective explains the social and cultural origins of the kinds of mental disorders that emerge in particular contexts.

4.2.2 Social constructionist

The social constructionist approach asserts that abnormality and normality are products of cultural constructions of acceptable behavior. This perspective directly challenges the view that psychiatric symptoms are purely properties of individuals. The history of the DSM categories exemplifies how social conditions form the perceptions of mental illness. For example, several diagnoses have recently been added or deleted due to changes beyond evidence-based scientific findings, such as the changing definitions of schizophrenia, the elimination of homosexuality as a mental illness, the elimination of neurasthenia as a diagnostic category, and the emergence of eating disorders. The problems studied with this approach are concerned with how these rules of pathology arise and change from one time period to the next and who has the power to effect these changes (Kutchins & Kirk, 1997; Rogler, 1997).

5. SYNTHESIS OF STRONG CULTURAL RELATIVISM AND INDIGENOUS CONCEPTS OF THE SELF

Although the models of psychopathology and mental distress described above in Horwitz's (1999) categories have been widely used, none appears to resolve the tension created by ignoring the indigenous constructions of the self. The theoretical model proposed in this chapter moves beyond Horowitz's (1999) sociologic models to explicitly integrate the contextual nature of culture. We combine Fabrega's (1987) strong cultural relativist model that supports the perspective of biologic similarities and cultural shaping of psychological distress with theories supporting indigenous constructions of the self. This synthesis provides the basis for a model to study the effects of culture and ethnicity on mental distress. Lemelson (1999) states that:

> When a Western diagnostic framework (such as the DSM) is given theoretical primacy, local constructions of interpretation and meaning are often ignored or lost. They argue that any approach that begins with symptoms relevant to Western cultures and that seeks to find lexical or semantic equivalents in other cultures rather than identifying local idioms of distress and relating those to a Western nosologic system, will produce syndromes that are potentially meaningless to members of that culture and often irrelevant to potential treatment concerns. (p. 12)

Thus, Western trained clinicians find what they seek. The theoretical basis of their perspective determines what landmarks they use to chart the landscape of mental distress. If equal validity is not afforded to different goals or constructs of the self, these clinicians and researchers will continue to travel down different paths than Asian American clients may want to travel. Unless demonstrated to be cross-culturally valid, the validity of research findings and the efficacy of treatment will be of little use at best when based upon a Euro-centric monocultural theoretical framework.

The disease/illness differentiation provided by anthropologists helps to clarify the relationships of culture and psychopathology cross-culturally. The disease (the objective, measurable causative agent) that causes the illness (or the meaning of the disease to the individual) (Eisenberg, 1977; Fabrega, 1974; Kleinman, 1980) is perceived to have an identifiable cause, for example, alterations in neurotransmitter function, such as serotonin uptake. In the U.S., such identified disorders or diseases are perceived as separate from the self and amenable to specific, biomedical interventions to cure the disease. In the European American ethos the body is viewed mechanistically as a system with interchangeable and reparable parts or correctable chemical pathways. Most other cultures, however, classify the etiology of disease as physical, metaphysical or supernatural (Eisenberg et al., 1993), and use modes of intervention that are appropriate to treat the disorder depending upon the etiologic factor. Western biomedicine gives little credibility to the spiritual or metaphysical causes of disease, thus negating significant segments of cultural constructions of distress, and threatens the credibility of the therapist. The efficacy of indigenous treatments requires extensive study that has yet to be widely tested (Lemelson, 1999). We propose placing the synthesis of the strong cultural relativism perspective and indigenous constructs of the self into an ecologic framework using a cultural systems approach.

6. CULTURAL SYSTEMS APPROACH

The Cultural Systems Approach for Asian American mental health demonstrates that the expression of symptoms of psychological distress among ethnic minorities is greatly influenced by complex cultural interactions of numerous nested variables that interact synergistically (Fabrega, 1987; Kirmayer, 1989; Kleinman,1980; Tseng, 1990). Variables studied in isolation and out of context lose their salience, integrity, and uniqueness in their particular cultural configuration. Thus, they are not additive and do not have a linear relationship. The Cultural Systems Approach operationalizes the elements of culture in a fashion that provides a dynamic mechanism to identify the structural importance of a particular culture that shapes the mental health of its members, and, moreover, indicates malleable points of entry for intervention (Facione, 1993). The nested layers that comprise the elements of this model function in an integrated cultural system and are defined as follows.

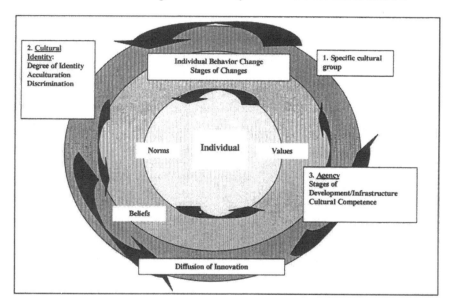

Figure 3. Cultural Systems Approach

7. SPECIFIC CULTURAL GROUPS

Culture provides the lens through which its members view reality and, for mental well-being, shapes the expectations of cure and the management of emotional distress. The structural content of beliefs, values, and practices form the cognitive map that creates the refraction through which its members see the world. Every culture creates reality for its members, ascribes meaning to events in that reality, and prescribes appropriate emotional and behavioral responses to those events. These norms of affect and behavior provide predictability, security, and rationale for everyday social interactions as well as for those inevitable stressful life events such as birth, sickness, and death (Hallowell, 1955). Culture also provides its members with some degree of personal and social meaning for human existence and suffering. Thus behaviors, which appear to be similar across cultures, may not have the same conceptual equivalence. The same stimulus in two different cultures may evoke different cognitive, affective and behavioral responses (Padilla, 1998). That is, the meaning and symbolic value of similar symptoms may be culture specific and thus are not interchangeable across cultures (Kleinman, 1978; Mechanic, 1980).

The majority of psychosocial research and practice, however, appears to treat the impact of culture on the processes of symptom recognition, labeling, and help seeking behavior as "nonproblematic" (Angel & Thoits,1987). That is, these underlying differences are considered epiphenomenal and ignored (Kleinman & Kleinman, 1991). Consequently, the premise and methodology used by Western and Western-trained researchers on most large-scale epidemiologic studies involving different ethnic groups reflect an ethnocentric bias that assumes that the attributions to stressors, the desired outcomes, and the means for adaptation to life stressors are universal (Horwitz, 1999; Kutchins & Kirk, 1997). The variability of the expressions of distress, however, strongly suggests that the search for universal similarities in psychiatric disorders may distort the actual pathology that exists (Castillo, 1996). Analyses conducted to investigate inter-group variation with this "universalist" premise, such as separating racial/ethnic subjects into dichotomous groups, usually results in the groups treated acontextually as homogeneous populations. Intra-group variation has seldom been analyzed, although recent studies on Asian Americans are beginning to analyze differences across various Asian ethnic groups with respect to language and acculturation (Chmielewski, Fernandes, Yee, & G. A. Miller, 1995).

Even these latter Asian American studies, though, operationalize culture with static and dichotomous cultural traits (e.g., fatalism, Confucian beliefs regarding authority, and shame) and use these traits acontextually as explanatory mechanisms to compare incidence, prevalence, and treatment responses. Three flaws, however, negate this approach. The first is that the validity of the diagnoses themselves (dependent variables) is rarely questioned (Huertin-Roberts, Snowden, & Miller, 1997). Second, the traits themselves are studied acontextually with minimal intra-group variation except along the poorly conceptualized axis of acculturation. Third, variations in incidence and prevalence are usually normed against the white populations. Little attention is directed towards understanding the fundamental cultural variances in the construct of the self (Charmaz, 1991; Kaufman, 1986). Culture and cultural traits must be recast from static, discrete traits to a contextualized, systems theory that encompasses these cultural characteristics within differing context dependent constructs of the self and acknowledges the effects of cultural expression, shaping, and meaning (Lin, Carter, & Kleinman, 1985).

Another way of examining the impact of culture on self is to operationalize the two main purposes of culture. The first purpose is integrative and consists of the beliefs and values that provide individuals their sense of identity, self-worth, and belonging. The second major purpose is functional: the rules of behavior for interpersonal interactions that enable the group to survive physically, provide for the welfare of its members, and prescribe rules for positive social interactions (Kagawa-Singer & Chung, 1994). These patterns of belief and rules for behavior enable its members to have a sense of security, predictability, and efficiency in communication. Members are recognizable to each other and social interactions and integration are facilitated. These two functions are analogous to the warp and woof or the perpendicularly woven threads of a tapestry. The technique of weaving is universal but the patterns that emerge from each group are culturally identifiable (Kagawa-Singer, 1988). That is, the concepts of beauty, (e.g., color, balance, symmetry) and the patterns chosen to display in the tapestries express the ethos of the culture and the message to be communicated through the tapestry. The significance of this analogy is that specific, discrete beliefs and behaviors are like the threads in the tapestry. A single thread of one cultural tapestry can be taken out and compared across cultural groups for its inherent characteristics (such as feeling alienated from one's group), but the usefulness and integrity of the thread as representative of the entire tapestry cannot be judged unless seen within the pattern of the entire cultural fabric within which it functions.

Taken in isolation and out of context, as the DSM-IV purports that syndromes of psychiatric disorders can be, leads to potential misinterpretation or misdiagnoses of culturally based behavior as maladaptive or pathologic. Difficulties in cross-cultural diagnoses occur when the pattern of the researcher's tapestry is used as the template to evaluate the behavior of an individual from a different culture. The essence of the client's pattern is not recognized as equally valid – or even existent.

8. CULTURAL AND ETHNIC IDENTITY

Cultural identity in a multicultural society becomes one's ethnicity. An ethnic group can be viewed as a self-perceived cultural group that resides within a power structure of a multicultural society (DeVos & Romanucci-Ross, 1982; Kagawa-Singer, 2000). Ethnicity and ethnic identity are more fundamental to an individual's identity than mere glossing by phenotype or particular beliefs and values and/or practices that are measured as static, dichotomous entities. Ishi, the last Yaqui Indian of California, stated this reality when he sadly commented on the death of his culture: "Ethnic identity is found in the 'cup of custom' passed on by one's parents from which one drinks the meaning of existence. Once the cup is broken, one can no longer taste of life" (DeVos & Romanucci-Ross, 1982, p. 364). One's ethnic group provides the individual a sense of identity, belonging, and ultimate loyalty (Berreman, 1982). Moreover, the effects of minority status are often overlooked in assessment strategies, yet the effects are well documented with poorer health outcomes (Dressler, 1996; Schulman et al., 1999).

8.1 Discrimination/Racism

Discrimination and racism, appears to be the underlying factor in the dynamic of differential assessment and treatment, and occurs when external group identifiers such as skin color, language, or religion is used within a power structure to judge the relative value of individuals and allocate resources based upon those criteria in a prejudicial manner (Kagawa-Singer, 2000; LaVeist, 1996; Williams, Yan, Jackson, and Anderson, 1997). In the U.S., discrimination based upon skin color appears to be a major influence on mental health status rather than the purported biologic construct of race per se (H. Myers & Rodriguez, 1998). The effects of society's racial attitudes on one's self-concept are apparent for Asian Americans as a **visible** minority (Ong, 1994; Sanjek, 1998). Consideration of their ethnic minority status is essential to understand their concept of self. The effects of racialized, color-conscious societies, like the U.S., engender self-hate and reduced self-esteem (Uba, 1994). These effects must be measured and included in any evaluation of normative levels of psychological distress.

8.2 Acculturation/Assimilation

The Asian American race/ethnic category is extremely heterogeneous. Over 30 distinct national groups comprise this category and multiple ethnic groups within each national group also exist, each with its own culture or subculture. Moreover, varying levels of acculturation and assimilation within each group also indicate differential expressions of cultural beliefs and practices and promote the need for assessment of individual variation within and between cultural groups. Within-group variation is significant. Varying levels of acculturation, age, education, income, family structure, gender, wealth, foreign versus U.S.-born status, and immigrant status all modify one's degree of ethnic identity and mental health status, as noted in Box 2 of Figure 3. Each of the variations must be accounted for in mental health assessment and research study sampling strategies by measuring these variations and interpreting them within their appropriate cultural tapestry (Kagawa-Singer, 1994). Lack of accountability of these differences perpetuates aggregating these groups and losing the ability to identify within and between group differences that may likely impact scientific findings. Variations in beliefs, attitudes and behaviors should be viewed as a kaleidoscope of changing relationships rather than as a static, homogenous, stereotypical caricature (Ying, Lee, Tsai, Yeh, & Huang, 2000).

8.3 Asian American Norms, Values, and Beliefs About Health and Illness

Asian nosology of health differs markedly from the European American concept. According to some Asian culture values, the individual is viewed as a microcosm of the universe and the unimpeded flow of *ki* or *chi*, (the vital life force within one's mind, spirit, and body) ensures well-being. The Western duality of mind and body does not exist and hierarchical structure of rational mind over emotional reality is not valued in the same manner in Asian cultures as it is in European American cultures. The objective in living a healthy life, according to some Asian cultural belief systems, is to constantly strive to seek a balance among the internal and external forces (Kagawa-Singer, 1994). Both health and illness are considered part of life, and perfect health is viewed as unattainable (Ohnuki-Tierney, 1984). For example, in the traditional Japanese world-view, the psyche, which in Western thought is half of the duality of mind and body, is relegated to one of the several equal forces at play in an individual's personal and social world. In more traditional Japanese and Japanese American[2] culture, for example, illness is perceived as a unique and changing constellation of imbalances in life forces and, therefore, medical intervention is directed towards pragmatic, symptom relief, not cure. Health is thus attained through perseverance and endurance of the person's will in conjunction with the facilitation and support of cosmopolitan medical intervention (Lock, 1982; Ito, Chung, & Kagawa-Singer, 1997).

In traditional Japanese American culture[2], one receives identity, a sense of worth, and security within the family, which is the primary group of allegiance. Psychotherapeutic alliances for Asian American clients appear to be facilitated if the traditional family structure is recreated rather than if individuation and autonomy are imposed (McGoldrick, Pearce, & Giordano, 1982; Shon & Ja, 1982). Asian American clients may feel torn between their values to obtain their support from within the natal or adopted family, and from "strangers" represented by the therapist.

Traditional Japanese culture recognizes the duality of the private/public (honne/tatemae) self and the necessity of it in order to maintain harmony in interpersonal relationships and family stability. In the dominant middle-class European American ethos, the emphasis on autonomy, honesty, and intimacy forces the individual to express his "Honne" in public interactions. The European American individual, however, might experience a greater sense of ambivalence than the Japanese American person, because as the European American tries to maintain a positive image inwardly and outwardly, the actual negative or unacceptable feelings in "Honne" must be kept from conscious awareness (Doi, 1985). In the West, the individual is expected to leave his original source of intimacy, (i.e., the family) and is expected to seek fulfillment of his needs for support and nurturance in other areas. For instance, the American culture expects the young adult to leave home and make it on his own in order to promote a positive sense of autonomy. In contrast, in the Japanese culture, the term for leaving home was reserved linguistically to mean severing ties with society and leaving, for example, to join a monastery.

This does not mean that awareness of unity of the "Honne/Tatemae" duality does not create tension for the traditional Japanese American, but the tension may be coped with differently—perhaps through somatization as the target of frustration and aggression that cannot be expressed emotionally against the offender in a socially acceptable manner (Lebra, 1984). This potential tension within the acculturative

---

[2] We define traditional Japanese-American in this chapter as follows: individuals who maintain a more traditional Japanese perspective on life compared to those who have adopted a more Western viewpoint.

process would be a fruitful area of study for the effects of chronic stress on Asian Americans as a minority group.

The behaviors of Asian Americans are often labeled as passive or unreflective. According to Western standards, such characteristics, such as passivity, inability to verbalize feelings, and being overly compliant are viewed as deviating from the ideal (i.e., having a weak ego). These criteria, however, are based on a Western European concept of self, and such assumptions would be ethnocentric and erroneous. An understanding of Asian American cultures would indicate that such categorizations would be premature at best, for the Asian ethos is based on quite different premises. For example, the U.S. health care system is founded on three basic values; inalienable rights of the individual, autonomous decision making ability, and the elimination of suffering. Most other cultures, however, are sociocentric or group-oriented. The three values that underlie the conceptualization of health in sociocentric cultures are the belief in the welfare of the group over individual needs, decision-making as consensus, and, importantly, the belief that suffering is an inevitable part of living that must be borne with strength and integrity (Kagawa-Singer, 1998; Padilla, 1998). Coping strategies would naturally vary (Kagawa-Singer, 1988).

9. PROFESSIONAL CULTURE

Each clinician also is a member of an ethnic culture(s) as well as a professional culture. Some Asian American clinicians have been trained in their native Asian cultures, and others have been trained in the U.S.. Each, therefore, comes with a different awareness as well as location in the intersection of cultures and assimilation and acculturation levels that will impact on the clinician in the same way as they do with the clients. Clear awareness of these differences and their effect on the therapeutic interaction has been discussed elsewhere (see Kagawa-Singer & Chung, 1994). The impact of the clinician's personal and professional culture on Western psychotherapy is also accounted for in the Cultural Systems Approach.

Analyses of the variables within a system context require capturing the dynamic nature of cultural shaping, and also require statistical applications that are beyond multilevel modeling. Perhaps the approach of chaos theory in physics would be a possible analogy. This theory states that the nature of the elements themselves changes depending upon the effect of the interaction of the constituent elements in time and space. Like the atomic periodic chart, each element is a system made up of similar parts as all other elements, but in very different configurations that create a totally different kind of matter: the essence differs. Such is the cultural construction of the self. The constituent molecules may be similar, but the make-up and configuration of the parts and the nature of their connections results in a totally different substance. Such is the nature of the self. Each culture constructs the self from similar compounds, but their configuration creates a different element or culturally identifiable self. Asian and Asian American cultures may create similar substances with similar molecular weights, but their configuration may create unique and identifiable elements (cultures).

TOWARD A NEW PARADIGM: A CULTURAL SYSTEMS APPROACH

Using the analogy of atomic particles and elements, mental health practice and research should focus on not only the general impact of culture on self, but also the intersect of culture, acculturation, and assimilation. In other words, the focus should be on the complexity of culture or its varying degrees and significance on and within the various domains of beliefs, values and norms of the individual as well as the degree of acculturation and assimilation. Each individual is unique, although certain patterns within ethnic groups may be similar.

10. IMPLICATIONS FOR ASIAN AMERICAN POLICY AND RESEARCH

The theoretical frameworks outlined by Horwitz (1999) and Fabrega (1992) provide different perspectives on the assessment of the mental health status of Asian Americans. The value of these frameworks is that it makes explicit the orientation used by each approach and provides a new basis for critique and testing. The cross-cultural Cultural Systems Approach, presented in this chapter provides a foundation to assess the shortcomings of the prevalent monocultural research paradigm. More effort must be directed to build upon this awareness and design studies that will further identify the underlying universal and culture specific patterns of distress.

Based upon the four propositions posed at the beginning of the chapter, the Cultural Systems Approach indicates three major strategies (theoretical, methodological, and culture-specific) for cross-cultural studies with Asian Americans. These strategies are not mutually exclusive. They should be addressed simultaneously, for they require different professional expertise to provide clarification at different levels of the model. The first is theoretical. The equal validity of indigenous constructs of the self should be explored, and cross-culturally valid methods should be designed to study the comparability of these constructs. Second is methodologic. Specifically, the construction of standardized tools and translation of concepts and instruments must be evaluated, recalibrated, and validated (Munet-Vilaro, 1994; Rogler & Cortes, 1993). Only a few studies have attempted to assure conceptual equivalence in cultural concepts as well as linguistic accuracy in the translations of standardized instruments, and even fewer of these have been conducted in Asian American populations (Canino & Bravo, 1994; Chung & Kagawa-Singer, 1994; Devins, Beiser, Dion, Pelletier, & Edwards, 1997; Ferketich, Phillips, & Verran, 1993; Jones & Kay, 1992; Jones & Korchin, 1982; Malgady, Rogler, & Tryon, 1992).

Most often, the measures used in studies of Asian Americans are symmetrically translated (Jones & Kay, 1992), that is, the standardized tools normed on U.S. or European populations are directly translated into the target Asian languages. The untested assumption is that the concepts developed in Western nosology are valid and reliable for Asian American populations. Yet in the majority of studies, variability in the conceptualization of psychological distress across specific ethnic nosologies such as in Cambodian, Laotian, Vietnamese, or Chinese- Vietnamese cultures have not been considered (Kirmeyer, 1989). An asymmetrical translation has not been conducted. In this latter technique, translation is conducted for conceptual accuracy in the target culture and language. For example, Western designed depression measures for Asians must be translated symmetrically, if not, the items on the depression measures makes no sense to that group. Items such as *feeling blue* is a concept unique to North Americans. Translating such a construct asymmetrically will only create confusion. Lack of awareness of these incompatible constructs will produce an inaccurate response for both practitioner and researcher.

The DSM-III categories were purported to be culture free and this edition was the first to make the paradigm shift from psychodynamic to biologic etiology of mental distress. Cultural differences were coded as *atypical* affective disorder or anxiety disorder (Lemelson, 1999). Kleinman and Kleinman (1991) noted that the *atypical* categories were the diagnoses most applicable to non-Western countries (where more than 80 percent of the world resides). In DSM-IV, the paradigm shifted again to recognize that complex social and cultural processes mediate the complex relation between brain biochemistry and major psychopathology. Acknowledgement of cross-cultural differences, however are still viewed as epiphenominal, and "atypical" categorizations were relabeled *Not Otherwise Specified* (NOS) (Agbayani-Siewert, Takeuchi, & Pangan, 1999). The logic of the cultural construction of reality presented thus far, however, makes it impossible to view the effects of cross-cultural differences as epiphenominal (Ots, 1990; Kawanishi, 1992). Castillo (1996) believes that the next paradigmatic shift, in the forthcoming DSM-V, will be strongly influenced by anthropological theory on the relation of culture to psychopathology.

The third strategy is to identify culture specific issues (e.g., constructs of the self or social network structure and function) that require modification and reorientation of psychotherapeutic assessment techniques to improve the mental health of Asian Americans. Assessing outcomes of therapy are dependent upon not only the means or techniques, but also assurance that the correct diagnosis was made. Both the destination and the means to get there must be negotiated between the patient, family and therapist.

All three strategies are necessary to increase the validity, reliability and appropriateness of mental health assessments for Asian Americans. The Cultural Systems Approach reveals the fundamental nature of cultural constructions of mental health. Use of this approach would explicitly acknowledge the validity of these cultural variations and deconstruct the current Western-based monocultural approach to mental health. The next task would be to develop methods to measure and evaluate the identified differences with conceptual equivalence and go beyond merely tailoring intervention to discrete *cultural* traits. This paradigm shift restructures our research models to refine assessments of psychological distress and to incorporate more appropriate and acceptable destinations. This shift also requires multidisciplinary research teams in order to analyze the effects of the complex, interrelated systems approach of culture on Asian American mental health.

11. REFERENCES

Agbayani-Siewert, P., Takeuchi, D. T., & Pangan, R. W. (1999). Mental illness in a multicultural context. In C. S. Aneshensel & J. C. Phelan (Eds.), *Handbook of the sociology of mental health* (pp. 19-36). New York: Kluwer Academic/Plenum Publishers.

Aneshensel, C. S. (1992). Social stress: Theory and research. *Annual Review of Sociology, 18,* 15-38.

Angel, R., & Thoits, P. (1987). The impact of culture on the cognitive structure of illness. *Culture, Medicine and Psychiatry, 11,* 465-494.

Averill, J., Opton, E., & Lazarus, R. (1969). Cross-cultural studies of psychophysiological response during stress and emotion. *International Journal of Psychology, 4*(2), 83-102.

Bellah, R., Madsen, R., Sullivan, W., Swidler, A., & Tipton, S. (Eds.). (1985). *Habits of the heart: Individualism and commitment in American life.* New York: Harper and Row.

Berreman, G. (1982). *Bazaar behavior: Social identity and social interaction in urban India* (1st ed.). Chicago: University of Chicago Press.

Canino, G., & Bravo, M. (1994). The adaptation and testing of diagnostic and outcome measures for cross-cultural research. *International Review of Psychiatry, 6,* 281-286.

Carroll, L. (1946). *Alice in wonderland.* New York: Grosset and Dunlap.

Castillo, R. (1996). *Culture and mental illness: A client centered approach.* New York: Brooks Cole.

Chang, S. C. (1988). The nature of the self: A transcultural view: I. Theoretical aspects. *Transcultural Psychiatric Research Review, 25*(3), 169-203.

Charmaz, K. (1991). *Good days, bad days: The self in chronic illness and time.* New Brunswick, NJ: Rutgers University Press.

Chmielewski, P. M., Fernandes, L. O., Yee, C. M., & Miller, G. A. (1995). Ethnicity and gender in scales of psychosis proneness and mood disorders. *Journal of Abnormal Psychology, 104*(3), 464-470.

Chung, R. C.-Y., & Kagawa-Singer, M. (1994). Predictors of psychological distress among Southeast Asian refugees. *Social Science and Medicine, 36*(5), 631-639.

Devins, G. M., Beiser, M., Dion, R., Pelletier, L. G., & Edwards, R. G. (1997). Cross-cultural measurements of psychological well-being: The psychometric equivalence of Cantonese, Vietnamese, and Laotian translations of the Affect Balance Scale. *American Journal of Public Health, 87*(5), 794-799.

DeVos, G., & Rommanucci-Ross, L. (1982). *Ethnic identity* (2nd ed.). Chicago: University of Chicago Press.

Doi, T. (1985). *The anatomy of self.* Tokyo: Kodansha International.

Dressler, W. W. (1996). Hypertension in the African American community: Social, cultural, and psychological factors. *Seminars in Nephrology, 16*(2), 1-12.

Edgerton, R. (1967). *The cloak of competence: Stigma in the lives of the mentally retarded.* Berkeley, CA: University of California Press.

Edgerton, R. (1985). *Rules, exceptions, and social order.* Berkeley, CA: University of California Press.

Eisenberg, D. M., Kessler, R. C., Foster, C., Norlock, F. E., Calkins, D. R., & Delbanco, T. L. (1993). Unconventional medicine in the United States: Prevalence, costs, and patterns of use. *New England Journal of Medicine, 328*(4), 246-252.

Eisenberg, L. (1977). Disease and illness. Distinctions between professional and popular ideas of sickness. *Culture, Medicine and Psychiatry, 1*(1), 9-23.

Ersak, M., Kagawa-Singer, M., Blackhall, L., Barnes, D., & Koenig, B. A. (1998). Multi-cultural considerations in the use of advance directives. *Oncology Nursing Forum 25*(10), 1683-1690.

Fabrega, H. (1974). *Disease and social behavior: An interdisciplinary perspective.* Cambridge, MA: MIT Press.

Fabrega, H. (1992). The role of culture in a theory of psychiatric illness. *Social Science of Medicine, 35,* 91-103.

Facione, N. C. (1993). The Triandis model for the study of health and illness behavior: A social behavior theory with sensitivity to diversity. *ANS: Advances in Nursing Science, 15*(3), 49-58.

Ferketich, S., Phillips, L., & Verran, J. (1993). Focus on psychometrics: Development and administration of a survey instrument for cross-cultural research. *Research in Nursing and Health, 16*(3), 227-230

Geertz, C. (1973). *The interpretation of cultures.* New York: Basic Books.

Gudykunst, W., & Ting-Toomey, S. (1988). *Culture and interpersonal communication.* Newbury Park, CA: Sage Publications.

Hallowell, A. I. (1955). *Culture and experience.* Philadelphia: University of Pennsylvania Press.

Heelas, P., & Lock, A. (1982). *Indigenous concepts of the self.* London: Academic Press.

Hinton, J. (1975). The influence of previous personality on reactions to having terminal cancer. *Omega, 6,* 95-111.

Hopper, K. (1992). Some old questions for the new cross-cultural psychiatry. *Medical Anthropology Quarterly, 7,* 299-330.

64 MARJORIE KAGAWA-SINGER AND RITA CHI-YING CHUNG

Horwitz, A. V. (1982). *The social control of mental illness.* New York: Academic Press.

Horwitz, A. V. (1999). Chapter 4: The sociological study of mental illness: A critique and synthesis of four perspectives. In C. S. Aneshensel & J. C. Phelan (Eds.), *Handbook of the sociology of mental health* (pp. 57-78). New York: Kluwer Academic/Plenum Publishers.

Heurtin-Roberts, S., Snowden, L. R., & Miller, L. (1997). Epressions of anxiety in African Americans: ethnography and the epidemiological catchment area studies. *Culture, Medicine and Psychiatry, 21*(3), 337-363

Ito, K., Chung, R. C.-Y., & Kagawa-Singer, M. (1997). Asian/Pacific American women: Health care issues of a multicultural group. In S. B. Ruzek, V. L. Olesen, & A. E. Clarke (Eds.), *Women's health: Complexities and differences* (pp. 300-328). Columbus, OH: Ohio State University Press.

Johnson, F. A., Marsella, A. J., & Johnson, C. L. (1974). Social and psychological aspects of verbal behavior in Japanese-Americans. *American Journal of Psychiatry, 131*(5), 580-583.

Jones, E. E., & Korchin, S. J. (Eds.). (1982). *Minority mental health perspectives.* New York: Praeger.

Jones, E. G., & Kay, M. (1992). Instrumentation in cross-cultural research. *Nursing Research, 41,* 186-188.

Kagawa-Singer, M. (1988). *Bamboo and oak: Differences in adaptation to cancer between Japanese-American and Anglo-American patients.* Unpublished doctoral dissertation, University of California, Los Angeles.

Kagawa-Singer, M. (1994). Cross-cultural views of disability. *Rehabilitation Nursing, 19*(6), 362-365.

Kagawa-Singer, M. (1998). Death rituals and mourning: A multicultural perspective. *Oncology Nursing Forum, 25*(10), 1752-1756.

Kagawa-Singer, M. (in press). Improving the cancer care outcomes of underserved U.S. populations: Expanding the research paradigm. *Annals of Epidemiology.*

Kagawa-Singer, M., & Chung, R. (1994). A paradigm for culturally based care for minority populations. *Journal of Community Psychology, 22*(2), 192-208.

Kaufman, J. S., & Cooper, R. S. (1999). Seeking causal explanations in social epidemiology. *American Journal of Epidemiology, 150*(2), 113-120.

Kaufman, S. (1986). *The ageless self: Sources of meaning in late life.* Madison, WI: University of Wisconsin Press.

Kawanishi, Y. (1992). Somatization of Asians: An artifact of Western medicalization? *Transcultural Psychiatric Research Review, 29,* 5-36.

Kleinman, A. M. (1980). *Patients and healers in the context of culture.* Berkeley, CA: of California Press.

Kleinman, A. M., Eisenberg, L., & Good, B. (1978). Culture, illness and care: Clinical lessons from anthropologic and cross-cultural research. *Annals of Internal Medicine, 88*(2), 251-258.

Kleinman, A. M., & Kleinman, J. (1991). Suffering and its professional transformation: Toward an ethnography of interpersonal experience. *Culture, Medicine and Psychiatry, 15*(3), 275-301.

Kutchins, H., & Kirk, S. A. (1997). *Making us crazy: DSM: The psychiatric bible and the creation of mental disorders.* New York: The Free Press.

LaVeist, T. A. (1996). Why we should continue to study race...but do a better job: An essay on race, racism and health. *Ethnicity & Disease, 6*(1-2), 21-29.

Lazarus, R. (1983). The costs and benefits of denial. In S. Breznitz (Ed.), *In the Denial of Stress* (pp. 1-30). New York: International Univeristy Press.

Lebra, T. (1976). *Japanese patterns of behavior.* Honolulu, HI: University of Hawai'i Press.

Lebra, T. (1984). Nonconfrontational strategies for management of interpersonal conflict. In E. S. Krauss, T. P. Rohlen & P. G. Steinhoff (Eds.), *Conflict in Japan* (pp. 41-84). Honolulu, HI: University of Hawai'i Press.

Lemelson, R. B. (1999). *Re-checking the color of chickens: Indigenous, ethnographic, and clinical perspectives on obsessive-compulsive disorder and Tourette's Syndrome in Bali.* Unpublished doctoral dissertation, University of Michigan, Ann Arbor.

Lin, E. H. B., Carter, W. B., & Kleinman, A. M. (1985). An exploration of somatization among Asian refugees and immigrants in primary care. *American Journal of Public Health, 75*(9), 1080-1084.

Lock, M. (1982). Models and practice in medicine: Menopause as syndrome or life transition? *Culture, Medicine and Psychiatry, 6*(3), 261-280.

Lukes, S. (1973). *Individualism.* New York: Harper and Row.

Malgady, R. G., Rogler, L. H., & Tryon, W. W. (1992). Issues of validity in the diagnostic interview schedule. *Journal of Psychiatric Research, 26*(1), 59-67.

TOWARD A NEW PARADIGM: A CULTURAL SYSTEMS APPROACH

McGoldrick, M., Pearce, J., & Giordano, J. (Eds.). (1982). *Ethnicity and family therapy*. New York: The Guilford Press.

Mechanic, D. (1980). *Mental health and social policy* (2nd ed.). Englewood Cliff, NJ: Prentice Hall.

Mechanic, D. (Ed.). (1987). *Improving mental health services: What the social sciences can tell us*. San Francisco: Jossey-Bass.

Munet-Vilaro, F. (1994). *Methodologic issues in the implementation of research with a Latino population (In nursing research in underserved populations)* (Special monograph No. 3072, pp. 39-43). Atlanta, GA: National American Cancer Society.

Myers, H., & Rodriguez, N. (1998, December). *Acculturation and physical health in racial/ethnic minorities*. Paper presented at the International Conference on Acculturation: Advances in Theory, Measurement, & Applied Research, San Francisco.

Ohnuki-Tierney, E. (1984). *Illness and culture in contemporary Japan: An anthropological view*. London: Cambridge University Press.

Ong, P. (1994). *The state of Asian Pacific America: Economic diversity, issues and policies*. Los Angeles: LEAP Asian Pacific American Public Policy Institute and UCLA Asian American Studies Center.

Ots, T. (1990). The angry liver, the anxious heart, and the melancholy spleen: The phenomenology of perceptions in Chinese culture. *Culture, Medicine and Psychiatry, 11*(1), 21-59.

Padilla, G., & Kagawa-Singer, M. (1998). Quality of Life and Culture. In C. R. King, & P. S. Hinds (Eds.), *Quality of life from nursing and patient perspectives: Theory, research, and practice* (pp. 74 - 92). Sudbury, MA: Jones and Bartlett Publishers.

Paul, B. D. (Ed.). (1955). *Health, culture and community; Case studies of public reactions to health programs*. New York: Russell Sage Foundation.

Pearlin, I. (1989). The sociological study of stress. *Journal of Health & Social Behavior, 30*, 241-256.

Rogler, L. H. (1997). Making sense of historical changes in the diagnostic and statistical manual of mental disorders: Five propositions. *Journal of Health and Social Behavior, 38*(1), 9-20.

Rogler, L. H., & Cortes, D. E. (1993). Help-seeking pathways: A unifying concept in mental health care. *American Journal of Psychiatry, 150*(4), 554-561.

Rosenberg, M. (1979). *Conceiving the self*. New York: Basic Books.

Sanjek, R. (1998). *The future of us all: Race and neighborhood politics in New York City*. Ithaca, NY: Cornell University Press.

Sartorius, N., Jablensky, A., Korten, A., Ernberg, G., Anker, M., Cooper, J. E., & Day, R. (1976). Early manifestations and first-contact incidence of schizophrenia in different cultures. *Psychological Medicine, 16*, 909-928.

Schulman, K. A., Berlin, J. A., Harless, W., Kerner, J. F., Sistrunk, S., Gersh, B. J., Dube, R., Teleghani, C. K., Burke, J. E., Williams, S., Eisenberg, J. M., & Escarce, J. J. (1999). The effect of race and sex on physicians' recommendations for cardiac catheterization. *The New England Journal of Medicine, 340*, 618-626.

Shon, S., & Ja, D. (1982). Asian families. In A. Gurman (Ed.), *Ethnicity and family therapy* (pp. 600). New York: The Guilford Press.

Smith, R. (1983). *Japanese society: Tradition, self, and the social order*. Cambridge, UK: Cambridge University Press.

Spiro, M. (1965). Religious systems as culturally constituted defense mechanisms. In M. Spiro (Ed.), *In context and meaning in cultural anthropology* (pp. 100-113). New York: The Free Press.

Tseng, W. S., Asai, M., Liu, J. Q., Wibulswasdi, P., Suryani, L. K., Wen, J. K., Brennan, J., & Heiby, E. (1990). Multicultural study of minor psychiatric disorders in Asia: Symptom manifestations. *International Journal of Psychology, 36*(4), 252-264.

Tursky, B., & Sternbach, R. (1967). Further physiological correlates of ethnic differences in responses to shock. *Psychophysiology, 4*(1), 67-74.

Uba, L. (1994). *Asian Americans: Personality patterns, identity, and mental health*. New York: The Guildford Press.

Waxler, N. E. (1974). Culture and mental illness: A social labeling perspective. *Journal of Nervous and Mental Disease, 159*, 379-395.

Wellenkamp, J. (1987). *The meaning of crying and wailing among the Toraja*. Paper presented at the meeting of the American Anthropological Association, Chicago, IL.

Wellesz, E., & Sternfeld, F. (1973). *The Age of Enlightenment - 1745-1790* (2nd ed.). London, New York: Oxford University Press.

Williams, D., Yan, Y., Jackson, J. S., & Anderson, N. B. (1997). Racial differences in physical and mental health: Socioeconomic status, stress and discrimination. *Journal of Health Psychology.*

Ying, Y., Lee, P. A., Tsai, J. L., Yeh, Y.-Y., & Huang, J. S. (2000). The conception of depression in Chinese American college students. *Cultural Diversity and Ethnic Minority Psychology* 6(2), 183-195.

KEH-MING LIN AND MARGARET LIN

CHAPTER 5

CHALLENGING THE MYTH OF A CULTURE FREE NOSOLOGICAL SYSTEM

1. INTRODUCTION: PROGRESS AND LIMITATIONS OF THE DSM-IV

Despite the existence of a voluminous and continuously growing literature indicating that cultural factors exert profound influences on psychopathology and psychiatric nosology, until most recently, culture had been practically completely neglected in most discussions on psychiatric diagnosis by the majority of psychiatric theorists, researchers and practitioners (Jensen & Hoagwood, 1997; Mezzich, Kleinman, Fabrega, & Parron, 1996). In this regard, the publication of the fourth version of the Diagnostic and Statistical Manual (DSM-IV) (American Psychiatric Association, 1994) represented a remarkable and encouraging departure. Thanks to the dedicated work of the Group on Culture and Diagnosis (GCD), and the receptive attitude of the leaders of the DSM-IV Task Force, the final version of the DSM-IV is indeed much more culturally informed and enriched as compared to its previous incarnations. As summarized in a recent article by Mezzich et al. (1997), although the Task Force's acceptance of GCD's recommendations was partial, inconsistent, and at times superficial, the final product does contain a substantial amount of cultural information that is overall useful for clinicians and researchers who consult the manual and related materials. These include: 1) the incorporation of a discussion on the role that culture plays in psychiatric diagnosis in the Introduction section of the Manual; 2) the inclusion of cultural information, where relevant, in most sections of the text; 3) outline for Cultural Formulation; 4) glossary of Culture Bound Syndromes (CBS). The last two are included in the DSM-IV as an Appendix.

It came as a surprise to the authors, and perhaps to other members of the GCD as well, that of the four areas, the last appears to have received most attention by professionals as well as the public, and perhaps has the most visible impact on the practice of transcultural psychiatry since the publication of the DSM-IV (Hughes, 1985). It is interesting and ironic that, due to concerns regarding the meaning of Cultural Bound Syndrome (CBS), especially the fear that the term might implicitly suggest that the other officially endorsed syndromes listed in the manual are not influenced by culture (that is, the Western professional culture), members of the GCD were reluctant to use the term. After much debate, the title of the Appendix was initially changed to "Glossary of Culturally-Related Idioms of Distress." However, for unclear reasons, the title of the glossary was eventually reverted back by the DSM Task Force to the more conventional although potentially misleading, "CBS," prior to the publication of the DSM IV (Mezzich et al., 1994; Mezzich, Kleinman, Fabrega, Good, et al., 1993; Mezzich, Kleinman, Fabrega, Parron et al., 1993).

Irrespective of the pros and cons for the continuing use of the term CBS, the inclusion of some of the better documented folk illness labels in the DSM-IV manual has helped to highlight the importance of culture in shaping and interpreting experiences of distress, in patterning its expression, and in providing a basis for the communication between patients and professionals or healers (Littlewood & Lipsedge, 1985; Kaplan & Sadock, 1988; M. Kleinman, Eisenberg, & Good, 1978). While highlighting the power of culture in shaping the experience and expression of distress, the term CBS can also be misleading in the sense that it implicitly endorses the deep-rooted bias that the current nosologic system is culture-free. Symptom clusterings divergent from those familiar to Western clinicians or that do not fit perfectly into the current Western categorical model of diagnosis are often labeled culturally unique, deviant, and less scientifically-valid. Yet these folk illness labels have endured the test of time and warrant further investigation as to their meaning and utility not only in a nosologic sense, but more importantly, in furthering our understanding of mental illness as it relates to the person afflicted and the most effective treatment for that individual (Lee & Wong, 1995; Zheng et al., 1994).

As the Introduction of the DSM IV points out, the limitation of the categorical approach becomes apparent where the members of a diagnostic class are not homogenous and there are no clear boundaries between the classes. Many of the so-called cultural-bound syndromes exemplify the heterogeneous nature of psychopathology. While most of the classic CBSs, such as *koro* and *amok,* were initially identified because of the dramatic nature of their manifestations, the majority of the more recently proposed CBSs capture patients who simultaneously suffer from prominent somatic, psychological, and behavioral symptoms. These syndromes are often conceptualized according to the indigenous systems of medical philosophy which sees the body and mind as unitary. In this sense, they often defy the contemporary psychiatric classification based on the Cartesian bias for the mind-body dicohotomy. For instance, brain fag, a condition initially described in West African students and entails somatic fatigue with symptoms of pain around the head and neck, pressure or tightness, blurring of vision is said to resemble certain anxiety, depressive, and somatoform disorders. Similarly, *shenjing shuairuo* (neurasthenia), a condition experienced by many Asian-Americans and non-American Asians, is characterized by physical and mental fatigue, dizziness, headaches, and sleep as well as concentration disturbance. Not unlike brain fag, neurasthenia also does not fit neatly into any diagnostic category, spanning over somatoform, anxiety, and depression spectrums (Cheung, 1989; Rin & Huang, 1989; M. Y. Zhang, 1989). Interestingly, data emerging in recent years have demonstrated that somatic and psychological symptoms usually co-occur, suggesting that the partitioning among mood, anxiety, and the so-called somatoform disorders may be largely artificial and a reflection of the Western Cartesian medical tradition (Chun, Enomoto, & Sue, 1996; Kirmayer, Young, & Allan, 1998). Ironically, the blurring of boundaries between categories of mental illness is not only limited to examples of non-Western

CHALLENGING THE MYTH OF A CULTURE FREE NOSOLOGICAL SYSTEM 69

psychopathologies. Chronic Fatigue Syndrome (CFS), a syndrome of physical fatigue and somatic symptoms has emerged in the Western culture in the mid-80's and has caused many to question whether or not this is the same entity as neurasthenia (Chun et al., 1996; Kirmayer & Young., 1998).

The authors challenge the reader to consider these outliers to the current categorical model of mental illness as not just exceptions to the cultural norm, but to consider them as possible diagnostic entities that may actually better reflect the meaning and phenomenology of the illnesses. As the following discussion hopes to demonstrate, the importance of culture as the diagnostic basis which leads to a comprehensive, dimensional model of mental illness is a crucial aspect in the assessment of not only Asian Americans or other non-Western patients, but indeed, is relevant to anyone whose experience of an illness takes place within the context of a culture.

2. THE ROLE OF CULTURE IN PSYCHIATRIC PHENOMENOLOGY AND NOSOLOGY

Any cursory review of the vast volume of cross-cultural literature would soon reveal that culture is one of the most important variables, which along with other factors such as age, gender and socioeconomic status, determines how the supposedly universal disease processes affect patients' well-being and ability to function (Alacron, 1995; Mezzich & Berganze, 1984; Mezzich et al., 1996; Rogler, 1989). As Jensen and Hoagwood point out, human behavioral and emotional symptoms often depends on the culture, history, and environment, but such complexity fails to be addressed by traditional approaches to disease and disorder classification (Jensen & Hoagwood, 1997). In attempting to classify disorders as universal entities across cultures, emphasis has traditionally been placed on treating disease processes as uniform and consistent so that the manifestation of the same disease in different persons, consists, for the most part, of the same symptoms. Difficulties are abound in applying this diagnostic approach across cultural boundaries including misdiagnosis, the frequent use of nonspecific categories such as NOS (not otherwise specified), and uncertainties regarding the specificity and meaning of diagnostic criteria (Jensen & Hoagwood, 1997; Kleinman, 1977; Kleinman, 1988; Perry, Cooper, & Michels, 1987; Schweder & Bourne, 1991), to name just a few.

Based on the categorical classification of disease processes, symptoms which do not fit neatly into any category are furthermore, either regarded as exceptions or primitive expressions of distress. For example, Asian American patients who present to their primary care physicians with somatic complaints are often regarded as not psychologically minded, or somatizers (Cheung, 1980; Jablesky & Sartorius, 1988; Kaplan & Saddock, 1988). In fact, recent epidemiological studies have shown that the rate of somatization disorders as defined by the DSM-IV is substantially lower in Taiwan and Korea compared to in the U.S. (Cheung & Lau, 1982; Lee et al., 1990; Yeh, Hwu, & Chang, 1989). Furthermore, many of these patients often spontaneously offer explanations for their symptoms such as a disturbance of the balance between the mind and the body. That is, psychological idioms of distress are expressed, but just not in ways traditionally classified in the Western culture (Fabrega, 1990; Kleinman & Kleinman, 1985; Lin, 1981). The greater tendency among Asians or Asian Americans to somatize may be a consequence of selective reporting, partially as a reflection of their belief in the unity rather than dichotomy between the body and the mind (Cheung, 1989). For example, studies on patient self-reports have shown that neurasthenia, or *shenjing shuairuo* in Mandarin, which literally means an exhaustion of the nerves, has been a popular diagnosis in Asia because of its implication that the physical manifestations of fatigue, insomnia, and nervousness, are a result of the nerves in the body being overspent. This explanation of the disease process which finds its basis in the indigenous belief that there is a continuous unity between the mind and the body is an example of how culture shapes one's understanding of an illness (Kleinman & Kleinman, 1985; Good & Kleinman, 1985). Knowing how a disease process is understood in a certain culture is crucial to accurate assessment and treatment of the patient. As in the case of the Asian American patient who presents with multiple nonspecific physical complaints, it helps to see that there may be an underlying psychological process involved such as depression and or anxiety, rather than classifying such patients as having a cultural-bound syndrome, or somatization disorder, NOS. CBS or somatization disorder NOS classifications provide little definitive treatment strategies, and often carry an overtone of stigma that these patients have no insight to their "mental illness" (whatever that may be) and/or are resistant to treatment.

The inclusion of "loss of interest or pleasure" as part of the depression diagnostic criteria resulted from observations that patients of ethnic minority and non-Western backgrounds frequently presented with these and other symptoms of major depression, but not depressive mood (Hughes, 1985). Although controversial at the time, this modification has consequently been found useful not only in non-Western settings, but also for a significant proportion of patients in Western societies that would have otherwise been difficult to classify. Consequently the schema has been retained in DSM-IV.

Hwa-byung, a common Korean folk illness label, represents another interesting challenge for the DSM classification system. Patients self-labeled as suffering from *hwa-byung* report prominent psychological as well as somatic symptoms, but regard them as secondary to chronic and unresolved anger often resulting from intense, ongoing interpersonal conflicts (Lin et al., 1992). Since the majority of these patients have been demonstrated to fulfill the diagnosis of major depression as defined by the DSMs, *hwa-byung* has been regarded as a culturally patterned form of major depression (Prince, 1989). However, it could be argued that such an approach may be unduly reductionistic. Instead of focusing only on the overlaps and similarities, it might be equally important, or even more so, to question if the concept of *hwa-byung* points to aspects of psychopathologies that have so far been neglected by the DSMs. Thus, one might question why phenomena related to anger and hostility have been so prominently absent in our current nosological systems. Is there a need to have a separate category of diagnosis with anger at the core, as we have done with depression and anxiety? Are some patients perhaps better described as suffering from problems related to anger rather than depression and/or anxiety?

CHALLENGING THE MYTH OF A CULTURE FREE NOSOLOGICAL SYSTEM

Do depressed patients with prominent symptoms of anger and hostility differ significantly in their clinical features, treatment responses and even neurobiologic correlates from those without such symptoms? Although little research efforts have been focused on these questions, some empirical data have indeed emerged in recent years to indicate that phenomena related to anger and hostility indeed deserve more attention than is currently acknowledged in our diagnostic systems (Fava & Rosenbaum, 1999; Kellner, J., & Pathak, 1992).

3. CONCLUSION

Having recognized that any classification of mental conditions cannot exist in the absence of culture, this chapter further points out that our current psychiatric diagnostic system evolved largely from Western intellectual traditions and is based on clinical experiences with limited number of patients treated mostly in Western Europe and North America over the past two centuries (Mezzich et al., 1996; Perry, Cooper, & Michels, 1987). Efforts have only recently begun to look at mental conditions which have been described in the rest of the world for centuries and which based on the current approach of classification, often fall into special categories that reflects little insight to whatever underlying mental phenomena there may be. Despite the often valiant efforts of several generations of ingenious pioneers in teasing out epiphenomena from what might be regarded as universal characteristics of mental conditions, much in the way we conceptualize and describe psychiatric phenomena still reflects deep-rooted influences by Western cultural traditions. This chapter presents the challenge that difficulties in applying our diagnostic systems to patients with non-Western backgrounds should not be limited to adjusting and modifying the concepts and criteria in order to derive at a diagnostic label. Even more importantly, they should be viewed as opportunities to highlight and critically examine biases inherent in our current conceptualization that may otherwise remain hidden. Seen in this way, cross-cultural studies may serve as an indispensable tool for the formulation of new criteria that can better define psychopathologic entities across cultures. While the universality of any of our diagnostic concepts may ultimately remain illusory, admittedly, systematic studies of cross-cultural clinical cases have been scarce. The future task would be to examine mental conditions more closely in the contexts of divergent cultures. The more we can understand and define an illness in a cultural setting, the more likely we may one day be able to regard it as being free of undue cultural biases.

4. REFERENCES

Alacron, R. D. (1995). Culture and psychiatric diagnosis: Impact on DSM-IV and ICD-10. *Psychiatric Clinics of North America, 18,* 49-465.

American Psychiatric Association. (1994*). Diagnostic and statistical manual of mental disorders* (4th ed.). Washington, DC: Author.

Cheung, F. M. (1980). The mental health status of Asian Americans. *Clinical Psychologist, 34,* 23-24.

Cheung, F. M. (1989). The indigenization of neurasthenia in Hong Kong. *Culture, Medicine, and Psychiatry, 13,* 227-241.

Cheung, F. M., & Lau, B.W. (1982). Situational variations of help-seeking behavior among Chinese patients. *Comprehensive Psychiatry, 23*, 252-262.

Chun, C.-A., Enomoto, K., & Sue, S. (1996). Health care issues among Asian Americans: Implications of somatization. In P. M. Kato (Ed.), *Handbook of diversity issues in health psychology* (pp. 347-364). New York: Plenum Press.

Demitrack, M. A., & Abbey, S. E. (1996). *Chronic Fatigue Syndrome.* New York: The Guilford Press.

Fava, M., & Rosenbaum, J. (1999). Anger attacks in patients with depression. *Journal of Clinical Psychiatry, 60* (Suppl. 15), 21-24.

Fabrega, H. (1990). The concept of somatization as a cultural and historical product of Western medicine. *Psychosomatic Medicine, 52,* 653-672.

Greenberg, D. B. (1990). Neurasthenia in the 1980's: Chronic mononucleosis, chronic fatigue syndrome, anxiety, and depressive disorders. *Psychosomatics, 31,*120-137.

Good, B., & Kleinman, A. M. (1985). Epilogue: Culture and depression. In A. Kleinman & B. Good (Eds.), *Culture and depression: Studies in the anthropology and cross-cultural psychiatry of affect and disorder* (pp. 491-505). Berkeley, CA: University of California Press.

Hughes, C. C. (1985). Culture-bound or construct-bound? The syndromes and DSM-III. In R. C. Simons & C. C. Hughes (Eds.), *The cultural-bound syndromes: Folk illnesses of psychiatric and anthropological interest.* Dordrecht, The Netherlands: D. Reidel.

Jablensky, A., & Sartorius N. (1988). Is schizophrenia universal? *Acta Psychiatrica Scandinavia, 344* (Suppl.), 65-70.

Jensen, P. S., & Hoagwood, K. (1997). The book of names: DSM-IV in context. *Development and Psychopathology, 9,* 231-249.

Kaplan, H. I., & Sadock, B. J. (1988). *Synopsis of psychiatry: Behavioral sciences and clinical psychiatry* (5th ed.). Baltimore: Williams & Wilkins.

Kellner, R., Hernandez, J., & Pathak, D. (1992). Self-rated inhibited anger, somatization and depression. *Psychotherapy Psychosomatics, 57,* 102-107.

Kleinman, A. M. (1977). Depression, somatization, and the new cross-cultural psychiatry. *Social Science in Medicine, 11,* 3-10.

Kleinman, A. M. (1988). *Rethinking Psychiatry.* New York: The Free Press.

Kleinman, A. M., & Kleinman, J. (1985). Somatization: The interconnections in Chinese society among culture, depressive experiences, and the meanings of pain. In A. Kleinman, & B. J. Goods (Eds.), *Culture and depression: Studies in the anthropology and cross-cultural psychiatry of affect and disorder* (pp. 429-490). Berkeley, CA: University of California Press.

Kleinman, M., Eisenberg, L., & Good, B. (1978). Clinical lessons from anthropologic and cross-cultural research. *Annals of Internal Medicine, 88,* 251-258.

Kirmayer, L. J., & Young, A. (1998). Culture and somatization: Clinical epidemiological and ethnographic perspectives. *Psychosomatic Medicine, 60,* 420-430.

Lee, C. K., Kwak, Y. S., Yamamoto, J., & Rhee, H., Kim, Y. S., Han, J. H., Choi, J. O., & Lee, Y. H. (1990). Psychiatric epidemiology in Korea: Urban and rural differences. *Journal of Nervous & Mental Disease, 178,* 247-252.

Lee, S., & Wong, K. C. (1993). Rethinking neurasthenia: The illness concepts of shenjing shuairuo among Chinese undergraduates in Hong Kong. *Culture, Medicine and Psychiatry, 19,* 91-111.

Lin, K.-M. (1981). Chinese medical beliefs and their relevance for mental illness and psychiatry. In A. Kleinman & T.Y. Lin, (Eds.), *Normal and abnormal behavior in Chinese culture* (pp. 95-111). Dordrecht, The Netherlands: D. Reidel.

Lin, K.-M., Lau, J. K. C., Yamamoto, J., Zheng, Y. P., Kim, H. S., Cho, K. H., & Nakasaki, G. (1992). Hwa-byung: A community study of Korean Americans. *The Journal of Nervous and Mental Disease, 180,* 386-391.

Littlewood, R., & Lipsedge, M. (1985). Culture-bound syndromes. In K. Granville (Ed.), *Recent advances in clinical psychiatry* (pp. 105-142). New York: Livingstone.

Mezzich, J. E., & Berganza C. E. (1984). *Culture and psychopathology.* New Yorkm NY: Columbia University Press.

Mezzich, J. E., Kleinman, A., Fabrega, H., Jr., Good, B. Johnson-Powell, G., Lin, K.-M., Manson, S., & Parron, D. (1993). *Cultural proposals for DSM-IV.* Submitted to the DSM-IV Task Force by the Steering Committee, NIMH-sponsored Group on Culture and Diagnosis. Pittsburgh, PA: National Institute of Mental Health.

CHALLENGING THE MYTH OF A CULTURE FREE NOSOLOGICAL SYSTEM 73

Mezzich, J.E., Kleinman, A., Fabrega, H., Jr., & Parron, D. (Eds.). (1996). *Culture & psychiatric diagnosis: A DSM-IV perspective.* Washington, DC: American Psychiatric Press.

Mezzich, J. E., Kleinman, A., Fabrega, H., Jr., Parron, D., Good, B. J., Lin, K.-M., & Manson, S. (1994). *Cultural issues and DSM-IV: Support papers.* Submitted to the DSM-IV Source Book by the Steering Committee, NIMH-sponsored Group on Culture and Diagnosis. Pittsburgh, PA: National Institute of Mental Health.

Mezzich, J. E., Kleinman, A., Fabrega, H., Jr., Parron, D. Good, B. Johnson-Powell, G., Lin, K.-M., Manson, S. (1993). *Revised cultural proposals for DSM-IV.* Submitted to the DSM-IV Task Force by the Steering Committee, NIMH-sponsored Group on Culture and Diagnosis. Pittsburgh, PA: National Institute of Mental Health.

Mezzich, J. E., Kleinman A., Fabrega, H., Jr., Parron, D., Good, B. J., Lin, K.-M., & Manson, S. (1997). Cultural issues for DSM-IV. In T. A. Wildiger, A. J. Frances, H. A. Pincus, R. Ross, M. B. First, & W. Davis (Eds.), *DSM-IV Source Book* (vol. 3, pp. 861-866). Washington, DC: American Psychiatric Press.

Perry, S., Cooper, A. M., & Michels, R. (1987). The psychodynamic formulation: Its purpose, structure, and clinical application. *American Journal of Psychiatry, 144,* 543-550.

Prince, R. (1989). Somatic complaint syndromes and depression: The problem of cultural effects on symptomatology. *Mental Health Research, 8,* 104-117.

Rin, H., & Huang, M. G. (1989). Neurasthenia as nosological dilemma. *Culture, Medicine and Psychiatry, 13,* 215-226.

Rogler, L. H. (1989). The meaning of culturally sensitive research in mental health. *American Journal of Psychiatry, 146,* 296-303.

Schweder, R. A., & Bourne, E. J. (1991). Does the concept of person vary cross-culturally? In R. A. Schweder (Ed.), *Thinking through cultures: Expeditions in cultural psychology* (pp. 113-155). Cambridge, MA: Harvard University Press.

Yeh, E. K., Hwu, H., & Chang L.Y. (1989). Mental Disorders in three types of Taiwan community: Urbanization hypothesis retested. *Chinese Psychiatry, 3,* 183-199.

Zhang, M. Y. (1989). The diagnosis and phenomenology of neurasthenia: A Shanghai study. *Culture, Medicine and Psychiatry, 13,* 147-161.

Zheng, Y. P., Lin, K.-M., Zhao, J. P., Zhang, M.Y., & Yong, D. (1994). Comparative study of diagnostic systems: Chinese Classification of Mental Disorders (2nd ed.) (CCMD-2) versus DSM-III-R. *Comprehensive Psychiatry, 35,* 441-449.

SECTION II: THEORIES OF RELEVANT SOCIOCULTURAL VARIABLES

6. **Assessing Acculturation and Cultural Variables**
   Gargi Roysircar
   Michael Lynch Maestas

7. **Models of Cultural Orientation: Differences Between American-born and Overseas-born Asians**
   Jeanne L. Tsai
   Yulia Chentsova-Dutton

8. **Cultural Variations in Self-Construal as a Mediator of Distress and Well-being**
   Sumie Okazaki

9. **The Use of Culturally-Based Variables in Assessment: Studies on Loss of Face**
   Nolan Zane
   May Yeh

GARGI ROYSIRCAR AND MICHAEL LYNCH MAESTAS[1]

CHAPTER 6

ASSESSING ACCULTURATION AND CULTURAL VARIABLES

1. BIDIRECTIONAL ACCULTURATION THEORY

Since the 1960's, the United States has had an influx of immigrants from South Asia and Southeast Asia, such as from the Indian subcontinent, the Philippines, Korea, Vietnam, Hong Kong, Taiwan, and mainland China (Kuo & Roysircar-Sodowsky, 1999; Rumbaut, 1997), contributing to a 35% increase among Asian Americans and Pacific Islanders in the 1990's (U.S. Bureau of the Census, 1999). This phenomenon of "new immigrants" or post-World War II immigrants from Asia and Latin America and the large birth rate of U.S.-born second generation children have begun to change U.S. society with the visibility of people of color who are different from even those who have been traditionally considered as minorities. New immigrants constitute the majority of immigrants to this country (Rumbaut, 1997). However, research has largely neglected them, perhaps because of their relative youth due to their post-1965 immigration; the obscurity of census and official data on them; and the relative invisibility of immigrants of color until recent times. There is limited research, both conceptual and empirical, that examines the acculturation process of immigrants, the ethnic identification process of children of immigrants, and the effects of such adaptations on their stress-related mental health. We attempt to address these issues conceptually and in measurement terms with regard to Asian Americans.

Acculturation has been delineated to encompass the collective or group level phenomenon as well as the psychological acculturation of the individual. Acculturation as a group level phenomenon involves a change in the culture of an ethnic minority group as it adapts to the mores, behaviors, and values of the dominant group, and psychological acculturation involves a change in the psychology of the ethnic individual. The distinction between levels is important in order to examine the systematic relationships between the individual and his or her ethnic minority group, because not all individuals participate to the same extent in the general acculturation being experienced by their group.

---

[1] We dedicate this chapter to our first- and second-generation immigrant families.

At the individual level, a person must confront **two general issues** that are in opposition and may create conflict: (1) the maintenance and development of one's ethnic distinctiveness by retaining one's cultural identity; and (2) the desire to seek interethnic contact by valuing and maintaining positive relations with the dominant society. These two general issues represent the dimensions of psychological acculturation (Berry, 1990). Subsumed in these dimensions are changes in multiple domains: physical changes, biological changes, social relationships, language change, cognitive processes, personality, identity, cultural attitudes and values, and acculturative stress (Berry, 1980). As indicated by later sections of this writing, acculturation studies to date have been involved in the measurement of language change, ethnic identity, social behaviors and orientation, cultural attitudes and values, acculturative stress, and related mental health and personality issues.

Responses to these two general issues lead to four modes of acculturation adaptations. The integration adaptation mode is characterized by an allegiance to cultural identity and involvement in the dominant culture. Those who use the assimilation mode relinquish their cultural identity and prefer to interact only with members of the dominant society. In contrast to assimilation, a separation mode involves the exclusive identification with and retention of one's cultural values and an avoidance of contact with the dominant society. Individuals who become marginal, the fourth adaptation mode, "lose cultural and psychological contact with both their traditional culture and the larger society" (Berry, Kim, Power, Young, & Bujaki, 1989, p. 188).

These acculturation modes, which are indicated by changes in multiple domains, also interface with various variables, as illustrated by Figure 1. This diagrammed multidirectional interface of acculturation is addressed in the rest of the writing.

2. MEASUREMENT OF ACCULTURATION

2.1 Methodological Issues

While the bidirectional theory of acculturation is popularly accepted, its measurement in quantitative terms is lagging. Several methodological questions are raised here. Each question is followed up with an analysis of how well it has been addressed by acculturation research.

2.1.1 Question 1

Is the bidirectional model of acculturation operationalized through independent measures that assess two opposing cultural experiences and commitments, one to the White dominant society and one to the individual's ethnic minority society?

The measurement of acculturation in the 70's and 80's largely proceeded along a linear theory (e.g., Szapocznik, Scopetta, Kurtines & Aranalde, 1978) which described acculturation as a process of relinquishing characteristics of the culture of

ASSESSING ACCULTURATION AND CULTURAL VARIABLES

origin and adopting characteristics of the dominant culture (the assimilation mode) as exposure to the dominant culture increases. There is indeed research indicating a linear relationship between time in the U.S. and behavioral acculturation (e.g., Sodowsky, Lai, & Plake, 1991; Sodowsky & Plake, 1992); however, with regard to self-labelling one's ethnicity and valuing one's ethnic identity retention, a linear decline has not been noted for later generation Japanese Americans (Connor, 1977), Chinese Americans (Ting-Toomey, 1981), Asian Indians (Hutnik, 1986; Kuo & Roysircar-Sodowsky, 2001), Canadian Jews (Isajiw, 1990), and Chinese Australians (Feldman, Mont-Reynaud, & Rosenthal, 1992a, 1992b).

Recently, pilot investigations have studied the bidirectional acculturation process. Readers are referred to the following measures: Acculturation Rating Scale for Mexican Americans II (ARSMA-II), which, when used in conjunction with the experimental orthogonal Marginality Scale, has created bicultural typologies (Cuéllar, Arnold, & Maldonado, 1995); the Acculturation Scale for Vietnamese Adolescents (Nguyen, Messe, & Stollak, 1999); the Bicultural Acculturation Scale developed on Puerto Ricans (Cortes, Rogler, & Malgady, 1994); and the Bidimensional Acculturation Scale for Hispanics (Marin & Gamba, 1996). As Nguyen et al. (1999) state, "cultural involvements are not necessarily bipolar and they can and should be measured separately" (p.9). Thus, Nguyen et al. for their instrument developed two subscales—*Involvement with U.S. Culture* and *Involvement with Vietnamese Culture*—and the two subscales showed a negative correlation with each other.

However, the assumed bidirectionality of these recent measures has not closely followed Berry's bidirectional model which asks two qualitatively different questions regarding retaining one's cultural identity and seeking relationships in the other cultural group. In these measures, the items are equivalent or comparable in nature except for the culture to which they are referred. That is, if an item assesses the ability to speak one's original language, another item assesses the ability to speak English. A more meaningful way to approach Berry's two questions is to use both an acculturation measure and an ethnic identity measure.

2.1.2 Question 2

Are there comparative studies examining various groups that identify common and different acculturation adaptations for diverse ethnic groups?

See Table 1 for representative studies of group comparisons. Has acculturation been studied at the group level and at the individual level? The measurement of acculturation to date has involved, for the most part, the ethnic individual as the unit of analysis, and individual acculturation has been related to the phenomena of group acculturation through multivariate statistics (e.g., Frey & Roysircar-Sodowsky, in press; Olmedo, Martinez, & Martinez, 1978; Osvold & Sodowsky, 1995; Sodowsky & Lai, 1997). Such studies in general have relied on the use of qualitative assessment of culture, operationalized as sociocultural variables (e.g., ethnicity, extent of ethnic friendships, country of origin, generation status, age of entry into the

U.S.), as well as quantitative measurement of values-oriented and behavioral variables. Ensuing investigations have shown many correlates of acculturation, such as self-esteem (Phinney, Chavira, & Williamson, 1992), collective group self-esteem and pride (Kwan, 1996; Rotheram-Borus, 1990), dissociative experiences and worldviews, (Frey & Roysircar-Sodowsky, 2000), and perceived prejudice, racial consciousness and coping (Roysircar-Sodowsky, 2001), as well as the relationship of these correlates to ethnic group membership.

Table 1. Findings of Acculturation Studies: Some Common Themes

Findings	Authors
1. Asian Americans perceived more prejudice than Hispanics.	Sodowsky et al., 1991
2. Vietnamese less acculturated than Japanese Americans and Koreans.	Sodowsky et al., 1991
3. Political refugees less acculturated than voluntary immigrants, such as Asian Indians.	Sodowsky et al., 1991
4. Those Asians who observed Eastern religions were the least acculturated, followed by Catholics, when these two groups were compared with Protestants who were the most acculturated.	Sodowsky et al., 1991
5. First-generation individuals perceived more prejudice, were less acculturated, and were less prone to use English than later generations.	Sodowsky et al., 1991
6. A linear relationship exists between time in the U.S. and acculturation.	Sodowsky et al., 1991; Sodowsky & Plake, 1992
7. Higher acculturation scores in a sample of Japanese American men predicted higher levels of gender-role conflict; as Japanese American males became more acculturated, they were more relaxed regarding emotional expression.	Kim, O'Neil, & Owen, 1996
8. Acculturation related to types of Asian Americans most likely to date outside one's race.	T. A. Mok, 1994
9. Differences in acculturation in the family.	Chambon, 1989; Connor, 1977; Rumbaut, 1994
10. Differences between Chinese immigrants in Australia and the U.S. and those who remained in the home country, with immigrants being more acculturated;	Feldman, Mont-Reynaud, & Rosenthal, 1992a,

Findings	Authors
immigrant families showed increased accommodation to autonomy-promoting norms, while still maintaining family values of structure, supervision, and family input across two generations.	1992b
11. Higher acculturation was related to years of U.S. schooling, younger age upon arriving in the U.S., language preferences, and ethnicity of friends.	Suinn, Ahuna, & Khoo, 1992
12. Feeling accepted by the dominant society, more years of U.S. residence, higher educational attainment and family income, higher level of pre-immigration adjustment, and being involved with the U.S. culture were related to better mental health for Asian Indian immigrants.	Mehta, 1998
13. Foreign-born Asian Americans more other-directed than American-born Asian Americans.	Abe & Zane, 1990
14. First generation Asian Indian immigrants are likely to sacrifice their personal desires and independence for the sake of maintaining their family obligations, avoiding loss of face, and bringing honor to the family name.	Sodowsky, 1991
15. Young Asian Indians wanted freedom with regard to dating and making their own choice with regard to marriage, without the imposition of their parents' traditional marriage values. Regarding marriage, second generation Asian Indians were more individualistic, while those in the first generation were more conservative and traditional.	Murthy, 1998
16. Second generation Asian Indians were more likely to associate with others outside their ethnic group than the first generation; the second generation also used ethnic languages and social customs less often.	Bufka, 1998
17. In a sample of Chinese Americans, the first generation mainly identified themselves with the Chinese culture, while second and third generations mainly identified themselves as bicultural.	Ting-Toomey, 1981
18. Self-assigned ethnic labels and ethnic self-descriptions were given by Asian Indian girls, Filipinos, three generations of Japanese, and three generations of Chinese who also showed White acculturated behaviors.	Connor, 1977; Hutnik, 1986; Masuda et al., 1970; Ting-Toomey, 1981
19. An integrated or bicultural attitude in Asian high schools and college students was related to higher levels	Phinney et al., 1992

Findings	Authors
of self-esteem; assimilation attitudes were negatively associated with self-esteem.	
20. Acculturation was related to world views: normativism and humanism.	Frey & Roysircar-Sodowsky, in press

2.1.3 Question 3

Has measurement identified the relationship of acculturation with mental health status?

Table 2 summarizes the findings with respect to this question. However, because it is difficult to pinpoint etiology, the findings have been complex. It has been shown that both high and low acculturation can have either positive or negative mental health effects (Berry & Kim, 1988; Cervantes & Castro, 1985; Frey & Roysircar-Sodowsky, in press; Moyerman & Forman, 1992; Osvold & Sodowsky, 1995; Negy & Woods, 1992a; Rogler, Cortes, & Malgady, 1991; Sodowsky et al., 1991).

Table 2. Findings of Acculturative Stress and Bicultural Stress: Some Common Themes

Findings	Authors
1. Involuntary groups experienced higher stress than the voluntary groups: Native people and refugees > Sojourners > Voluntary immigrants and ethnic groups; US < UK < India < Africa < South American < Hong Kong.	Berry & Kim, 1988; Berry et al., 1987
2. Chinese sojourner groups reported more problem areas with regard to work, family and children, language and communication, homesickness, loneliness, etc., as compared to Chinese Canadians and non-Chinese Canadian groups; 70% of the sojourner participants were considered "non-adapted."	Zheng & Berry, 1991
3. Hong Kong Chinese students had more trait anxiety, less perceived social support of friends, and greater problems with communication, prejudice, adaptation, and English language competence than French and English students.	Chataway & Berry, 1989
4. Compared to Black and Hispanic high school students, Asian Americans were more likely to express the desire to belong to a different ethnic group, and had the lowest ethnic identity search among all groups;	Phinney, 1989

Findings	Authors
author attributed this to lack of Asian American role models.	
5. Asian Americans, compared to other groups, perceived their ethnic group as having less power and had significantly less cross-ethnic contact; the higher the contact levels, the less the experience of stress.	Rotheram-Borus, 1990
6. Social support was negatively related to the experience of stress.	Berry et al., 1987
7. Asian Americans reported significantly more behavioral problems than other groups.	Rotheram-Borus, 1990
8. Interpersonal-Intercultural competence concerns; cultural distress.	Sodowsky & Lai, 1997
9. Career-choice indecision for Asian sojourning youth.	Sodowsky, 1991
10. Traditional Asian cultural orientation, young age, immigration at an older age, social network that excludes White Americans, limited family kinship, low income, and higher levels of perceived prejudice contributed to acculturative stress.	Sodowsky & Lai, 1997
11. For Japanese Americans, the best predictors of stress among first, second, and third/later generations were: low acculturation level, first generation status, and low self-esteem.	Padilla et al., 1985
12. For early and late immigrants and second and third generations, the first generation scored higher on stress and lower on self-esteem; late immigrants experienced the greatest stress. Early immigrants were more similar to second and later generations.	Mena, Padilla, & Maldonado, 1987
13. Foreign-born Asian high school students felt more separated from White society than U.S.-born second generation Asians.	Phinney et al., 1992
14. When compared to American-born Chinese students, foreign-born Chinese students reported greater socioemotional distress.	Sue & Zane, 1985
15. Stress experienced by first generation is a function of cultural alienation; stress experienced by second generation is a function of cultural marginality.	Masuda, G. H. Matsumsoto, & Meredith, 1970
16. Acculturation was related to ratings of dissociative experiences.	Frey & Roysircar-Sodowsky, 2000

Findings	Authors
17. Ethnic identity and bicultural stress were related to perceived prejudice, Asian racial consciousness, and coping.	Kuo & Roysircar-Sodowsky, 2000
18. Acculturation-related family conflicts decreased across three generations of Japanese American families.	Connor, 1977
19. Higher amounts of family acculturation conflicts were observed for Filipino, Vietnamese, and Cambodians than for Hispanic/Latino immigrant adolescents.	Rumbaut, 1994
20. Middle school Chinese immigrant students reported higher scores on the SCL-90-R that were associated with low acculturation, more cultural adjustment difficulties, and low cross-cultural adaptability.	Yeh, Chiang, & Wang, 1998
21. Second generation, late adolescent Asian Americans reported more depressive symptoms and a less favorable view of their family relationships than White college students.	Greenberger & Chen, 1996
22. Second generation, early adolescent Asian Americans reported less maternal warmth and acceptance than White early adolescents.	Greenberger & Chen, 1996

2.1.4 *Question 4*

Have acculturation instruments been used as moderator variables to examine the interface between an ethnic individual's responses and mainstream diagnostic systems (e.g., DSM-IV) or tests (e.g., MMPI-2, WISC-III)?

First, it is important to note that "neither the DSM-IV nor standard psychological tests and structured interviews have adequately recognized and described the potential confound between culture and psychopathology" (Dana, 1996, p. 322). Second, while professional psychology recognizes the need to incorporate acculturation as a moderator variable in clinical diagnosis and assessment, the practice has yet to become routine. Acculturation instruments have been developed with the specific purpose of being used as moderator variables, as the ARSMA and ARSMA II were intended to be (Cuéllar, Harris & Jasso, 1980; Cuéllar et al., 1995). Yet, most instruments have been used in research, and they have not been used clinically for interpretation, treatment, and client-feedback purposes.

However, there is a caveat to using acculturation measures clinically. Before clinicians use the instruments or assess the client's acculturation through open-ended questions, they must have a competent understanding of the research showing a complex link between acculturation and mental health status (see Figure 1). In addition, unraveling "mixed results" in acculturation research (see Question 3) must precede clinical interpretation of an ethnic minority individual's intake and test data vis-a-vis his or her acculturation level. Clinicians need to keep in mind Rogler et al.'s (1991) statement that acculturation "has been hypothesized to relate linearly both negatively and positively with psychological distress, and also to relate in curvilinear fashion to psychological distress" (p. 588). For example, Burnam, Hough, Karno, Escobar, and Telles (1987a) found that higher levels of acculturation were related to certain types of psychopathology in Mexican Americans. Padilla, Wagatsuma, and Lindholm (1985) reported that highly acculturated third and later generation Japanese Americans tended to experience the least stress. Frey and Roysircar-Sodowsky (in press) showed that low acculturated Asian Americans and Latinos, compared to White Americans, gave higher ratings to dissociative experiences. Lang, Munoz, Bernal, and Sorenson (1982) showed that healthy psychological adjustment for Latinos was related to biculturalism with an orientation toward one's ethnic group. Kuo and Roysircar-Sodowsky (1999) have discussed that foreign-born, first generation Asian immigrants experience acculturative stress, while second-generation U.S.-born Asian Americans experience bicultural stress. Thus, high and low acculturation may be related to different types of disorders, and adaptation modes have different types of positive and negative effects.

2.1.5 Question 5

Is the inquiry on acculturation framed within a social context, and can adaptations vary by context?

The linear emphasis of the measurement of acculturation (high acculturation versus low acculturation) has resulted in a limited understanding of contextual variations in acculturation adaptations. Mendoza (1989) and Sodowsky, Kwan, and Pannu (1995) have conceptualized that an ethnic individual may be affected by contextual factors that make acculturation a dynamic process. For example, a highly acculturated second-generation individual may find himself or herself in a situation in which a strong ethnic identity and low acculturation is most adaptive. This person may temporarily adopt the rejection mode to deal with a current pressing situation. Such data on individual acculturation dynamics are perhaps best documented in clinical cases and need to be collected through open-ended clinical interviews. To do this, clinicians might turn to some instruments that have an interview format.

Examples of such instruments are: Acculturation Scale for Southeast Asians (ASSA) (J. Anderson et al., 1993), Brief Acculturation Scale for Hispanics (BASH) (Norris, Ford, & Bova, 1996), Los Angeles Epidemiologic Catchment Area-Acculturation Scale (LAECA-AS) (Burnam, Telles, Karno, Hough, & Escobar, 1978b), and Psychological Acculturation Scale for Puerto Ricans (PAS) (Tropp, Erkut, Garcia-Coll, Alarcon, & Vasquez-Garcia, 1999). There are some instruments that may also be completed by raters (e.g., Children's Acculturation Scale, Franco, 1983). Such measures for interviewers and raters might be adapted for clinical interviews to assess the individual dynamics of a client. For instance, to follow up with the previously mentioned case, a few interview questions adapted from acculturation measures might suggest high acculturation in a U.S.-born, second generation client, who, nonetheless, presents a rejection mode with regard to particular occupational or work-related issues. This might cue the clinician to explore with the client his or her unique current conflict, such as the experience of job discrimination and an increase in ethnic sociopolitical consciousness in an otherwise highly acculturated individual.

2.1.6 Question 6

Do varying measurements of acculturation (unidimensional scales, classifications, factorial dimensions, short scales, multiple choice format for sociocultural variables, various Likert and semantic differential scales) differ in the amount, kind, and quality of information they provide?

Clearly, the four-item Language Acculturation Scale for Mexican Americans (LASMA, Deyo, Diehl, Hazuda, & Stern, 1985), applicable to indigent, less-educated clients in clinical settings, provides different information from multidimensional measures such as the 76-item Acculturation Scale for Vietnamese Americans (Nguyen et al., 1999), the 38-item Minority-Majority Relations Scale (Sodowsky et al., 1991), and the 155-item Cultural Awareness-Ethnic Loyalty Scale (Padilla, 1980). However, scales that are brief, non-threatening, and independent of interviewers' subjectivity are potentially useful for clinical purposes, particularly with regard to test data interpretation and provision of test feedback to clients.

Initially, acculturation measures employed a single index with a heavy emphasis on language usage/preference (e.g., ARSMA, Cuéllar et al., 1980). Many instruments continue to do the same, such as the 10-item ARSMA-Short Form (Dawson, Crano, & Burgoon, 1996), the 13-item ASSA (J. Anderson et al., 1993), and the four-item BASH (Norris, Ford, & Bova, 1996). When investigating acculturation level with such instruments, one would conclude that an ethnic minority individual who uses English fluently would be highly acculturated. This unidimensional conceptualization of acculturation does not provide a complete understanding of the phenomena.

Acculturation has come to be conceptualized as a multidimensional construct. Through factor analysis, Padilla (1980) identified five dimensions important in the measurement of acculturation, and Sodowsky and Plake (1991) identified three dimensions that have withstood the inquiry of several studies. Negy and Woods (1992b) held that "acculturation's multidimensional nature may preclude ever having one scale capable of adequately and sufficiently capturing it, thus requiring multi-measures and multimethods of assessment" (p. 242). Indeed, almost all of the acculturation instruments include items related to linguistics, culture-specific knowledge and behavior, and sociocultural variables, and to a lesser extent, original culture-affiliation and cultural value adherence (Olmedo, 1979; Roysircar-Sodowsky & Maestas, 2000). Although the number of dimensions of acculturation varies across instruments, certain dimensions consistently account for a large percentage of variance. In 98% of instrument-development studies, language use/preference accounted for the largest amount of variance, the mean contribution being 48.7% (Roysircar-Sodowsky & Maestas, 2001). For a review and metanalysis of acculturation instruments, see Roysircar-Sodowsky and Maestas (2001).

3. CULTURAL STRESS

3.1 Acculturative Stress

Acculturative stress refers to a specific kind of stress directly related to the process of acculturation and can be distinguished from general life stress and hassles (Sodowsky & Lai, 1997; Kwan & Sodowsky, 1997). Dressler and Bernal (1982) state that acculturative stress occurs "when an individual's adaptive resources are insufficient to support adjustment to a new cultural environment" (p. 34). The stress is elicited by drastically new life events, and the stress of the new life events cues the acculturating individual to possible dangers or opportunities. While a certain amount of stress may be necessary or helpful in alerting the individual to respond to new situations, too much stress can threaten healthy adaptation, such as inhibiting responses to acculturation or resulting in disintegration. Thus, acculturative stress could result in a "reduction in health status (including psychological, somatic, and social aspects) of individuals" (Berry, Kim, Minde, & D. Mok, 1987, p. 491), and it has been related to psychopathology, cultural marginalization, poor self-concept, disordered eating attitudes and behaviors, and career choice indecision (see review by Roysircar-Sodowsky & Maestas, 2000).

Figure 1 illustrates how acculturative stress results from the multidirectional interaction of acculturation, pulls toward identification with one's own ethnic group, extracultural stressors in the environment (e.g., low income, unfamiliar educational system), and mediating variables. The eventual outcome of stress is mediated by complex sociocultural and personal characteristics. The list of mediating variables has been derived from both theoretical and empirical literature referenced in this writing. Figure 1 is a fully recursive model (that is, it is not unidirectional) which represents influences from two or three directions. For example, for an ethnic individual, certain mediating variables (e.g., generation status, religion, personality characteristics) affect acculturation to White society. Acculturation, in turn, impacts extracultural stressors (e.g., educational experiences). Extracultural stressors also affect an individual's acculturation to White society and are themselves impacted by specific mediating variables. The recursive influence of acculturation, ethnic identity, extracultural stressors, and mediating variables on an acculturating individual creates the experience of acculturative stress, which varies from individual to individual.

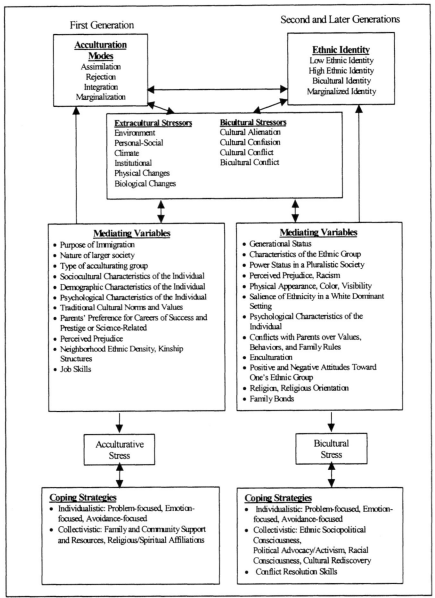

Figure 1. An integrated model of acculturation and ethnic identity that shows their multidirectional interfaces with mediating variables, stress, and coping strategies. While acculturation and ethnic identity interact and are influenced by some common variables, their respective experiences for individuals are relatively independent.

Dressler and Bernal (1982) state that individuals cope with acculturative stress with personal and social resources. Similarly, we propose that ethnic minority individuals use two broad types of coping strategies: individualistic coping and collectivistic coping. Individualistic-oriented coping includes dimensions addressed in the mainstream literature on coping strategies, for example, problem-focused, emotion-focused, and avoidance-focused strategies (Lazarus & Folkman, 1984). Collectivistically-oriented coping represents the in-group resources and support available to Asian and Latino families and ethnic groups (see Cervantes & Castro, 1985; Colombo, Santiago, & Rossello, 1999; Dyal, & Dyal, 1981; Oleh, 1995), given the notable collectivism of these people. Figure 1 links acculturative stress with coping.

3.2 Bicultural Stress

U.S.-born second and later generation ethnic minorities experience bicultural stress owing to the conflicts that arise out of their bicultural socialization (De Anda, 1984). Biculturalism refers to the orientation of minorities who inherit two different cultural traditions. U.S.-born Asian Americans undergoing a bicultural socialization process must negotiate between two disparate cultures, their ethnic culture and the White dominant culture. An Asian American may be highly conflicted when finding oneself sandwiched between two contrasting value systems, whereas the key to positive mental health may be accommodation and integrative adaptation (Sodowsky, 1991). Figure 1 illustrates a fully recursive model of a U.S.-born individual's ethnic identity, acculturation to the dominant society, ethnic identity stressors, and mediating variables that finally influence bicultural stress. The list of mediating variables (e.g., physical visibility, collective self-esteem) has been derived from the theoretical and empirical literature on ethnic identity, as reviewed by Roysircar-Sodowsky and Maestas (2000) and Sodowsky et al. (1995). It has been suggested that coping responses to ethnic identity issues include sociopolitical consciousness, activism (Phinney & Chavira, 1995; Smith, 1985), and cultural rediscovery (Sodowsky et al., 1995). Figure 1 links bicultural stress with coping.

Ethnic identity is understood to entail retention of cultural heritage and a sense of belonging and significance attached to a reference group (see Sodowsky et al., 1995). Kiefer (1974) identifies three types of ethnic identity conflict experienced by later generation Asian Americans that might act as ethnic identity stressors. **Cultural alienation** refers to a sense of personal discontinuity that occurs across time and as a result of disruption in cultural patterns. Cultural alienation experienced by Asian Americans is compounded by racial and ethnic stereotypes which denies one's individuality. **Cultural confusion** occurs as a result of being confronted with multiple norms (e.g., norms of Asian cultures; norms of Western cultures), and the inability to identify and associate with a definite norm within a given context. Thus, there is an incongruence between one's experiences and his or her assumptions. **Cultural conflict** occurs when one's values are perceived to be incompatible with a given social interaction. Sodowsky and Lai (1997) stated that as a result of living with two sets of opposing norms and attitudes with regard to interpersonal behaviors, Asian Americans' cultural conflict appears to involve interpersonal and intrapersonal dimensions (Sodowsky & Lai, 1997). The interpersonal dimension involves having cultural conflicts with one's own ethnic group and/or with members of the dominant culture. The intrapersonal dimension includes identity crisis, a personal sense of inferiority as a member of one's cultural group, lack of ethnic differentiation due to feeling marginalized from both cultural groups, and feelings of anger and guilt toward one or both cultural groups.

Table 2 is a summary of results of studies on acculturative and bicultural stress of Asian Americans. Table 2 provides an understanding of the nature of culturally-related stress.

4. CONCLUSION

Earlier knowledge of Asian Americans was based upon the study of domestic-born Chinese and Japanese Americans. The demographic landscape, however, of persons of Asian ancestry in the U.S. is changing rapidly with new immigration post-World War II and since 1965 occurring from various Asian countries. With two-thirds (66%) of Asian Americans being foreign-born, conceptualizations and empirical studies are needed to understand the cultural issues of new immigrants and of their U.S.-born second-generation children.

Acculturation involves a minority individual's behavioral, cultural, and social adaptations that take place as a result of contact between the individual's ethnic society and the White dominant society. Acculturative stress is the direct result of the acculturation adaptation process for first generation immigrants, and bicultural stress is a response to the pulls of maintaining ethnic ties in second and later generations. Moderating variables, such as generational status, differentially impact these processes. Empirical studies have measured these variables individually, in isolation of the other related cultural variables. Now that we have a broader picture of acculturation, more complex measurement models can be hypothesized and tested.

5. REFERENCES

Abe, J. S., & Zane, N. W. S. (1990). Psychological maladjustment among Asian and White American students: Controlling for confounds. *Journal of Counseling Psychology, 37*(4), 437-444.

Anderson, J., Moeschberger, M., Chen, M. S., Jr., Kunn, P., Wewers, M. E., & Guthrie, R. (1993). An acculturation scale for Southeast Asians. *Social Psychiatry and Psychiatric Epidemiology, 28*, 134-141.

Berry, J. W. (1980). Acculturation as varieties of adaptation. In A. M. Padilla (Ed.), *Acculturation: Theory, models and some new findings* (pp. 9-25). Boulder, CO: Westview.

Berry, J. W. (1990). Psychology of acculturation. In J. J. Berman (Ed.), *Cross-cultural perspectives* (pp. 201-234). Lincoln, NE: University of Nebraska Press.

Berry, J. W., & Kim, U. (1988). Acculturation and mental health. In P. Dasen, J. W. Berry, & N. Sartorius (Eds.), *Health and cross-cultural psychology: Towards applications* (pp. 207-236). Newbury Park, CA: Sage Publications.

Berry, J. W., Kim, U., Minde, T., & Mok, D. (1987). Comparative studies of acculturative stress. *International Migration Review, 21*, 491-511.

Berry, J. W., Kim, U., Power, S., Young, M., & Bujaki, M. (1989). Acculturation attitudes in plural societies. *Applied Psychology: An International Review, 38*(2), 158-206.

Bufka, L. F. (1998, August). *Family factors, acculturation, and identity in second generation Asian Indian*. Paper presented at the annual convention of the American Psychological Association, San Francisco, CA.

Burnam, M. A., Hough, R. L., Karno, M., Escobar, J. I., & Telles, C. A. (1987). Acculturation and lifetime prevalence of psychiatric disorders among Mexican Americans in Los Angeles. *Journal of Health and Social Behavior, 28,* 89-102.

Burnam, M. A., Telles, C. A., Karno, M., Hough, R. L., & Escobar, J. I. (1987). Measurement of acculturation in a community population of Mexican Americans. *Hispanic Journal of Behavioral Sciences, 9*(2), 105-130.

Cervantes, R. C., & Castro, F. G. (1985). Stress, coping, and Mexican American mental health. *Hispanic Journal of Behavioral Sciences, 7*(1), 1-73.

Chambon, A. (1989). Refugee families experiences: Three family themes—family disruption, violent trauma, and acculturation. *Journal of Strategic and Systemic Therapies, 8,* 3-3.

Colomba, M. I., Santiago, E. S., & Rossello, J. (1999). Coping strategies and depression in Puerto Rican adolescents: An exploratory study. *Cultural Diversity and Ethnic Minority Psychology, 5,* 65-75.

Connor, J. W. (1977). *Tradition and change in three generations of Japanese Americans.* Chicago: Nelson-Hall.

Cortes, D. E., Rogler, L. H., & Malgady, R. G. (1994). Biculturality among Puerto Rican adults in the United States. *American Journal of Community Psychology, 22*(5), 707-721.

Chataway, C. J., & Berry, J. W. (1989). Acculturation experiences, appraisal, coping, and adaptation: A comparison of Hong Kong Chinese, French, and English students in Canada. *Canadian Journal of Behavioural Science, 21*(3), 295-309.

Cuéllar, I., Arnold, B., & Maldonado, R. (1995). Acculturation Rating Scale for Mexican Americans-II: A revision of the original ARSMA scale. *Hispanic Journal of Behavioral Sciences, 17*(3), 275-304.

Cuéllar, I., Harris, L. C., & Jasso, R. (1980). An acculturation scale for Mexican American normal and clinical populations. *Hispanic Journal of Behavioral Sciences, 2*(3), 199-217.

Dana, R. H. (1996). Assessment of acculturation in Hispanic populations. *Hispanic Journal of Behavioral Sciences, 18*(3), 317-328.

Dawson, E. J., Crano, W. D., & Burgoon, M. (1996). Refining the meaning and measurement of acculturation: Revisiting a novel methodological approach. *International Journal of Intercultural Relations, 20*(1), 97-114.

De Anda, D. (1984). Bicultural socialization: Factors affecting the minority experience. *Social Work, 29,* 101-107.

Deyo, R. A., Diehl, A. K., Hazuda, H. & Stern, M. P. (1985). A simple language-based acculturation scale for Mexican Americans: Validation and application to health care research. *American Journal of Public Health, 75*(1), 51-55.

Dressler, W. W., & Bernal, H. (1982). Acculturation and stress in a low-income Puerto Rican community. *Journal of Human Stress, 8*(3), 32-38.

Dyal, J. A., & Dyal, R. Y. (1981). Acculturation, stress, and coping. *International Journal of Intercultural Relations, 5,* 301-328.

Feldman, S. S., Mont-Reynaud, R., & Rosenthal, D. A. (1992a). The acculturation of Chinese immigrants: Perceived effects on family functioning of length of residence in two cultural contexts. *Journal of Genetic Psychology, 151,* 495-514.

Feldman, S. S., Mont-Reynaud, R., & Rosenthal, D. A. (1992b). When east moves west: The acculturation of values of Chinese adolescents in the U.S. and Australia. *Journal of Research on Adolescence, 2,* 147-143.

Franco, J. N. (1983). An acculturation scale for Mexican-American children. *The Journal of General Psychology, 108,* 175-181.

Frey, M. & Roysircar-Sodowsky, G. (in press). Relationships of acculturation, worldview, and environmental perceptions. *Journal of Multicultural Counseling and Development.*

Greenberger, E., & Chen, C. (1996). Perceived family relationships and depressed mood in early and late adolescence: A comparison of Europeans and Asian Americans. *Developmental Psychology, 32*(4), 707-716.

Hutnik, N. (1986). Patterns of ethnic minority identification and modes of social adaptation. *Ethnic and Racial Studies, 2,* 150-167.

Isajiw, W. W. (1990). Ethnic-identity retention. In R. Breton, W. W. Isajiw, W. E. Kalbach, & J. G. Reitz, (Eds.), *Ethnic identity and equality* (pp. 34-91). Toronto, Canada: University of Toronto Press.

Kiefer, C. W. (1974). *Changing cultures, changing lives: An ethnographic study of three generations of Japanese Americans*. San Francisco: Jossey & Bass.

Kim, E. J., O'Neil, J. M., & Owen, S. V. (1996). Asian American men's acculturation and gender-role conflict. *Psychological Reports, 79*, 95-104.

Kuo, P. Y., & Roysircar-Sodowsky, G. (1999). Cultural ethnic identity versus political ethnic identity: Theory and research on Asian Americans. In D. S. Sandhu (Ed.), *Asian and Pacific Islander Americans: Issues and concerns for counseling and psychotherapy* (pp. 71-90). New York: Nova Sciences.

Kwan, K.-L. K. (1996). *Ethnic identity and cultural adjustment difficulties of Chinese Americans*. Unpublished doctoral dissertation. University of Nebraska-Lincoln.

Lang, J. G., Munoz, R. F., Bernal, G., & Sorensen, J. L. (1982). Quality of life and psychological well-being in a bicultural Latino community. *Hispanic Journal of Behavioral Sciences, 4*, 433-450.

Lazarus, R. S., & Folkman, S. (1991). The concept of coping. In A. Monat & R. S. Lazarus (Eds.), *Stress and coping: An anthology* (3rd ed.). New York: Columbia University Press.

Marin, G., & Gamba, R. J. (1996). A new measurement of acculturation for Hispanics: The Bidimensional Acculturation Scale for Hispanics (BAS). *Hispanic Journal of Behavioral Sciences, 18*(3), 297-316.

Masuda, M., Matsumoto, G. H., & Meredith, G. M. (1970). Ethnic identity in three generations of Japanese Americans. *Journal of Social Psychology, 81*(2), 199-207.

Mehta, S. (1998). Relationship between acculturation and mental health for Asian Indian immigrants in the United States. *Genetic, Social, and General Psychological Monographs, 124*, 61-78.

Mena, F. J., Padilla, A. M., & Maldonado, M. (1987). Acculturative stress and specific coping strategies among immigrant and later generation college students. *Hispanic Journal of Behavioral Sciences, 9*, 207-225.

Mendoza, R. H. (1989). An empirical scale to measure type and degree of acculturation in Mexican-American adolescents and adults. *Journal of Cross-Cultural Psychology, 20*(4), 372-385.

Mok, T. A. (1994, August). Looking for love: Factors influencing Asian Americans' choice of dating partners. In J. Y. Fong (Ed.), *Proceedings of the Asian American Psychological Association 1994 Convention*, Los Angeles, CA.

Murthy, K. (1998, August). *Implications for counseling Asian Indian: Second generation perceptions of the American milieu*. Paper presented at the annual convention of the American Psychological Association, San Francisco, CA.

Negy, C., & Woods, D. J. (1992a). A note on the relationship between acculturation and socioeconomic status. *Hispanic Journal of Behavioral Sciences, 14*(2), 248-251.

Negy, C., & Woods, D. J. (1992b). The importance of acculturation in understanding research with Hispanic-Americans. *Hispanic Journal of Behavioral Sciences, 14*(2), 224-247.

Nguyen, H. H., Messe, L. A., & Stollak, G. E. (1999). Toward a more complex understanding of acculturation and adjustment: Cultural involvements and psychosocial functioning in Vietnamese youth. *Journal of Cross-Cultural Psychology, 30*(1), 5-31.

Norris, A. E., Ford, K., & Bova, C. A. (1996). Psychometrics of a Brief Acculturation Scale for Hispanics in a probability sample of urban Hispanic adolescents and young adults. *Hispanic Journal of Behavioral Sciences, 18*(11), 29-38.

Olah, A. (1995). Coping strategies among adolescents: A cross-cultural study. *Journal of Adolescence, 18*, 491-512.

Olmedo, E. L. (1979). Acculturation: A psychometric perspective. *American Psychologist, 34*(11), 1061-1070.

Olmedo, E. L., Martinez, J. L., Jr., & Martinez, S. R. (1978). Measure of acculturation for Chicano adolescents. *Psychological Reports, 42*, 159-170.

Osvold, L. L., & Sodowsky, G. R. (1995). Eating attitudes of Native American and African American women: Differences by race and acculturation. *Explorations in Ethnic Studies, 18*, 187-210.

Padilla, A. M. (1980). The role of cultural awareness and ethnic loyalty in acculturation. In A. M. Padilla (Ed.), *Acculturation: Theory, models and some new findings* (pp. 47-84). Boulder, CO: Westview.

Padilla, A. M., Wagatsuma, Y., & Lindholm, K. J. (1985). Acculturation and personality as predictors of stress in Japanese and Japanese-Americans. *Journal of Social Psychology, 125*, 295-305.

ASSESSING ACCULTURATION AND CULTURAL VARIABLES

Phinney, J. S. (1989). Stages of ethnic identity development in minority group adolescents. *Journal of Early Adolescence, 6*(1-2), 34-49.

Phinney, J. S., & Chavira, V. (1995). Parental ethnic socialization and adolescent coping with problems related to ethnicity. *Journal of Research on Adolescence, 5*, 31-53.

Phinney, J. S., Chavira, V., & Williamson, L. (1992). Acculturation attitudes and self-esteem among high school and college students. *Youth and Society, 23*, 299-312.

Rogler, L. H., Cortes, D. E., & Malgady, R. G. (1991). Acculturation and mental health status among Hispanics. *American Psychologist, 46*(6), 585-587.

Rotheram-Borus, M. J. (1990). Adolescents' reference-group choices, self-esteem, and adjustment. *Journal of Personality and Social Psychology, 59*(5), 1075-1081.

Rumbaut, R. G. (1994). The crucible within: Ethnic identity, self-esteem and segmented assimilation among children of immigrants. *International Migration Review, 28*, 748-794.

Rumbaut, R. G. (1997). Ties that bind: Immigration and immigrant families in the United States. In A. Booth, A. C. Crouter, & N. Landale (Eds.), *Immigration and the family: Research and policy on U.S. immigrants* (pp. 3-46). Mahwah, NJ: Lawrence Erlbaum Associates.

Roysircar-Sodowsky, G. (2001). *A within-group comparative analysis of Asian Indian: Ethnic identity, perceived prejudice, acculturative stress, and coping.* Manuscript submitted for publication.

Roysircar-Sodowsky, G. R., & Maestas, M. V. (2000). Acculturation, ethnic identity, and acculturative stress: Evidence and measurement. In R. H. Dana (Ed.), *Handbook of cross-cultural and multicultural personality assessment.* (pp. 131-172). Mahwah, NJ: Lawrence Erlbaum Associates.

Roysircar-Sodowsky, G., & Maestas, M. V. (2001). *Acculturation and ethnic idenity measures: Analyses of methdology and psychometrics.* Book submitted for publication.

Smith, E. M. J. (1985). Ethnic minorities: Life stress, social support and mental health issues. *The Counseling Psychologist, 13*, 537-579.

Sodowsky, G. R. (1991). Effects of culturally consistent counseling tasks on American and international student observers' perception of counselor credibility: A preliminary investigation. *Journal of Counseling and Development, 69*, 253-256.

Sodowsky, G. R., Kwan, K.-L. K., & Pannu, R. (1995). Ethnic identity of Asians in the United States: Conceptualization and illustrations. In J. Ponterotto, M. Casas, L. Suzuki, & C. Alexander (Eds.), *Handbook of multicultural counseling* (pp. 123-154). Newbury Park, CA: Sage.

Sodowsky, G. R., & Lai, E. W. M. (1997). Asian immigrant variables and structural models of cross-cultural distress. (pp. 211-234). In A. Booth, A. C. Crouter, & N. Landale (Eds.), *Immigration and the family: Research and policy on U.S. immigrants*. Mahwah, NJ: Lawrence Erlbaum Associates.

Sodowsky, G. R., Lai, E. W. M., & Plake, B. S. (1991). Moderating effects of sociocultural variables on acculturation attitudes of Hispanics and Asian Americans. *Journal of Counseling and Development, 70*, 194-204.

Sodowsky, G. R., & Plake, B. S. (1991). Psychometric properties of the American-International Relations Scale. *Educational and Psychological Measurement, 51*(1), 207-216.

Sodowsky, G. R., & Plake, B. (1992). A study of acculturation differences among international people and suggestions for sensitivity to within-group differences. *Journal of Counseling and Development, 71*, 53-59.

Sue, S., & Zane, N. W. S. (1985). Academic achievement and socioemotional adjustment among Chinese university students. *Journal of Counseling Psychology, 32*(4), 570-579.

Suinn, R. M., Ahuna, C. Khoo, G. (1992). The Suinn-Lew Asian Self-Identity Acculturation Scale: Concurrent and factorial validation. *Educational and Psychological Measurement, 52*(4), 141-146.

Szapocznik, J., Scopetta, M. A., Kurtines, W., & Aranalde, M. A. (1978). Theory and measurement of acculturation. *International Journal of Psychology, 12*, 113-130.

Ting-Toomey, S. (1981). Ethnic identity and close relationships in Chinese-American college students. *International Journal of Intercultural Relations, 5*, 383-406.

Tropp, L. R., Erkut, S., Garcia-Coll, C., Alarcon, O., & Vazquez-Garcia, H. A. (1999). Psychological acculturation: Development of a new measure for Puerto Ricans on the U.S. mainland. *Educational and Psychological Measurement, 59*(2), 351-367.

U.S. Bureau of the Census, Population Division (1999). *United States Population estimates by age, sex, race, and Hispanic origin.* URL: http://www.census.gov/population/estimates/nation/intfile3.

Yeh, C., Chiang, L., & Wang, Y. W. V. (1998, August). *Cultural adjustment and mental health of Chinese immigrant adolescents.* Paper presented at the annual convention of the American Psychological Association, San Francisco, CA.

Zheng, X., & Berry, J. W. (1991). Psychological adaptation of Chinese sojourners in Canada. *International Journal of Psychology, 26*(4).

JEANNE L. TSAI AND YULIA CHENTSOVA-DUTTON

CHAPTER 7

MODELS OF CULTURAL ORIENTATION: DIFFERENCES BETWEEN AMERICAN-BORN AND OVERSEAS-BORN ASIANS

1. INTRODUCTION

Being American means...just living here, assimilating to their culture. Sometimes I don't consider myself American...I look at myself as more Hmong (Overseas-born Hmong American)

Being American means...being whoever I want to be, whatever makes me happy, whatever I do, just exploring my possibilities and not being limited... (American-born Hmong American)

The above quotes are the responses of two Hmong college students, one born in Laos and the other born in the United States, to the question, "What does being American mean to you?" (Tsai, Wong, Mortensen, & Hess, in press). The first respondent describes "being American" in relation to "being Hmong," whereas the second respondent describes "being American" without making any reference to Hmong culture. In this chapter, we argue that these two responses represent the different models of cultural orientation held by overseas- and American-born Asians. Although a considerable body of research has focused on models of cultural orientation across groups, few scholars have examined how these models might vary *within* cultural groups. Uncovering sources of variation within groups is becoming increasingly important, particularly in multicultural societies such as the United States, where differences within cultural groups may be as large as differences between them.

2. WHAT IS CULTURAL ORIENTATION?

Cultural orientation is the degree to which individuals are influenced by and actively engage in the traditions, norms, and practices of a specific culture. This chapter examines the models of cultural orientation held by Asian Americans who were born in the United States and those who were born overseas (i.e., immigrants). Therefore, we have chosen to use the term "cultural orientation" rather than acculturation, which refers to the cultural adaptation and adjustment of immigrants only (Berry, 1980, 1995). According to Ying (1995), cultural orientation should be distinguished from ethnic identity, which refers to one's conscious identification with a cultural group (Tajfel, 1981). That is, individuals may be strongly influenced by and oriented to their cultures without explicitly identifying with their cultural groups. Despite their disparate meanings, these terms have been used interchangeably in the literature. For example, Rosenthal (1989) uses the term "cultural identity" to refer to cultural knowledge, feelings about one's culture, and participation in cultural activities. Similarly, Phinney (1990)'s definition of "ethnic identity" includes components of ethnic identity as defined by Tajfel (e.g., the ethnic labels used when describing oneself) and of cultural orientation as defined by Ying (e.g., language proficiency, participation in cultural activities, and affiliation with other cultural group members). In this chapter, we focus on cultural orientation rather than ethnic identity.

2.1 Domains of Cultural Orientation

In the literature, scholars have studied levels of cultural orientation in various life domains. The main domains that have been examined include social affiliation, participation in cultural activities, language use and proficiency, and feelings about one's culture.

2.1.1 Social affiliation

Social affiliation refers to the cultural composition of individuals' social networks, including friendships, dating relationships, and marriages. Social affiliation has been found to be an important indicator of cultural orientation, even among children and grandchildren of immigrants (Constantinou & Harvey, 1985).

2.1.2 Activities

Activities and participation in other cultural practices are also an important domain of cultural orientation. Examples of such activities include traditional holidays, rites of passage, and forms of entertainment and recreation. For example, Birman and Tyler (1994) found that the more Russian Jewish female refugees living in the United States participated in activities associated with Russian Jewish culture (e.g., attending synagogue; listening to Russian music), the more alienated they felt by American society.

2.1.3 Language

Language has long been viewed as an important indicator of cultural orientation. For example, Olmedo and Padilla (1978) argue that among Latinos, language is the strongest predictor of cultural orientation. This domain typically includes spoken and written language proficiency as well as preferred language use in different social situations.

2.1.4 *Feelings about one's culture*

Feelings about one's culture refers to individuals' attitudes toward and feelings about their native and host cultures (Boski, 1991; Der-Karabetian & Ruiz, 1997). These feelings may be either positive (e.g., proud, satisfied) or negative (e.g., ashamed, disappointed, critical). As individuals have less direct contact with their native cultures, their cultural orientation may become based more on this domain (S. E. Keefe & Padilla, 1987; Tsai, Ying, & Lee, 2000b).

2.2 Models of Cultural Orientation

Although a number of models of cultural orientation have been proposed, the unidimensional and bidimensional models are the most widely studied.

2.2.1 *Unidimensional models*

Unidimensional (or linear) models were first developed to explain immigrants' adjustment to their host cultures. These models consider orientation to native and host cultures as opposite ends of the same continuum (Stonequist, 1964). Thus, according to these models, becoming more oriented to American host culture by definition requires Asian immigrants to become less oriented to their Asian native culture. As Figure 1 illustrates, the unidimensional model allows for several types of cultural orientation. An individual may be: (a) more oriented to her native culture (N) than her host culture (H), (b) more oriented to her host culture than her native culture, or (c) equally oriented to both her host and native cultures.

Unidimensional models have been criticized for several reasons. First, these models assume that bicultural or multicultural orientation is psychologically unhealthy, particularly if the host and native cultures hold opposing world-views (Stonequist, 1964). For example, Park (1928) described an individual who is suspended between two cultures as "marginal," or unable to function in either culture. Increasing evidence, however, contradicts this assumption (LaFromboise, Coleman, & Gerton, 1993). Second, unidimensional models assume that the more oriented individuals are to their host cultures (and the less oriented they are to their native cultures), the healthier they are. For example, Gordon (1964) explicitly outlined several stages of cultural adjustment, of which the most optimal is the "identificational" stage, during which one's native culture is abandoned in favor of orientation to one's host culture. Findings from several studies, however, suggest that higher orientation to the host culture is not associated with more positive health outcomes. For example, Vega et al. (1998) and Burnam et al. (1987) found that compared to their more Americanized U.S.-born Mexican peers, less Americanized Mexican immigrants had *lower* levels of depression and other mental disorders. Other studies suggest that individuals born in the United States have higher rates of suicide (Sorenson & Shen, 1996), drug and alcohol use (Gilbert, 1989; Vega, Kolody, Hwang, Noble, & Porter, 1997), and anxiety disorders (Karno et al., 1989) than their immigrant peers. Thus, assuming that individuals born in the United States are more oriented to American culture than immigrants, these findings suggest that orientation to the host culture may result in negative rather than positive mental health. In fact, Escobar (1998) suggests that retaining a strong orientation to one's native culture may protect one against stress and may lead to positive health outcomes. Third, unidimensional models typically focus on only one or two domains of life experience (e.g., language proficiency), although a growing number of scholars is acknowledging that levels of cultural orientation may vary by life domain (Olmedo & Padilla, 1978; Szapocznik, Kurtines, & Fernandez, 1980; Tsai et al., 2000b).

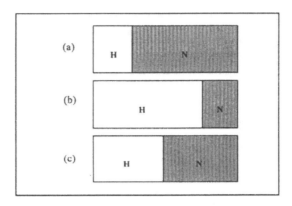

Figure 1. Types of cultural orientation according to the unidimensional model. "H" refers to the host culture; "N" refers to the native culture.

2.2.2 Bidimensional models

In response to these criticisms, *bidimensional (or orthogonal) models* have been proposed (Berry, 1995; LaFromboise et al., 1993; Oetting & Beauvais, 1991; Sayegh & Lasry, 1992; Zak, 1973). These models view orientation to native and host cultures as separate processes that develop independently. Figure 2 illustrates several different possible types of bidimensional cultural orientation. An individual may be: (a) highly oriented to the host culture, but only slightly oriented to the native culture, (b) not oriented to either culture, (c) highly oriented to both cultures, or (d) highly oriented to the native culture, but only slightly oriented to the host culture. In each case, host and native cultural orientations are not related to each other. Berry (1980, 1995) has used the following terms to describe each of these types of orientations: (a) assimilated, (b) marginal, (c) integrated, and (d) separated.

Bidimensional models do not assume that high orientation to the host culture coupled with low orientation to the native culture is the optimal outcome. Nor do they view high levels of orientation to both host and native cultures as psychologically unhealthy. However, the primary criticism waged against bidimensional models is that they do not describe the experiences of certain groups, such as immigrants. That is, by definition, adjusting to a new culture requires some degree of change in one's previous practices and beliefs; therefore, it seems unlikely that immigrants' orientations to their native and host cultures are completely unrelated to each other.

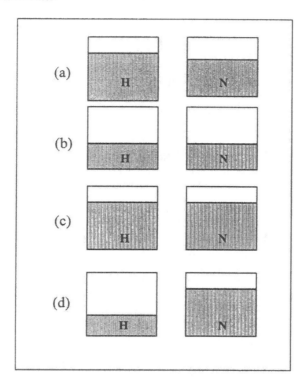

Figure 2. Types of cultural orientation according to the bidimensional model. "H" refers to the host culture; "N" refers to the native culture.

3. EMPIRICAL EVIDENCE FOR UNIDIMENSIONAL AND BIDIMENSIONAL MODELS

Empirical support exists for both models. For example, in support of the unidimensional model, Cuéllar, Nyberg, Maldonado, and R.E. Roberts (1997) found that for a culturally diverse sample of college students, orientation to American culture was negatively correlated with orientation to one's native culture. Other studies, however, suggest that while individuals become less oriented to their native culture for some domains of cultural orientation, such as language proficiency, they remain highly oriented to their native culture in other domains, such as social affiliation (Constantinou & Harvey, 1985).

In support of bidimensional models, some studies demonstrate that cultural orientation does not diminish with time spent in the host country (Boski, 1992), but instead remains stable among subsequent generations (Der-Karabetian & Ruiz, 1997). Also in support of the bidimensional model, scholars have found that orientation to one's native culture is unrelated to orientation to the host culture (Der-Karabetian & Ruiz, 1997; Phinney & Devich-Navarro, 1997; Sayegh & Lasry, 1992; Suleiman & Beit-Hallahmi, 1997). For example, Der-Karabetian and Ruiz (1997) found that for first- and second-generation Mexican American adolescents, feelings about Latino culture and feelings about American cultures (e.g., pride) were not related to each other.

Both the unidimensional and bidimensional models have been used to describe Asian American cultural orientation. For example, the most widely used measure of cultural orientation for Asian Americans, the Suinn-Lew Asian Self-Identity Acculturation Scale, is based on a unidimensional model. This instrument has been found to be a reliable and valid measure of cultural orientation for a variety of Asian American samples (Ownbey & Horridge, 1998; Ponterotto, Baluch, & Carielli, 1998). However, other findings suggest that Asian American cultural orientation is bidimensional (Krishnan & Berry, 1992; Wong-Rieger & D. Quintana, 1987; Ying, Coombs, & Lee, 1999).

Given that both the unidimensional and bidimensional models have received empirical support, scholars have suggested that the characteristics and circumstances of a particular cultural group determine which model best describes the cultural orientation of that group (Ghuman, 1998; Oetting & Beauvais, 1991; Sayegh & Lasry, 1992). However, none of these scholars has explicitly identified what these particular characteristics or circumstances are or how they might result in a unidimensional or bidimensional model of cultural orientation. In Tsai et al. (2000b), we argued that one's place of birth and concomitant cultural experiences would determine which model holds and that this would explain differences in models of cultural orientation among individuals within the same cultural group. In the next section, we discuss this argument in greater detail, focusing on Asian Americans.

4. DIFFERENT MODELS OF CULTURAL ORIENTATION FOR AMERICAN- AND OVERSEAS BORN ASIANS

Among Asian Americans, 60 percent were born overseas; the remaining 40 percent were born in the United States (U.S. Bureau of the Census, 1999). As mentioned above, place of birth may assume an important role in determining individuals' cultural experiences, which may in turn affect individuals' models of cultural orientation. In the next section, we describe this process for American-born and overseas-born Asians.

Until they arrive in the United States, most Asian immigrants and refugees primarily have experience with and exposure to their native Asian cultures. As a result, until the time of migration, individuals may be entirely unaware of the degree to which their values, behaviors, and ideas are influenced by their native culture. When they arrive in the United States, immigrants are confronted with the task of adapting to a culture that differs greatly in its values, norms, and beliefs. At this point, immigrants may become acutely aware of their cultural orientation, or how strongly tied they are to the values, norms, and traditions of their native culture. In order to function effectively in their new environments, immigrants must learn the values, norms, and beliefs of their host cultures, even if they do not internalize them. Age of migration (e.g., before or after age 12), reason for migration (e.g., education or economic advancement, political refuge), and mode of migration (e.g., with or without parents) are factors that may influence this process of cultural adaptation and change. However, in most cases, immigrants must relinquish aspects of their native culture for aspects of their host culture, particularly in school and work contexts. In home contexts, immigrants may retain their connections to the native culture; however, this may become increasingly difficult over time.

By being born and raised in the United States, American-born Asians have first-hand knowledge of American culture. Like their immigrant counterparts, they may first be exposed to Asian practices (depending on whether their parents retain connections to their native culture); however, outside of the home, their environments are American. Thus, although to some extent American-born Asians may have to adapt to mainstream American culture, this adaptation process may be much easier and more natural than that of immigrants. American-born Asians can retain ties to their parents' native Asian culture at home, and, at the same time, develop an American orientation in school, work, or other contexts. Over time, American-born Asians may struggle with their status as ethnic minorities in American society; however, this challenge is considerably different from that of immigrants, who must learn and master American customs and traditions.

The different cultural experiences of immigrant and American-born Asians may result in distinct models of cultural orientation. Because immigrants must relinquish aspects of their native culture in order to acquire those of their host culture, their model of cultural orientation may be *unidimensional*. In contrast, American-born Asians are able to develop different cultural orientations in different contexts. As a result, their model of cultural orientation may be *bidimensional*. To date, we have conducted two studies that support this hypothesis. In the first study, we compared the cultural orientation of a group of American-born and overseas-born Chinese American college students living in the multicultural San Francisco Bay Area (Tsai et al., 2000b). The second study compared the cultural orientation of a group of American-born and overseas-born Hmong college students living in the Midwest (Tsai, 2001). In both studies we administered the General Ethnicity Questionnaire, an instrument that measures orientation to American and Asian cultures separately across a variety of life domains (e.g., language use and proficiency, social affiliation, cultural pride, cultural exposure, media, and cultural activities) (Tsai et al., 2000b). We examined the correlation between overall levels of orientation to American and

Asian cultures and found that for Chinese and Hmong born overseas, orientation to Asian culture was negatively correlated with orientation to American culture, supporting a *unidimensional* model of cultural orientation. For Chinese and Hmong born in the United States, overall levels of orientation to Asian and American cultures were not correlated with each other, supporting a *bidimensional* model of cultural orientation.

5. DIFFERENT EFFECTS OF CULTURAL ORIENTATION ON ASPECTS OF PSYCHOLOGICAL WELL-BEING

Given their different experiences with Asian and American cultures, American-born and immigrant Asians face somewhat different cultural challenges. Whereas the psychological well-being of Asian immigrants may be related to the process of cultural adaptation (Berry & Kim, 1988; Furnham & Bochner, 1986), the psychological well-being of American-born Chinese may be related more to their minority status in American society. In two studies that compared the relationship between cultural orientation and measures of psychological well-being for American-born and immigrant Chinese, we found evidence that supports this hypothesis. Tsai et al. (2000a) found that cultural orientation was related to self-esteem for overseas-born Chinese. This finding was similar to that of Chentsova (1996), who found that for a sample of international students, one-third of which were Asian, positive attitudes toward and identification with their native culture were positively correlated with self-esteem. Ying, Lee, & Tsai (in press) found that cultural orientation was significantly related to sense of coherence (the feeling that one's world is meaningful, manageable, and comprehensible) (Antonovsky, 1979, 1987) for overseas-born Chinese. However, for American-born Chinese, cultural orientation was not related to self-esteem (Tsai et al., 2000a) or sense of coherence (Ying et al., in press). Moreover, Ying et al. (in press) found that while the experience of racial discrimination was related to sense of coherence for American-born Chinese, it was not related to sense of coherence for immigrant Chinese. Across the studies described above, no group differences were found in overall levels of self-esteem, sense of coherence, or racial discrimination. These findings support our contention that the psychological well-being of American-born Chinese and overseas-born Chinese is affected by different cultural challenges. Although these findings are by no means comprehensive, they do have important implications for clinical interventions and future research with American-born and immigrant Asian groups.

6. CLINICAL AND COUNSELING IMPLICATIONS

Guidelines regarding the assessment and treatment of members of different cultural groups emphasize the importance of assessing the client's current level of cultural orientation (Okazaki & Sue, 1995). Our findings, however, suggest that within groups, there are systematic differences in models of cultural orientation.

MODELS OF CULTURAL ORIENTATION: DIFFERENCES BETWEEN AMERICAN-BORN AND OVERSEAS-BORN ASIANS

These systematic differences may result in the same intervention having very different meanings for American-born and immigrant Asian Americans. For example, to increase a client's level of comfort with American culture, a clinician may ask the client to participate in more American activities. This intervention may be perceived as threatening to an immigrant Asian American, who may equate increased participation in American activities with decreased participation in Asian activities. As a result, immigrant Asian Americans may not comply with this intervention. In contrast, this suggestion may be viewed positively by an American-born Asian, who may view increased participation in American activities as not affecting his/her participation in Asian activities. Thus, compliance with this intervention may be high for this group.

Moreover, the life challenges that may lead American-born and immigrant Asian Americans to seek treatment may be qualitatively different. As mentioned above, immigrant Asian Americans face stresses due to the process of cultural adaptation, and therefore, their psychological well-being is based on their orientation to their native and host cultures. American-born Asians, however, face stresses due to their minority status. As a result, their psychological health is based less on their cultural orientation and more on their direct experiences of racial prejudice and discrimination. Clinicians should keep these differences in mind when treating each Asian American group.

7. FUTURE RESEARCH ON ASIAN AMERICAN CULTURAL ORIENTATION

Identifying differences within cultural groups in models of cultural orientation is essential in order to understand how cultural variables mediate the expression and subjective experience of emotional distress and psychological health. Although we are beginning to learn more about sources of difference within groups, more research is clearly needed. First, our findings are based on college student samples of Chinese Americans living in the San Francisco Bay Area and of Hmong Americans living in the Midwest. Despite variation in their migration histories and in the diversity of their current environments, differences between American-born and overseas-born individuals were comparable for these two groups. However, future research must determine whether the differences between American-born and immigrant Asian groups discussed in this chapter apply to other Asian American samples living in other regions of the United States. Second, these findings are based on inventories of cultural orientation that sample some, but not all, domains of life experience. Future research should include other life domains. For example, very few studies have directly examined the political and ideological component of cultural orientation (Constantinou & Harvey, 1985). However, research on political behavior of immigrant and minority groups suggests that political awareness and group ideology are more salient among American-born than immigrant generations. For example, American-born members of ethnic minorities are more likely to be involved in political and organizational activity than their naturalized counterparts (DeSipio, 1996). Participation in a range of political activities such as voting, campaigning and working to solve community problems continues to increase from the first to the second and third generations of Asian American immigrants (Junn, 1999; Lien, 1994). Immigrants are struggling with cultural adjustment, and therefore, they may have less time to spend on politics than American-born Asians. In addition, compared to immigrants, American-born Asians may be more aware of and more likely to protest discrimination and prejudice because they are citizens of the United States by birth.

A third direction of future research should focus on other sources of difference within cultural groups. For example, Manaster, Rhodes, Marcus, and Chan (1998) examined the relationship between cultural orientation and birth order. They found that among second and third generation Japanese Americans, first-borns were more oriented to Japanese culture (as measured by traditional religious affiliation, adherence to traditional values, cultural knowledge and language competence) than were later-born Japanese Americans. Parents may spend less time with their second- and third-born children than with their first-born children; as a result, first-borns may have more contact with their native culture (through their parents) than their younger siblings. In addition, the parents themselves may be less oriented to their native culture by the time they raise their second and third children. Therefore, they may transmit less of their native culture to their later-born children than they did to their first-born child. Other sources of within cultural group variation include age of migration and the diversity of individuals' immediate environments.

Finally, research should focus on the mechanisms by which variations within cultural subgroups result in different models of cultural orientation. For example, how do differences in place of birth influence models of cultural orientation? We suggested that place of birth influences the ease of adjustment to a different culture by determining the nature of the cultural environments that individuals are exposed to early in their lives. However, there may be other mechanisms by which place of birth influences models of cultural orientation. Future research must examine such mechanisms.

8. REFERENCES

Antonovsky, A. (1979). *Health, stress, and coping.* San Francisco: Jossey-Bass.
Antonovsky, A. (1987). *Unraveling the mystery of health: How people manage stress and stay well.* San Francisco: Jossey-Bass.
Berry, J. W. (1980). Acculturation as varieties of adaptation. In A. M. Padilla (Ed.), *Acculturation: Theory, models and some new findings* (pp. 9-25). Colorado: Westview Press, Inc.
Berry, J. W. (1995). Psychology of acculturation. In N. Goldberg and J. Veroff (Eds.), *The culture and psychology reader* (pp. 457-488). New York: New York University Press.
Berry, J. W., & Kim, U. (1988). Acculturation and mental health. In P. R. Dasen, J.W. Berry, and N. Sartorius (Eds.). *Health and cross-cultural psychology: Towards applications* (pp. 207-236). London: Sage Publications.
Birman, D., & Tyler, F. B. (1994). Acculturation and alienation of Soviet Jewish refugees in the United States. *Genetic, Social, and General Psychology Monographs, 120* (1), 101-115.
Boski, P. (1991). Remaining a Pole or becoming a Canadian: National self-identity among Polish immigrants to Canada. *Journal of Applied Social Psychology, 21* (1), 41-77.
Boski, P. (1992). In the homeland: National self-identity and well-being of Poles in Poland and in America. In S. Iwawaki, Y. Kashima & K. Leung (Eds.), *Innovations in cross-cultural psychology* (pp. 199-213). Amsterdam: Swets and Zeitlinger.

MODELS OF CULTURAL ORIENTATION: DIFFERENCES BETWEEN AMERICAN-BORN AND OVERSEAS-BORN ASIANS

Burnam, M. A., Hough, R. L., Karno, M., Escobar, J. I., & Telles, C. A. (1987). Acculturation and lifetime prevalence of psychiatric disorders among Mexican Americans in Los Angeles. *Journal of Health & Social Behavior, 28* (1), 89-102.

Chentsova, Y. E. (1996). *International students: Identity and well-being in cross-cultural transitions.* Unpublished manuscript.

Constantinou, S. T., & Harvey, M. E. (1985). Dimensional structure and intergenerational differences in ethnicity: The Greek Americans. *Sociology and Social Research, 69* (2), 234-254.

Cuéllar, I., Nyberg, B., Maldonado, R. E., & Roberts, R. E. (1997). Ethnic identity and acculturation in a young adult Mexican-origin populations. *Journal of Community Psychology, 25* (6), 535-549.

Der-Karabetian, A., & Ruiz, Y. (1997). Affective bicultural and global-human identity scales for Mexican-American adolescents. *Psychological Reports, 80* (3), 1027-1039.

DeSipio, L. (1996). Making citizens or good citizens? Naturalization as a predictor of organizational and electoral behavior among Latino immigrants. *Hispanic Journal of Behavioral Sciences, 18* (2), 194-213.

Escobar, J. I. (1998). Immigration and mental health: Why are immigrants better off? *Archives of General Psychiatry, 55* (9), 781-782.

Furnham, A., & Bochner, S. (1986). *Culture shock: Psychological reactions to unfamiliar environments.* London: Methuen.

Ghuman, P. A. S. (1998). Ethnic identity and acculturation of South Asian adolescents: A British perspective. *International Journal of Adolescence and Youth, 7,* 227-247.

Gilbert, M. J. (1987). Alcohol consumption patterns in immigrant and later generation Mexican American women. *Hispanic Journal of Behavioral Sciences, 9* (3), 299-313.

Gordon, M. M. (1964). *Assimilation in American life.* New York: Oxford University Press.

Junn, J. (1999). Participation in liberal democracy: The political assimilation of immigrants and ethnic minorities in the United States. *American Behavioral Scientist, 42* (9), 1417-1438.

Karno, M., Golding, J. M., Burnam, M. A., Hough, R. L., Escobar, J. I., Wells, K. M., & Boyer, R. (1989). Anxiety disorders among Mexican Americans and non-Hispanic Whites in Los Angeles. *Journal of Nervous and Mental Disease, 177* (4), 202-209.

Keefe, S. E., & Padilla, A. M. (1987). *Chicano ethnicity.* Albuquerque: University of New Mexico Press.

Krishnan, A. & Berry, J. W. (1992). Acculturative stress and acculturation attitudes among Indian immigrants to the United States. *Psychology & Developing Societies, 4* (2), 187-212.

LaFromboise, T., Coleman, H. L. K., & Gerton, J. (1993). Psychological impact of biculturalism: Evidence and theory. *Psychological Bulletin, 114* (3), 395-412.

Lien, P. (1994). Ethnicity and political participation: A comparison between Asian and Mexican Americans. *Political Behavior, 16*(2), 237-264.

Manaster, G. J., Rhodes, C., Marcus, M. B., & Chan, J. C. (1998). The role of birth order in the acculturation of Japanese Americans. *Psychologia, 41,* 155-170.

Oetting, E. R., & Beauvais, F. (1991). Orthogonal cultural identification theory: The cultural identification of minority adolescents. *The International Journal of the Addictions, 25* (5A & 6A), 655-685.

Okazaki, S., & Sue, S. (1995). Cultural considerations in psychological assessment of Asian Americans. In J. Butcher (Ed.), *Clinical personality assessment: Practical approaches* (pp. 107-119). New York: Oxford University Press.

Olmedo, E. L., & Padilla, A. M. (1978). Empirical and construct validation of a measure of acculturation for Mexican Americans. *Journal of Social Psychology, 105,* 179-187.

Ownbey, S. F. & Horridge, P. E. (1998). The Suinn-Lew Asian Self-identity Acculturation Scale: Test with a Non-student, Asian-American sample. *Social Behavior & Personality, 26* (1), 1998, 57-68.

Park, R. E. (1928). Human migration and the marginal man. *The American Journal of Sociology, 33,* 881-893.

Phinney, J. S. (1990). Ethnic identity in adolescents and adults: Review of research. *Psychological Bulletin, 108,* 499-514.

Phinney, J. S., & Devich-Navarro, M. (1997). Variations in bicultural identification among African American and Mexican American adolescents, *Journal of Research on Adolescence, 7* (1), 3-32.

Ponterotto, J. G., Baluch, S., & Carielli, D. (1998). The Suinn-Lew Asian Self-Identity Acculturation Scale (SL-ASIA): Critique and research recommendations. *Measurement & Evaluation in Counseling & Development, 31* (2), 109-124.

Rosenthal, D. A. (1989). Psychological development of second-generation immigrant adolescents. In D. M. Keats, D. Munro, & L. Mann (Eds.), *Heterogeneity in cross-cultural psychology* (pp. 157-163). Amsterdam: Swets and Zeitlinger.

Sayegh, L., & Lasry, J. (1992). Immigrants' adaptation in Canada: Assimilation, acculturation, and orthogonal cultural identification. *Canadian Psychology, 34* (1), 98-109.

Sorenson, S. B., & Shen, H. (1996). Youth suicide trends in California: An examination of immigrant and ethnic group risk. *Suicide and Life-Threatening Behavior, 26*(2), 143-154.

Stonequist, E. V. (1964). The marginal man: A study in personality and culture conflict. In E. Burgess, & D. J. Bogue (Eds.), *Contributing to urban sociology* (pp. 115-127). Chicago: University of Chicago Press.

Suleiman, R., & Beit-Hallahmi, B. (1997). National and civic identities of Palestinians in Israel. *Journal of Social Psychology, 137*(2), 219-228.

Szapocznik, J., Kurtines, W. M., & Fernandez, T. (1980). Bicultural involvement and adjustment in Hispanic-American youths. *International Journal of Intercultural Relations, 4*, 353-365.

Tajfel, H. (1981). Human groups and social categories. Cambridge: Cambridge University Press.

Tsai, J. L. (2001). Cultural orientation of Hmong young adults. *Journal of Human Behavior and the Social Environment, 3-4*, 99-114.

Tsai, J. L., Wong, Y., Morstensen, H., & Hess, D. (in press). What does "being American" mean? Differences between Asian American and European American adults. *Cultural Diversity and Ethnic Minority Psychology*.

Tsai, J. L., Ying, Y., & Lee, P. A. (2000a). *Cultural orientation and self-esteem: Variation between American-born and immigrant Chinese.* Manuscript submitted for publication.

Tsai, J. L., Ying, Y., & Lee, P. A. (2000b). The meaning of "being Chinese" and "being American": Variation among Chinese American young adults. *Journal of Cross-Cultural Psychology, 31*(3), 302-322.

U.S. Bureau of the Census (1995). *Population profile of the United States.* Washington, D.C.: U.S. Government Printing Office.

U.S. Bureau of the Census (1999). *Statistical abstract of the United States.* Washington, D.C.: U.S. Government Printing Office.

Vega, W. A., Kolody. B., Hwang, J., Noble, A. & Porter, P. A. (1997). Perinatal drug use among immigrant and native-born Latinas. *Substance Use & Misuse, 32*(1), 43-62.

Vega, W. A., Kolody, B., Aguilar-Gaxiola, S., Alderete, E., & Catalano, R., & Caraveo-Anduaga, J. (1998). Lifetime prevalence of DSM-III-R psychiatric disorders among urban and rural Mexican Americans in California. *Archives of General Psychiatry, 55*, 771-778.

Wong-Rieger, D. & Quintana, D. (1987). Comparative acculturation of Southeast Asian and Hispanic immigrants and sojourners. *Journal of Cross-Cultural Psychology, 18*(3), 345-362.

Ying, Y. (1995). Cultural orientation and psychological well-being in Chinese Americans. *American Journal of Community Psychology, 23*(6), 893-911.

Ying, Y., Coombs, M., Lee, P. A. (1999). Family intergenerational relationship of Asian American adolescents. *Cultural Diversity & Ethnic Minority Psychology, 5* (4), 350-363.

Ying, Y., Lee, P. A., & Tsai, J. L. (2000). Cultural orientation and racial discrimination: Predictors of coherence in Chinese American young adults. *Journal of Community Psychology, 28*, 427-442.

Zak, I. (1973). Dimensions of Jewish-American identity. *Psychological Reports, 33*, 891-900.

SUMIE OKAZAKI

CHAPTER 8

CULTURAL VARIATIONS IN SELF-CONSTRUAL AS A MEDIATOR OF DISTRESS AND WELL-BEING

1. INTRODUCTION

Cultural models have yet to gain an equal footing with other psychological and biological models of normal and abnormal behavior (Miller, 1999). Ethnic minorities continue to be under-represented in behavioral psychology research (Iwamasa & Smith, 1996), and there exist a paucity of high quality research concerned with culture and ethnicity (Sue, 1999). These conditions remain despite a consensus in cross-cultural psychology that cultural factors are inextricably linked to the etiology, prevalence, symptom manifestations, and course and outcome of psychopathology (Marsella, 1985). One likely reason that cultural models of psychopathology have not garnered wider acceptance is that cross-cultural and ethnic research are often criticized as lacking grounding in sophisticated theoretical framework. In an effort to advance the field, Betancourt and López (Betancourt & López, 1993) challenged both mainstream and cross-cultural investigators to conduct hypothesis-driven research that identify and measure directly the aspect of a group variable (e.g., specific cultural element such as religiosity) that could predict specific behavior of interest (e.g., content of delusions). In this regard, the self has taken a center stage in the past decade in psychology as a key variable in explaining the influence of culture on human behavior. Theorists have offered various models of cultural variations in the self to explain differences in the clinical phenomenology across ethnic minority and cultural groups (e.g., Landrine, 1992; Markus & Kitayama, 1991; Marsella, 1985). This chapter discusses the usefulness of culturally-based self-construal variables in mental health research with Asian Americans, with an emphasis on the assessment issues involved in this line of research.

2. SELF AS THE LINK BETWEEN CULTURE AND DISTRESS

Anthropologists have long acknowledged that the view of the person as independent, self-contained, and autonomous is a perspective limited to Western cultures (Hollan, 1992). That there are cultural differences in the fundamental notions about selfhood, and that such differences would then be reflected in concepts of well-being and mental health, appear self-evident in retrospect. However, psychology and psychiatry have only recently begun to recognize that much

107

knowledge about human nature and mental health derived from American and Western European psychological tradition is not necessarily universal (Thakker, Ward, & Strongman, 1999). It is only within the past decade and a half that analyses of cultural variations in human functioning have placed the notion of the culturally-variant self at the crux of these formulations.

Marsella's paper in 1985 was one of the first to articulate the theoretical importance of the self as the critical link between cultural variables and symptom manifestations. In his paper, Marsella characterized the "unindividuated" self-structure of non-Western cultures, which arises from interdependencies in human relations and their consequent de-emphasis on individual autonomy and independence. This was contrasted with the "individuated" self-structure common in the West, where independence, autonomy, and separateness of individuals are valued. Marsella contended that such cultural variations in self-structure likely reflect a continuum of cultural variations in epistemology, from the more objective epistemic orientation of the West (with a preference for abstract language and lexical mediation of reality) to the more subjective epistemic orientation of the East (with its preference for metaphorical language and imagistic mediation of reality). Significantly, he asserted that "the self provides the bridge between culture and mental disorder, a bridge for understanding why disorders assume certain forms of expression and content" (Marsella, 1985, p. 299). According to this framework, these fundamental differences in the self-structure may explain why non-Western individuals are likely to experience depression primarily through somatic terms, as non-Western cultural self is not construed in existential and affective terms.

In the same vein, a recent integrative analysis of cross-cultural literature surrounding subjective well-being reiterated the argument that the self holds a key to understanding cultural differences in reported levels subjective well-being (Suh, 2000). Suh's analysis was motivated by the widely documented phenomenon of North Americans reporting being more happy and positive about the self on average than East Asians. Suh lays out the evidence that psychological constructs such as self-esteem and self-congruence, which have been viewed as essential characteristics of mental health in the West, appear less central to the mental health of East Asians. That is, self-esteem and identity consistently are less powerful predictors of mental health in collectivistic cultures than in individualistic cultures. Additionally, members of collectivistic cultures tend to base judgments of their life satisfaction on social norms as well as their own emotions, whereas members of individualistic cultures tend to judge their life satisfaction based primarily on their emotions (Suh, E. Diener, Oishi, & Triandis, 1998). Suh argues that because achievement of personal happiness is a less salient goal in East Asian cultures and because the self-appraisals of East Asians are based relatively more on external social standards (which are less flexible to be tailored in service to the self), these motivational and cognitive features of East Asian cultures restrict how positively individuals can view themselves. Conversely, because Western cultures highly regard the achievement of personal happiness as an individual right and an important goal, and because Western cultures foster self-judgment based on private standards that are flexibly geared toward confirming pre-existing beliefs about the self, Westerners are socialized to view themselves positively and to feel happy. Suh presents an

CULTURAL VARIATIONS IN SELF-CONSTRUAL AS A MEDIATOR OF DISTRESS AND WELL-BEING

intriguing argument for using self-processes to understand cultural differences in the levels of reported well-being.

Perhaps the most influential argument for the centrality of the self in cross-cultural analysis of human behavior has been offered by Markus and Kitayama (1991). Their seminal paper on independent and interdependent self-construal has received wide attention in psychology and energized the field of cross-cultural psychology as well as ethnic psychology. The authors distinguished between an independent construal of the self, a view held primarily by those in Western European and American cultures, and an interdependent construal of the self, a view held primarily by non-Western European (e.g., Asian, African, Latin-American, and southern European) cultures. The independent self-construal emphasizes individual as independent and autonomous, and internal aspects of the self (e.g., desires, preferences, attributes, or abilities) are considered to be the most significant factors regulating behavior and are assumed to be relatively stable and invariant. In contrast, those who hold interdependent self-construal recognize that their behavior is governed by what they perceive to be the thoughts, feelings, and actions of others in the relationship. To that end, relationships with other people are used to define the self, and people derive self-worth through their abilities to adjust themselves to the social climate, to restrain expressions of their selves, and to maintain harmony with others. Markus and Kitayama examined a number of documented cross-cultural differences in cognition, emotion, and motivation that are consistent with the differing cultural conceptions of the self.

The ideas put forth by Markus and Kitayama (1991) were similar to those offered by others (Landrine, 1992; Marsella, 1985; see also Matsumoto, 1999 for other related concepts). However, the notion of independent and interdependent self-construals has held an enormous appeal as a theoretical framework that has a potential to explain a wide array of cross-cultural psychological differences (e.g., Chao, 1995). Since its publication, Markus and Kitayama's paper has been cited in close to 800 publications to date and has spawned a number of attempts to empirically test the notion of culturally variant self-construal to explain observed cultural differences in psychological behavior.

3. QUESTIONNAIRE MEASURES OF SELF-CONSTRUAL

Although Markus and Kitayama's (1991) theory has enjoyed a wide conceptual influence on psychology and related disciplines, only a relatively small number of empirical studies have examined independent and interdependent self-construals as *a priori* explanatory variables. One methodological limitation contributing to the paucity of such studies is the lack of reliable measure to assess independent and interdependent self-construal. As detailed below, the majority of studies have operationalized the self-construal variables using a questionnaire format.

To date, at least five different questionnaires have been developed to assess independent and interdependent self-construal, as conceptualized by Markus and Kitayama (1991). Of these, only one scale (Singelis, 1994) has undergone extensive

110   SUMIE OKAZAKI

psychometric validation whereas the other scales remain unpublished. These measures of independent and interdependent self-construal have been used in a number of cross-cultural communication research as well as research in personality, social, and clinical psychology. The following is a brief review of the five scales and their use in empirical studies involving individuals from American and Asian cultural backgrounds.

3.1 Self-Construal Scale

Singelis (1994) constructed a 24-item Self-Construal Scale (SCS) to assess the strength of an individual's independent and interdependent self-construals. Notably, Singelis premised the development of his scale on the notion that individuals in any culture simultaneously hold both independent (or private) and interdependent (or collectivist) self-concepts but are emphasized and supported to different degrees in various ethnocultural groups. This was in contrast to most prior attempts to measure the related concept of individualism-collectivism as a single bipolar dimension. The resulting 24-item scale (12 for each factor) has been used by Singelis and his colleagues in cross-cultural studies of embarrassability (Sharkey & Singelis, 1995; Singelis, Bond, Sharkey, & Lai, 1999; Singelis & Sharkey, 1995), predictors of life satisfaction (Kwan, Bond, & Singelis, 1997), communication (Singelis & Brown, 1995), and biculturalism (Yamada & Singelis, 1999). The SCS has also been used in a study of Asian American-White American differences in reporting of depressive and social anxiety symptoms (Okazaki, 2000), a cross-cultural study of attitudes toward affirmative action (Ozawa, Crosby, & Crosby, 1996), a cross-cultural study of social phobia in the U.S. and Japan (Kleinknecht, Dinnel, Kleinknecht, Hiruma, & Harada 1997), and a cross-cultural study of self-esteem in the U.S. and Japan (Sato & Cameron, 1999).

Cronbach alpha reliabilities for the independent and interdependent subscales in the original psychometric studies with multiethnic undergraduates in Hawai'i ranged from .69~.70 and .73~.74, respectively (Singelis, 1994). In a sample of Asian American and White American college students (Okazaki, 2000), alpha coefficients ranged from .51 ~ .71 for the independent scale and from .57 ~ .66 for the interdependent scale. A recent study reported even lower reliability estimates (.58 ~ .66 for independence, .53 ~ .64 for interdependence) in samples of U.S. European American, Hawai'i Asian American, and Hong Kong Chinese college students (Singelis et al., 1999). Acknowledging the SCS scales' less than ideal internal reliability estimates, Singelis et al. (1999) noted that an updated version of the SCS has been developed. The new version has additional 6 items, with internal reliabilities in the mid .70's (Singelis, personal communication, February 19, 2000).

3.2 Takata's scale

Takata constructed a 40-item Japanese measure of independent and interdependent self-construal and used it in the studies of self-concept (Takata, 1993) and self-assessment behavior (Seike & Takata, 1997) among Japanese college

CULTURAL VARIATIONS IN SELF-CONSTRUAL AS A MEDIATOR OF DISTRESS AND WELL-BEING 111

students. Okazaki (1997) used an abbreviated (29 item) English translation of the Takata measure in a study of Asian American-White American differences on measures of depression and social anxiety. Asian American college students in Okazaki's sample endorsed higher interdependent self-construal and lower independent self-construal than their White American counterparts. Cronbach alpha reliabilities for the independent and interdependent scales were .86 and .68, respectively (Okazaki, 1997).

3.3 Independence/Interdependence Scale

Markus and a colleague (Kato & Markus, 1993) developed the Interdependence/Independence Scale (IIS), a 31-item measure consisting of four subscales, two that reflect interdependence (Concern with Others' Evaluation, Maintaining Self-Other Bonds) and two that reflect independence (Self-Other Differentiation and Self-Knowledge). An abbreviated (25-item) version of the IIS was used by Hetts, Sakuma, and Pelham (1999) in a recent study of cultural variations in the self-concept, with Cronbach alpha reliabilities for the independent and interdependent scales reported as .79 and .86, respectively.

3.4 Gudykunst et al.'s scale

Gudykunst and his colleagues (Gudykunst et al., 1996) combined items from various scales (including Singelis' SCS) as well as additional newly-written items to assess independent and interdependent self-construals in their research to test a mediational model of cultural effects on communication styles. The pool of 94 items was administered to college students from the U.S., Japan, Korea, and Australia. The results were submitted to a factor analysis with forced two-factor orthogonal solution, and the 29 items that loaded onto the factors were used to form the independent and interdependent self-construal scales. Cronbach's alpha coefficients for the 15-item independent scale were reported to range between .77 and .83, and between .80 and .85 for the 14-item interdependent scale. A modified version of this scale was also used in a series of cross-ethnic studies of decision-making and conflict styles in college students with reliability estimates of .76~79 and .72~.80 for independent and interdependent scales (Oetzel, 1998a, 1998b, 1998c, 1999).

3.5 Kim and Leung's scale

Kim and Leung developed a 29-item Revised Self-construal Scale, which combined items from other self-construal scales (Singelis, 1994; Gudykunst et al., 1996) and scales of related constructs used by (Cross, 1995; Kim, Sharkey, & Singelis, 1994) with some newly-written items. The scale (Kim & Leung, 1997), with reported reliability estimates of .87 for independence scale and .82 for interdependence scale, has been used primarily by Kim and her colleagues in

112   SUMIE OKAZAKI

intercultural communication research. In a recent study of depression and social anxiety among Asian American and White American college students (Okazaki, 1999), Cronbach's alpha coefficients for the independent scale ranged from .78 to .83 and from .74 to .76 for the interdependent scale.

In sum, researchers who wish to assess independent and interdependent self-construal may choose from a small selection of questionnaires that have been developed to date. The next section reviews the empirical studies positing self-construals as mediator of cultural differences in psychological well-being between Asians or Asian Americans and White Americans.

4. SELF-CONSTRUAL AND DISTRESS AND WELL-BEING INDICES

Several studies have examined the relationship between self-construal and some indices of distress or well-being across ethno-cultural groups. In two studies, Okazaki (1997, 2000) examined the relationship between independent and interdependent self-construals and symptoms of depression and social anxiety. In a large survey of White and Asian American college students (Okazaki, 1997), self-construals were assessed using the translated version of the Takata scale (1993). In this sample, independent self-construal was found to be negatively correlated with a measure of depression ($r = -.27$) and with two measures of social anxiety ($r = -.37$ and -.48). Interdependent self-construal was found to be positively correlated with a measure of depression ($r = .20$) and with two measures of social anxiety ($r = .24$ and .53). The levels of self-construal were found to explain additional variance in the levels of social anxiety beyond those explained by ethnicity and by covariance between the measures of social anxiety and depression. Specifically, those who were more concerned with asserting one's own judgment and emphasizing autonomy from others (i.e., individuals with higher independent self-construal) were less likely to be socially avoidant, distressed in social situations, and fearful of social evaluations. In another study with White and Asian American students (Okazaki, 2000), self-construals were assessed using the Self-Construal Scale (Singelis, 1994). Although the levels of interdependent self-construal were not significantly associated with the measures of depression and social anxiety in this sample, independent self-construal was negatively correlated with a depression measure ($r = -.27$) as well as a social anxiety measure ($r = -.55$). Thus both studies conducted by Okazaki found that levels of self-construals appear to be closely related to levels of mental health symptoms reported by college students.

Singelis, Bond, and their colleagues (Kwan et al., 1997; Singelis et al., 1999) have conducted a series of cross-cultural investigations examining the relation between independent and interdependent self-construals (as assessed by SCS, Singelis, 1994) and indices of well-being, such as self-esteem, life satisfaction, and embarrassability. In a study comparing these indices across three ethno-cultural groups (European American, Asian American in Hawai'i, and Hong Kong Chinese), Singelis et al. found the expected differences across the groups on levels of independence and interdependence. However, contrary to their expectations, the correlation between self-construal and self-esteem measures did not vary across the

CULTURAL VARIATIONS IN SELF-CONSTRUAL AS A MEDIATOR OF DISTRESS AND WELL-BEING

three groups. That is, within each ethno-cultural group, a more independent and less interdependent self-construal was associated with higher levels of self-esteem. In another study, Kwan et al. found that self-construals were significantly related to life satisfaction ratings in both U.S. and Hong Kong students. More specifically, the researchers found that the effect of the independent self-construal on life satisfaction was mediated through self-esteem, whereas the effect of the interdependent self-construal was mediated through "relationship harmony," or the degree to which individuals reported harmony across five most important dyadic relationships in their lives. Of note, Kwan et al. also found no cultural differences in this study in these mediating processes of self-construal in predicting life satisfaction. Thus the relationship between self-construal measures and indices of well-being (e.g., self-esteem and life satisfaction) appear to hold across cultures.

In a similar vein, Sato and Cameron (1999) examined the relationship between self-construal (also assessed by SCS, Singelis, 1994) and collective self-esteem (i.e., the positivity of one's generalized group-based identity) in Japanese and Canadian students. This study found that Canadians scored higher than Japanese on interdependent self-construal as well as on positive collective self-esteem, and the groups did not differ in the level of independent self-construal. Nonetheless, the researchers found that the pattern of relationships among self-construal and collective self-esteem variables were similar in the two cultural groups.

Kleinknecht et al. (1997) compared two forms of culturally-defined social anxiety (DSM-IV social phobia vs. a Japanese variant) in Japanese and U.S. students in relation to self-construal (assessed by SCS, Singelis, 1994). In both cultural groups, independent self-construal was negatively correlated with all measures of social anxiety. Interdependent self-construal was positively correlated with social anxiety only in the U.S. sample but not in the Japanese sample. In a slightly different use of self-construal as a mediator variable, Brockner and Y. Chen (1996) tested the cross-cultural validity of a finding that people with high self-esteem are more self-protective than people with low self-esteem (Crocker, Thompson, McGraw, & Ingerman, 1987). The researchers found that the positive relationship between trait self-esteem and self-protection in response to negative feedback typically found in the U.S. was not generally found among their Chinese research participants in mainland China except for those Chinese individuals who were high in independent self-construal (as assessed by Triandis et al.'s (1986) measure of individualism and collectivism).

In sum, findings from the various cross-cultural and cross-ethnic studies of self-construals and psychological adjustment (e.g., self-esteem, social anxiety) appear to converge. Most studies have found a positive relationship between independent self-construal and well-being and a negative relationship between interdependent self-construal and well-being. That is, regardless of one's ethno-cultural background, those who hold more independent self-construal tend to report being less depressed, less socially anxious, think more highly of themselves, and protect their self-concepts against threats. Conversely, those who hold more interdependent self-construal tend to appear more depressed, more socially anxious, and have lower self-esteem.

5. CRITIQUE OF SELF-CONSTRUAL RESEARCH

The foregoing review suggests that higher independence was consistently associated with indices of well-being whereas higher interdependence was associated with indices of poor well-being. Moreover, Asian Americans tend to score as more interdependent and less independent than White Americans, although cross-national comparisons between Japan and North America have failed to show that Japanese are more interdependent and that North Americans are more independent. These findings raise some important questions regarding the nature as well as the measurement of these constructs.

Specifically, the patterns of associations between the two forms of self-construal and indices of well-being warrant further scrutiny. In Markus and Kitayama's (1991) paper, independent self-construal and interdependent self-construal were conceptualized as normative models of the self that vary across cultures. Consequently, we would not expect that individuals from a collectivistic culture holding an interdependent self-construal would be any more maladjusted on average than individuals from an individualistic culture holding an independent self-construal. Then why is it that highly interdependent individuals appear to be more depressed, more socially anxious, and have lower self-esteem (i.e., high on negative affect)? Is there something about interdependent self-construal that promotes a general tendency toward negative affect?

Recent evidence suggests that people from different cultures vary in the predictors of general positive and negative affect. For example, E. Diener and M. Diener (1995) found that self-esteem is strongly related to subjective well-being in individualistic cultures but only modestly so in collectivistic cultures. Heine and Lehman (1999) showed that the magnitude of actual-ideal self-discrepancy was larger for Japanese than it was for both Asian Canadian and White Canadian subjects. The researchers interpreted this finding as consistent with the notion that Japanese are more likely to focus on their shortcomings in order to fit in better with their in-groups and thus rate themselves as further away from their personal goals. However, Heine and Lehman also found that actual-ideal discrepancies were not as strongly related to depression for Japanese as they were for White Canadians. They argued that because Japanese culture may view self-critical stance as a normative behavior, viewing oneself as inadequate may not have as much negative psychological consequence as it would in a Western culture that emphasizes attaining one's own goals and ideals. And most recently, Kitayama, Markus, and Kurokawa (2000) reported that correlates of general good feelings (e.g., calm, elated) were different across cultural groups; general good feelings felt by Japanese subjects were most closely related to interpersonally engaged positive emotions (e.g., close, friendly feeling), whereas general good feelings felt by American subjects were most closely related to interpersonally disengaged positive emotions (e.g., proud, feel good about the self).

As revealing as these findings regarding cross-cultural differences in emotion and self processes, they do not directly answer the previous question about the relationship between independent or interdependent self-construal and positive or negative affect. Although Kitayama et al. (2000) stated that their intent was to test

CULTURAL VARIATIONS IN SELF-CONSTRUAL AS A MEDIATOR OF DISTRESS AND WELL-BEING

the hypothesis that "good feelings" are associated with interdependence in Japan and independence in the U.S., they did not directly assess independent or interdependent self-construals in their subjects. Thus all we know at this point is that the Japanese (and sometimes other East Asians or Asian Americans) tend to report more general negative affect (e.g., more depression, more social anxiety, lower self-esteem, lower subjective well-being) compared to North Americans, but that negative affectivity may have culturally variant meanings. However, we do not know whether the cultural variation in independent and interdependent self-construals is the critical variable operating in these instances.

Further, to fully examine the utility of the self-construal variables for assessing and understanding the psychological well-being of Asian Americans, we must examine carefully the potential problems that exist in the conceptualizations and measurements of self-construal and indicators of distress and well-being. The final section of this chapter re-evaluates Markus and Kitayama's (1991) model of independent and interdependent self-construal, points to some unresolved problems in the assessment of self-construal, and offer some future directions.

5.1 Criticism of the self-construal model

Although Markus and Kitayama's (1991) paper has made an extraordinary impact in the cross-cultural and Asian American personality and mental health research, it has not been without its critics. Notably, Matsumoto (1999) questioned the evidentiary bases for their models of self-construal. He first outlined the following assumptions underlying their model: 1) cultures being compared (e.g., Japan and U.S.) must differ in level of individualism-collectivism, which is presumably the underlying cultural characteristic that differentially fosters independent or interdependent self-construal, 2) individuals from those cultures must hold differing self-construals, 3) collectivism must correspond to interdependent self-construal in a culture and individualism must correspond to independent self-construal in the contrasted culture, and 4) cultural differences in behavior (e.g., communication style) must be explained by the cultural differences in self-construal. Matsumoto argued that these assumptions have not been tested directly by Markus, Kitayama, and their colleagues. Further, most cross-cultural studies conducted by Markus and Kitayama's team or the studies used to support the model have only demonstrated that cross-national differences exist on the psychological variables of interest. Finally, Matsumoto reviewed 18 cross-national studies involving the U.S. and Japan that directly measured individualism-collectivism and found that 17 of them provided little or no support for the contention that Americans are individualistic and Japanese collectivistic. In fact, a significant number of studies found that the Japanese tended to be more individualistic and less collectivistic than Americans. Matsumoto also reviewed studies that directly compared independent and interdependent self-construal between individuals from U.S. and East Asian countries (e.g., Gudykunst et al., 1996; Kleinknecht et al., 1997; Kim et al., 1996) that failed to find predicted patterns

116   SUMIE OKAZAKI

of cross-cultural differences in the levels of self-construal. Matsumoto used these findings to question the basic assumptions underlying Markus and Kityama's model.

5.2 Unresolved problems in assessing self-construal

It is possible that model of cultural variations in the self, as conceptualized by Markus and Kitayama (1991), is flawed in ways that Matsumoto (1999) criticized. However, it is important to keep in mind that what Markus & Kitayama proposed were conceptual models regarding the **structure** of the self. In contrast, the prevailing approaches to assessing self-construals share a methodological commonality in the questionnaire format. Although various methodological approaches have been offered to examine the structural aspects of the self (Markus, 1990; Ogilvie & Ashmore, 1991), none have been attempted in the assessment of independent and interdependent self-construal. Consequently, the questionnaire items tend to assess the presumed affective, cognitive, and behavioral consequences of holding each form of self-construal, rather than the structural aspects of the self-construals. For example, an item for interdependent subscale of the SCS, "I will sacrifice my self-interest for the benefit of the group I am in" (Singelis, 1994), is a logically derived behavioral and attitudinal consequence of holding an interdependent self-construal. The questionnaire methods do not involve a direct measurement of the permeability of the boundary between self and others.

An advantage, of course, to the questionnaire approach to assessing self-construals is the relative ease of data collection and analyses. However, as reviewed above, two main problems have emerged: (1) the various questionnaires of independent and interdependent self-construals have suffered from low internal consistency, and (2) there are close associations between measures of self-construal and well-being or distress. With regard to the poor internal reliability estimates, Singelis (T. M. Singelis, personal communication, February 19, 2000) as well as Kim (personal communication, December 16, 1998) have revised the original SCS (Singelis, 1994) to improve on its reliability estimates. The second problem regarding the correlation between interdependent self-construal and indices of general negative affect and the correlation between independent self-construal and general positive affect is one that was initially detected by Okazaki (1997) in using the English translation of a Japanese scale of self-construal (Takata, 1993). Okazaki had found that some of the items that loaded onto the interdependent self factor (e.g., "I am often sensitive to how others see me because they may be evaluating me") resembled items for assessing social anxiety. Although other self-construal scales (e.g., Kim & Leung, 1997; Singelis, 1994) do not contain such obvious overlaps in item face content with scales of psychopathology, the scales of interdependent self contain multiple items with negative content (e.g., "If my brother or sister *fails*, I feel responsible," "I feel *uncomfortable disagreeing* with my group") whereas the scales of independent self-construal have no item with clear negative content. It is thus possible that the items for the interdependent self scale are more biased toward the negative content than the items assessing independent self scale. Such bias in the affective valence of the two scales may have resulted from the researchers' attempts

CULTURAL VARIATIONS IN SELF-CONSTRUAL AS A MEDIATOR OF DISTRESS AND WELL-BEING

to improve internal reliability, as items worded with similar affective content tend to cohere together. Further efforts are necessary to examine whether it is possible to construct scales to assess independent and interdependent self-construals that are orthogonal to positive and negative affectivity.

5.3 Implicit measurement of the self

Many of the problems discussed above are not unique to the assessment of self-construal but are inherent problems in constructing reliable and valid questionnaires. A viable alternative to self-report is to assess self-construal implicitly. In discussing the extent to which automatic processes involved in human perception, cognition, affect, and behavior may be enculturated, Cohen (1997) argued that research methods that examine automatic, preconscious processes hold promise in bypassing the problems of verbal reports. Cohen (1997) noted that people may not be able to introspect accurately, and even if they could, there are likely to be distortions in reporting their subjective experience. As noted by Brislin (1993), elements of a culture are often unarticulated among its members. Cohen argues that cultural patterns may be so overlearned as to bypass conscious processing. Further, verbal reports may not only be the weakest indicator of cultural differences, verbal reports sometimes show cultural differences in the "wrong" direction (Peng, Nisbett, & Wong, 1997). For many reasons, then, it makes sense to expand the methodological repertoire for assessing various cultural elements beyond the questionnaire format.

Recently, Pelham and Hetts (1999) made a case for distinguishing between explicit and implicit self-evaluation in cross-cultural studies of the self and self-related processes. They contend that the traditional measurement approach to self-evaluation such as the questionnaires only assess explicit, consciously-considered evaluations of selves that are responsive to the normative demands of the respondents' current cultural contexts. Thus a reason why some researchers fail to find ethnic differences between Asian Americans and White Americans on explicit measures of the self may be because their responses are largely reflections of normative cultural demands placed by the cultural context in which all respondents reside (in this case, middle-class American culture). In contrast, implicit or indirect measurement of self-concept, such as response latency to identity-relevant primes, are thought to be relatively immune to self-presentational concerns. Further, implicit self-concept may be slower to change in response to cultural context, presumably because nonconscious beliefs are assumed to reflect the long-term influence of the respondents' cultural upbringing.

Hetts and colleagues conducted a series of studies in which implicit and explicit self-concepts of people who differed in their degree of exposure to an individualistic culture were assessed (Hetts et al., 1999; Pelham & Hetts, 1999). Two of their studies involved comparing recently immigrated Asian Americans, U.S.-born Asian Americans, and U.S.-born White Americans all currently residing in the U.S., and one study compared Japanese students currently living in Japan who either had or had not lived in North America. Two of the studies used response latency to a word

118 SUMIE OKAZAKI

identification task (good or bad) following collectivistic and individualistic primes (me vs. us) as an index of implicit self-regard, and another study used a word-fragment completion task with positive and negative words following collectivistic and individualistic primes to assess implicit self-regard. The studies showed that subjects tended to endorse explicit self-evaluations that were consistent with their current cultural context, but that implicit self-evaluations mirrored prior cultural socialization. Specifically, on an explicit measure of independent and interdependent self (IIS, Kato & Markus, 1993), recently immigrated Asian Americans appeared to endorse the kind of favorable conceptions of the self promoted by individualistic cultures. However, on implicit measures, the same recently immigrated Asian Americans tended to show relatively higher positive group regard and relatively lower individual self-regard compared to American-born Asian Americans and White Americans. These findings point to a pattern of dissociation between implicit and explicit self-construals of Asian Americans, especially the recent immigrants who are in the midst of learning to adapt to a new individualistic cultural setting. Implicit self-regard, or the evaluation of the individualistic or group-based self-concept, appear slower to acculturate than explicit self-construals.

Finally, a recent study that implicitly primed independent and interdependent self-construals have produced intriguing results. Gardner, Gabriel, and Lee (1999) used a word search task (subject searches for independent pronouns such as "I" or "mine" in a text passage) or a story task (subject reads a story with an independent or interdependent theme) to prime the self-construals among European American and Hong Kong Chinese subjects. In this study, the number of independent or interdependent self-descriptors generated in response to an open-ended Twenty Statements Test (TST; Kuhn & McPartland, 1954) was used as indices of independent or interdependent self-construal. Gardner et al. demonstrated that priming of self-construal influenced the extent to which subjects endorsed individualistic and collectivistic values, and that this effect was mediated by self-construals (as measured by the TST).

The social cognition research tradition, in which studies by Hetts and colleagues (Hetts et al., 1999; Pelham & Hetts, 1999) and Gardner et al. (1999) were conducted, represents a promising avenue for exploring the nature of self-construals held by bicultural individuals such as Asian Americans. Importantly, they offer an alternative approach to the measurement of the enculturated self that are worthy of further development.

6. CONCLUSION

We are far from knowing exactly how cultural variations in self-construal influence the experience and manifestation of well-being and distress. To advance our knowledge, better assessments of both the self-construal and distress among Asian Americans are needed. Specifically, we need further research to improve the tools for assessing self-construals. In addition, it is important to examine whether we are accurately assessing distress and well-being among Asian Americans and to enhance our understanding of the essentially cultural nature of widely-accepted

CULTURAL VARIATIONS IN SELF-CONSTRUAL AS A MEDIATOR OF DISTRESS AND WELL-BEING

psychological constructs such as self-esteem and negative affect. And finally, we must continue to investigate whether a construct derived from cross-cultural contrasts, such as the independent and interdependent self-construals, is a culturally valid conceptual tool for understanding the psychological functioning of Asian Americans.

7. REFERENCES

Betancourt, H., & López, S. R. (1993). The study of culture, ethnicity, and race in American psychology. *American Psychologist, 48*(6), 629-637.

Brislin, R. (1993). *Understanding culture's influence on behavior*. New York: Harcourt, Brace Jovanovich College Publishers.

Brockner, J., & Chen, Y. (1996). The moderating roles of self-esteem and self-construal in reaction to a threat to the self: Evidence from the People's Republic of China and the United States. *Journal of Personality & Social Psychology, 71*(3), 603-615.

Chao, R. K. (1995). Chinese and European American cultural models of the self reflected in mothers-childrearing beliefs. *Ethos, 23*(3), 328-354.

Cohen, D. (1997). Ifs and thens in cultural psychology. In R. S. J. Wyer (Ed.), *The automaticity of everyday life: Advances in social cognition, Vol. 10* (pp. 121-131). Mahwah, NJ: Lawrence Erlbaum Associates

Crocker, J., Thompson, L. L., McGraw, K. M., & Ingerman, C. (1987). Downward comparison, prejudice, and evaluations of others: Effects of self-esteem and threat. *Journal of Personality & Social Psychology, 52*(5), 1907-1916.

Cross, S. E. (1995). Self-construals, coping, and stress in cross-cultural adaptation. *Journal of Cross-Cultural Psychology, 26*(6), 673-697.

Diener, E., & Diener, M. (1995). Cross-cultural correlates of life satisfaction and self-esteem. *Journal of Personality & Social Psychology, 68*(4), 653-663.

Gardner, W. L., Gabriel, S., & Lee, A. Y. (1999). "I" value freedom, but "we" value relationships: Self-construal priming mirrors cultural differences in judgment. *Psychological Science, 10*, 321-326.

Gudykunst, W. B., Matsumoto, Y., Ting-Toomey, S., Nishida, T., Kim, K., & Heyman, S. (1996). The influence of cultural individualism-collectivism, self construals, and individual values on communication styles across cultures. *Human Communication Research, 22*(4), 510-543.

Heine, S. J., & Lehman, D. R. (1999). Culture, self-discrepancies, and self-satisfaction. *Personality and Social Psychology Bulletin, 25*, 915-925.

Hetts, J. J., Sakuma, M., & Pelham, B. W. (1999). Two roads to positive regard: Implicit and explicit self-evaluation and culture. *Journal of Experimental Social Psychology, 35*, 512-559.

Hollan, D (1992). Cross-cultural differences in the self. *Journal of Anthropological Research, 48*, 283-300.

Iwamasa, G. Y., & Smith, S. K. (1996). Ethnic diversity in behavioral psychology: A review of the literature. *Behavior Modification, 20*(1), 45-59.

Kato, K., & Markus, H. R. (1993). *Development of the Interdependence/Independence Scale: Using American and Japanese samples*. Paper presented at the 5th annual convention of the American Psychological Society, Washington, DC.

Kim, M. S., Hunter, J. E., Miyahara, A., & Horvath, A. M. (1996). Individual- vs. -level dimensions of individualism and collectivism: Effects on preferred conversational styles. *Communication Monographs, 63*(1), 1928-1949.

Kim, M. S., & Leung, T. (1997). *A Revised Self-Construal Scale*. Unpublished scale, University of Hawai'i at Manoa.

Kim, M. S., Sharkey, W. F., & Singelis, T. M. (1994). The relationship between individuals' self-construals and perceived importance of interactive constraints. *International Journal of Intercultural Relations, 18*(1), 117-140.

Kitayama, S., Markus, H. R., & Kurokawa, M. (2000). Culture, emotion, and well-being: Good feelings in Japan and the United States. *Cognition and Emotion, 14*, 93-124.

120 SUMIE OKAZAKI

Kleinknecht, R. A., Dinnel, D. L., Kleinknecht, E. E., Hiruma, N., & Harada, N. (1997). Cultural factors in social anxiety: A comparison of social phobia symptoms and Taijin Kyofusho. *Journal of Anxiety Disorders, 11*(2), 157-177.

Kuhn, M. H., & McPartland, T. (1954). An empirical investigation of self-attitudes. *American Sociological Review, 19,* 69-76.

Kwan, V. S. Y., Bond, M. H., & Singelis, T. M. (1997). Pancultural explanations for life satisfaction: Adding relationship harmony to self-esteem. *Journal of Personality & Social Psychology, 73*(5), 1038-1051.

Landrine, H. (1992). Clinical implications of cultural differences: The referential versus the indexical self. *Clinical Psychology Review, 12*(4), 401-415.

Markus, H. (1990). Unresolved issues of self-representation. *Cognitive Therapy & Research, 14*(2), 241-253.

Markus, H. R., & Kitayama, S. (1991). Culture and the self: Implications for cognition, emotion, and motivation. *Psychological Review, 98*(2), 224-253.

Marsella, A. J. (1985). Culture, self, and mental disorder. In A. J. Marsella, G. DeVos, & F. L. K. Hsu (Eds.), *Culture and self: Asian and Western perspectives* (pp. 281-307). New York: Tavistock Publications.

Matsumoto, D. (1999). Culture and self: An empirical assessment of Markus and Kitayama's theory of independent and interdependent self-construals. *Asian Journal of Social Psychology, 2*(3), 289-310.

Miller, J. G. (1999). Cultural psychology: Implications for basic psychological theory. *Psychological Science, 10*(2), 85-91.

Oetzel, J. G. (1998a). Culturally homogeneous and heterogeneous groups: Explaining communication processes through individualism-collectivism and self-construal. *International Journal of Intercultural Relations, 22*(2), 135-161.

Oetzel, J. G. (1998b). The effects of self-construals and ethnicity on self-reported conflict styles. *Communication Reports, 11*(2),133-144.

Oetzel, J. G. (1998c). Explaining individual communication processes in homogeneous and heterogeneous groups through individualism-collectivism and self-construal. *Human Communication Research, 25*(2), 202-224.

Oetzel, J. G. (1999). The influence of situational features on perceived conflict styles and self-construals in work groups. *International Journal of Intercultural Relations, 23*(4), 679-695.

Ogilvie, D. M., & Ashmore, R. D. (1991). Self-with-other representation as a unit of analysis in self-concept research. In R. C. Curtis (Ed.), *The relational self: Theoretical convergence in psychoanalysis and social psychology.* New York: Guilford.

Okazaki, S. (1997). Sources of ethnic differences between Asian American and White American college students on measures of depression and social anxiety. *Journal of Abnormal Psychology, 106*(1), 52-60.

Okazaki, S. (1999). [Independent and interdependent self-construals in Asian American and White American university students.] Unpublished raw data.

Okazaki, S. (2000). Asian American-White American differences on affective distress symptoms: Do symptom reports differ across reporting methods? *Journal of Cross-Cultural Psychology, 31*(5), 603-625.

Ozawa, K., Crosby, M., & Crosby, F. (1996). Individualism and resistance to affirmative action: A comparison of Japanese and American samples. *Journal of Applied Social Psychology, 26*(13), Jul 1996, 1138-1152.

Pelham, B. W., & Hetts, J. J. (1999). Implicit and explicit personal and social identity: Toward a more complete understanding of the social self. In T. R. Tyler, R. M. Kramer, & O. P. John (Eds.), *The psychology of the social self: Applied social research* (pp. 115-143). Mahwah, NJ: Lawrence Erlbaum Associates.

Peng, K., Nisbett, R. E., & Wong, N. Y. C. (1997). Validity problems comparing values across cultures and possible solutions. *Psychological Methods, 2*(4), 329-344.

Sato, T., & Cameron, J. E. (1999). The relationship between collective self-esteem and self-construal in Japan and Canada. *Journal of Social Psychology, 139*(4), 426-435.

Seike, M., & Takata, T. (1997). Cultural views of self and self-assessment behavior: Empirical findings in Japanese culture. *Japanese Journal of Social Psychology, 13*(1), Sep 1997, 23-32.

Sharkey, W. F., & Singelis, T. M. (1995). Embarrassability and self-construal: A theoretical integration. *Personality & Individual Differences, 19*(6), Dec 1995, 919-926.

CULTURAL VARIATIONS IN SELF-CONSTRUAL AS A MEDIATOR OF DISTRESS AND WELL-BEING

Singelis, T. M. (1994). The measurement of independent and interdependent self-construals. *Personality & Social Psychology Bulletin, 20*(5), 580-591.

Singelis, T. M., Bond, M. H., Sharkey, W. F., & Lai, C. S. Y. (1999). Unpackaging culture's influence on self-esteem and embarrassability: The role of self-construals. *Journal of Cross-Cultural Psychology, 30*(3), 315-341.

Singelis, T. M., & Brown, W. J. (1995). Culture, self, and collectivist communication: Linking culture to individual behavior. *Human Communication Research, 21*(3), 354-389.

Singelis, T. M., & Sharkey, W. F. (1995). Culture, self-construal, and embarrassability. *Journal of Cross-Cultural Psychology, 26*(6), 622-644.

Sue, S. (1999). Science, ethnicity, and bias: Where have we gone wrong? *American Psychologist, 54*, 1070-1077.

Suh, E. M. (2000). Self, the hyphen between culture and subjective well-being. In E. Diener & E. M. Suh (Eds.), *Subjective well-being across cultures* (pp. 63-86). Cambridge, MA: MIT Press.

Suh, E., Diener, E., Oishi, S., & Triandis, H. C. (1998). The shifting basis of life satisfaction judgments across cultures: Emotions versus norms. *Journal of Personality & Social Psychology, 74*(2), 482-493.

Takata, T. (1993). Social comparison and formation of self-concept in adolescent: Some findings about Japanese college students. *Japanese Journal of Educational Psychology, 41*(3), 339-348.

Thakker, J., Ward, T., & Strongman, K. T. (1999). Mental disorder and cross-cultural psychology: A constructivist perspective. *Clinical Psychology Review, 19*(7), 843-874.

Triandis, H. C., Bontempo, R., Betancourt, H., Bond, M., et al. (1986). The measurement of the etic aspects of individualism and collectivism across cultures. *Australian Journal of Psychology, 38*(3), 1257-1267.

Yamada, A. M., & Singelis, T. M. (1999). Biculturalism and self-construal. *International Journal of Intercultural Relations, 23*(5), 697-709.

NOLAN ZANE AND MAY YEH

CHAPTER 9

THE USE OF CULTURALLY-BASED VARIABLES IN ASSESSMENT: STUDIES ON LOSS OF FACE

1. INTRODUCTION

Invariably, clinicians find themselves in the predicament of prescribing what constitutes appropriate assessment for Asian American clients. On the one hand, many culturally sensitive and culturally competent clinicians think and go about doing assessment in certain ways to account for and incorporate the cultural background and experiences of Asian American clients into the diagnostic, case conceptualization, and treatment planning processes. Sometimes certain procedural and stylistic changes are indicated while at other times completely different assessment strategies and approaches are necessary to achieve effective outcomes. We also know with a fair degree of confidence that such changes in the traditional Western therapy regimen have an ameliorative effect, which result in clinically significant improvements in treatment efficacy. On the other hand, when asked to describe the manner by which these clinicians come to select a particular strategy or to implement a certain procedure, we frequently experience difficulty in articulating this process. This difficulty cannot be solely attributed to language problems. American-born, primarily English-speaking Asian American therapists also may find it difficult to explain the process by which they account for and use cultural information to enhance interventions. Rather, the problem results more from the use of a Western-based "therapeutic language" that prevents us from expressing the cultural dynamics involved in a particular case.

2. ORIGINS OF CULTURAL BIAS IN ASSESSMENT AND PSYCHOTHERAPY

It is proposed that a major source of cultural bias in psychotherapy centers on the lack of adequate descriptive and explanatory concepts that can be used to construct a meaningful and valid assessment of an Asian American client's bicultural experiences. In order to formulate effective treatment strategies, therapists must first conceptualize how clients experience and respond to their interpersonal environment. Common conceptual schemata for capturing such experiences have been referred to as worldviews, personal constructs, interpersonal dynamics (e.g. transference, countertransference), coping styles (e.g. sensitization versus repression), perceptual sets (e.g. field dependence/independence), and problem-solving strategies. In essence, these various approaches are diverse attempts to describe the salient cognitive, affective, and behavioral aspects of a client's psychological functioning that are operative in his or her efforts to effectively negotiate the interpersonal environment. Case conceptualization (not synonymous with diagnosis) uses certain of these schemata to reconstruct what and how clients are experiencing their problems within the context of their particular cultural milieu. Adequate case conceptualization enhances the formulation of appropriate treatment strategies and goals. In this context, appropriateness refers to the extent to which such interventions are culturally syntonic with client needs, values, and coping styles. Indeed, it can be argued that adequate case conceptualization in part reflects the degree to which the therapist can empathize with the client that, in turn, subsequently affects the development of rapport in therapy.

It is in the process of case conceptualization that cultural information can have its most significant impact. The crucial task is to utilize various constructs that do not violate the phenomenological validity of the client's experience. Previous work on cultural bias in mental health practice tends to focus on such issues as misdiagnosis, over-diagnosis, over-pathologization, over-medication, and the use of treatment approaches that are unfamiliar to Asian American clients. Many of these problems result from inadequate case conceptualization. Cultural bias in psychotherapy may develop less out of therapist neglect or prejudice but out of the use of conceptual frameworks that fail to comprehensively account for the bicultural experiences of the Asian American individual. From a bicultural perspective the descriptive and explanatory constructs proffered by the various schools of Western psychotherapy comprise a valid but incomplete set of conceptual tools for assessment. What is needed are alternative ways of viewing and interpreting human behavior from different cultural vantage points. Such conceptual tools can supplement, complement, and at times completely supplant more Western-based constructs frequently used for such tasks. The purpose of this chapter is to examine one such construct, loss of face, which possesses the potential to lend descriptive and explanatory breadth for understanding the clinical experiences of Asian American individuals. One study investigating the loss of face construct is presented followed by a discussion of how the application of this construct can facilitate effective assessment and treatment with Asian American clients.

3. AN ALTERNATIVE CONCEPTUAL TOOL: LOSS OF FACE

The development of assessment and treatment approaches that are more culturally-responsive to the mental health needs and issues of ethnic minority clients has been a challenging and, at times, frustrating undertaking. Problems in conducting culturally-sensitive assessments have been attributed to methodological difficulties such as the conceptual non-equivalence of measures (Brislin, Lonner, & Thorndike, 1973), culturally-specific response sets (Kleinman, 1977), cultural differences in handling contextualized versus non-contextualized information (Lynch & Hanson, 1992), clinician bias (López, 1989), and distortions that occur when clients describe problems using English as their second language (Marcos, Urcuyo, Kesselman, & Alpert, 1973). However, in addition to methodological limitations, there are serious conceptual difficulties that constrain the valid and comprehensive assessment of human behavior as framed from different cultural contexts.

One major conceptual lacuna involves the lack of constructs that characterize and explain certain types of interpersonal dynamics that may be more salient in one culture than in another. In other words, cultures differ in the extent to which certain types of interpersonal dynamics can predict and account for variation in interpersonal relationships.

Tracking and assessment of the attitudes and orientations that people have in and toward their relationships are critical for several reasons. First, relational issues tend to be at the core of many problems that clients present in psychotherapy, and much of the time spent in therapy focuses on how clients can better manage and cope with their interpersonal problems (Horowitz, 1979). Second, change in therapy is primarily mediated through the client-therapist relationship so that it is important to examine certain interpersonal constructs that may be relatively more culturally-salient for different ethnic groups. Such variables may directly affect the relationship between client and therapist or what clinical researchers have called the working alliance between the client and the therapist. Finally, the assessment of a specific psychological dimension such as a particular interpersonal orientation provides for stronger explanatory models by allowing clinicians and researchers to determine *what it is specifically about culture* that accounts for a certain behavior or clinical problem. The deconstruction of culture into specific psychological elements enhances assessment efforts by providing more testable hypotheses (in terms of specific constructs) concerning the influence of culture on the client's behavior, symptoms, and/or psychosocial functioning (Betancourt & López, 1993).

Ho (1976) has noted that East Asian cultures, given their collectivist emphasis, are rich in relational constructs such as *on, amae,* filial piety, and "face." Moreover, the lack of emphasis on relational constructs in Western psychology has hindered our understanding of the role of culture in psychotherapy—given its interpersonal nature. One such construct that is definitely more salient in East Asian cultures is face. Face has been identified as a key and often-dominant interpersonal dynamic in Asian social relations (Sue & Morishima, 1982), particularly when the relationship involves seeking help for personal issues (Shon & Ja, 1982).

Based on various accounts of face in both East Asian and Western psychology, it appears that face has the following psychosocial parameters: First, as social beings, people are invested in presenting to others, either implicitly or explicitly, certain claims about their character in terms of traits, attitudes, and values. Others come to recognize and accept the person's "face" or "line" that the person claims for her or himself. This set of claims constitutes that person's face (Ho, 1991). Second, face is not simply prestige or social reputation obtained through success and personal achievements. Rather, according to Hu (1944) face represents the person's social position or prestige gained by performing one or more specific social roles that are well recognized by others or as Goffman (1955) notes, "face is an image of self

126   NOLAN ZANE AND MAY YEH

delineated in terms of approved social attributes" (p. 213). The line or face that one can claim is constrained or parameterized by the social roles ascribed and assumed by that person. Third, as Ho (1991) has observed, face is very salient in East Asian social relations whereas it has less social significance in more individualistic-oriented societies such as in the United States. The importance of face in East Asian cultures lies in its function as a mechanism that maintains group harmony. Reflecting a collective emphasis, great value is placed on maintaining harmonious relationships among in-group members and protecting the integrity of the group. Face-saving behaviors and the avoidance of face loss interactions enhance smooth relations among group members and help minimize disruptions to the social order. In this way, face concerns (especially for those with East Asian cultural heritage) are tied to *both* individual and group integrity. Thus, face can be defined as essentially a person's set of socially-sanctioned claims concerning one's social character and social integrity in which this set of claims or this "line" is largely defined by certain prescribed roles that one carries out as a member and representative of a group. The fact that face has esteem implications that extend beyond the individual to that individual's reference group is probably the main reason it has such psychological power in certain shame-based societies such as East Asian cultures.

The decision was made to focus on loss of face in this chapter because it appears to have more serious effects on one's social behavior. "Basic differences are found between the processes involved in gaining and losing face. While it is not a necessity to strive to gain face, losing face is a serious matter which will in varying degrees affect one's ability to function effectively in society" (Ho, 1974). Face loss is more serious because it tends to disrupt the interpersonal harmony within the group that is often a strong behavioral norm among East Asian societies (Ho, 1991). Moreover, it appears that face loss concerns and shame issues may be especially salient for Asian American clients seeking help for mental health problems that tend to be highly stigmatized issues in their communities and families (Uba, 1994).

In the following study, a measure assessing loss of face was developed and validated. In addition to concurrent and discriminant validity concerns, we also determined if the measure could account for ethnic variance above and beyond that accounted for by existing personality measures of more person-centered constructs.

4. DEVELOPMENT AND VALIDATION OF THE LOSS OF FACE MEASURE

4.1 Scale development

Using the rational development approach, a 21-item, 7-point Likert scale measure assessing loss of face (LOF) was constructed. An item pool was generated following an extensive review of available literature on the concept of loss of face, resulting in a list of 45 face-related behaviors and face-threatening situations. A research team of five persons including one clinical psychologist, one social psychologist, and three research assistants, using the following criteria, evaluated these items: (a) The item must involve a face-threatening behavior in one of the following four areas which have been suggested by the literature to be the most common face-threatening situations (Hu, 1944; Ho, 1976; Hwang, 1987), and these are social status, ethical behavior, social propriety, or self-discipline; (b) the item must not be highly related to maladjustment; and (c) the item must be easily translated into Japaese and Chinese for cross-national research purposes. Decisions on the items using these criteria were reached by the unanimous agreement of all five researchers. Consequently, 21 items (for example, "I am more affected when someone criticizes me in public than when someone criticizes me in private") were selected for inclusion in the Loss of Face Scale (see Appendix A). Each statement was rated on a 7-point Likert scale, from 1 (*Strongly Disagree*) to 7 (*Strongly Agree*). All items were scored in the direction of face loss concern.

4.2 Sample

The participants were 158 undergraduate students at a major research university in California. There were 77 Caucasian Americans (42 males, 35 females) and 81 Asian Americans (37 males, 44 females) in this sample. The Asian American sample consisted of 34 Chinese (42%), 10 Filipino (12%), 7 Japanese (7%), 22 Korean (22%), and 8 Vietnamese (8%). Because there were no significant differences between Chinese, Korean, and other Asian American groups on the variables of interest (described below), the Asian American groups were combined for the subsequent analyses. There were no significant differences between males and females on all variables so that the groups were combined for all analyses. There were 29 Asian Americans (35.8%) born in the United States and 52 foreign-born Asian Americans (64.2%). For the foreign-born Asian Americans, the average number of years living in the United States was 12.5 ($SD = 3.9$).

4.3 Validation Study Design

The Self-Consciousness Scale (Fenigstein, Scheier, & Buss, 1975), the Self-Monitoring Scale (Snyder, 1974), the Social Desirability Scale (Edwards, 1957), and an acculturation scale were chosen for inclusion in the validation study with the expectation that they would be related to the Loss of Face measure.

4.4 Concurrent Validity

Yang (1945) has suggested that there are several factors that influence face loss concerns. These include the degree of equality or inequality of status between the persons involved, the presence of another individual, the type of social relationship, social sanctions, age of the interactants, and sensibility. Therefore, it is expected that face loss concerns would involve awareness of one's own feelings, actions, and social status, indicated by a high level of self-consciousness. In addition, the control of self that an individual must exhibit to maintain and avoid losing face necessitates a degree of self-monitoring. Thus, the Self-Consciousness Scale and the Self-Monitoring Scale were chosen to test concurrent validity.

It was expected that the public self-consciousness and private self-consciousness factors of the Self-Consciousness Scale and the other-directedness factor of the Self-Monitoring Scale would positively correlate with the Loss of Face Scale. It has been noted that face serves both the function of "a social sanction for enforcing moral standards" as well as that of "an internalized social sanction" (Hu, 1944, p. 62). Hwang (1987) has also indicated that face loss concern involves awareness of norms, the structure of social relationship networks within the society, and social obligations that are "incurred through a self-conscious manipulation of face and related symbols." As stated earlier, interactions of face include awareness of one's own social prestige, social relationship, and the social status of others as compared to the self (Yang, 1945). Thus, awareness of one's role in society, as measured by the public self-consciousness and other-directedness scales, and an awareness of one's internal state, as indicated by the private self-consciousness scale, would be expected to correlate with the face concerns.

Although a concern for face exists in every culture (Hu, 1944), the salience of face in the social interactions individuals from East Asian cultures has been well-documented (Chen-Louie, 1981; Goffman, 1955; Yang, 1945; Zane, Enomoto, & Chun, 1994). However, Chen-Louie (1981) has noted that face is important in "traditional Chinese culture, but esteemed in varying degrees by generations [in the United States] less steeped in the old ways" (p. 232). Thus, it is expected that high cultural identification with Asian American cultures would correlate positively with face loss concerns while high identification with White American culture would correlate negatively with loss of face.

4.5 Discriminant Validity

Loss of Face involves both an awareness of social norms as well as a consciousness of one's own internal state (Hu, 1944). We would expect that face loss would be distinguishable from simple conformity to social norms, namely, social desirability. It was expected that the Loss of Face measure would correlate somewhat with both the Social Anxiety subscale of the Self-Consciousness Scale and the Social Desirability Scale. As indicated by Yang (1945), the age of the persons involved, the presence of another individual, and the social status of the participants are all factors that influence face interactions. Face loss concern includes responsiveness to the status of the persons involved in the interaction beyond that of behaving in a strictly socially desirable manner. Thus, it was expected that although social desirability and social anxiety would correlate to some extent with loss of face, these relationships would not be so strong as to suggest that the constructs would be indistinguishable. Because all the items in the Loss of Face Scale are worded in the direction of face loss, a Response Acquiescence scale was also included in this study to control for this tendency. Finally, as noted earlier, items were selected so that they would not reflect a maladjusted, insecure behavioral style associated with individuals who are simply too concerned about what others think or feel about them. To determine if the Loss of Face measure assessed individual tendencies independent of poor psychological functioning, a measure of maladjustment was included.

4.6 Incremental Validity

If indeed the Loss of Face Scale measures a salient construct that reflects important ethnic and cultural differences, ethnic differences on face loss should be evident beyond that which are registered by existing personality measures. First, ethnic comparisons between Asian and Caucasian American groups were conducted on all the personality variables assessed in the study including face loss. Second, to determine if face loss contributed to ethnic variance above and beyond what was accounted for by other personality variables, ethnic differences on face loss were examined after controlling for all other personality variables for which significant Asian-White differences were found.

4.7 Instruments

4.7.1 Self-Consciousness Scale
The Self-Consciousness Scale consists of 23 items designed to measure individual tendencies of self-attention (Fenigstein et al., 1975). The Self-Consciousness construct involves 3 factors: private self-consciousness, public self-consciousness, and social anxiety (Fenigstein, et al., 1975). Private self-consciousness measures attention to one's internal state of thoughts and feelings (e.g., "I'm constantly examining my motives"), while public self-consciousness concerns awareness of oneself as a social object, which affects others (e.g., "I'm concerned about what other people think of me"). Social anxiety refers to discomfort in the presence of others that may result from focusing attention on one's self through private self-consciousness or public self-consciousness (e.g., "I have trouble working when someone is watching me"). Items are rated on a 5-point Likert scale from 0 (*Extremely uncharacteristic*) to 4 (*Extremely characteristic*). Substantial evidence for the construct, convergent, and discriminant validity of the public and private self-consciousness scales has been found (Fenigstein et al., 1975; Carver & Glass, 1976; Carver & Scheier, 1978; Turner, Scheier, Carver, & Ickes, 1978). Previous studies on the Self-Consciousness Scale have found 4 of the 23 items to be "conceptually inconsistent with the underlying dimensions and/or did not load onto the identified factors" (Abe & Zane, 1990). Thus, these four items were omitted in the study, resulting in the administration of a 19-item scale.

4.7.2 Self-Monitoring Scale
The Self-Monitoring Scale is a 25-item, true-false measure developed to assess "self-observation and self-control guided by situational cues to social

appropriateness" (Snyder, 1974, p. 526). The Self-Monitoring Scale has been found to have at least three factors (Briggs, Check, & Buss, 1980) that include: other-directedness (11 items), acting (5 items), and extraversion (6 items). Other-directedness refers to changing one's behavior to please other people (e.g., "In order to get along and be liked, I tend to be what people expect me to be rather than anything else"); acting involves the ability to do and enjoyment of speaking and entertaining (e.g., "I have considered being an entertainer"); and extraversion deals with being the center of attention and confidence in social skills (e.g., "At a party I let others keep the jokes and stories going"). Nunnally (1978) found alpha coefficients for the subscales of the Self-Monitoring Scale as well as for the full scale itself that meet acceptable standards of internal consistency. The Kuder-Richardson reliability of the whole scale has ranged from .63 to .70 (Snyder, 1974), and the test-retest reliability after one month was found to be .83.

4.7.3 Cultural Identification

Two measures of cultural identification were used in this study, one of which was designed to assess identification with White American culture and the other which measured identification with Asian American cultures (Oetting & Beauvais, 1991). Each measure includes four questions involving adherence and an attachment to a particular cultural lifestyle and orientation (e.g., "Do you live by or follow the White-American way of life?" "Does your family live or follow the Japanese American way of life?"). Respondents indicate on a 4-point Likert scale the extent to which they have been involved in a particular cultural lifestyle varying from 1 (*Not at all*) to 4 (*Most of the time*). It was hypothesized that the Loss of Face measure would be correlated negatively with White cultural identification and positively with Asian American identification.

4.7.4 Social Desirability

The Social Desirability Scale (Edwards, 1957) is a 39-item, true-false inventory drawn from the Minnosota Multiphasic Personality Inventory, which is designed to assess "the tendency to endorse statements on the basis of their implicit social desirability rather than their actual explicit content" (e.g., "I dream frequently about things that are best kept to myself"). A corrected split-half reliability of .83 was reported and this measure has been correlated with other measures of social desirability such as the Marlow-Crowne Scale (Edwards, 1957).

4.7.5 Response Acquiescence and Maladjustment

The Minnesota Multiphasic Personality Inventory (MMPI) contains 79 true-false items designed to assess personality styles that can be factored into what Welsh and Dahlstrom (1956) have called the A and R scales. The R scale (40 items) has been shown to measure response acquiescence (e.g., "Sometimes, when embarrassed, I break out in a sweat which annoys me greatly"). The A scale (39 items) contains statements that generally have socially undesirable attributes (e.g., "I feel anxiety about something or someone almost all the time"). The A scale generally correlates negatively with the Social Desirability Scale from -0.81 to -0.91 (Edwards, 1957).

4.8 Procedure

Subjects were scheduled in groups of 2 to 12, and the time for survey completion was generally 15 to 40 minutes. The surveys were administered by one of four female Asian American research assistants. Subjects were instructed to respond to each question and were permitted to leave after completing the survey. Explanations of the purpose of the survey were offered and given on request after the completion of the questionnaire.

Table 1. Reliability Alphas for Loss of Face Questionnaire for Total Sample

Subscales	α ($n = 231$)
Acting	.64
Other-directedness	.63
Extraversion	.63
Loss of Face	.83
Private Self-Consciousness	.72
Public Self-Consciousness	.77
Social Anxiety	.77
White-American Cultural Identity	.83
Asian Ethnic Cultural Identity	.87
Social Desirability	.78
Response Acquiescence	.60
Maladjustment	.81

4.9 Results and Discussion

The LOF measure was internally consistent with an alpha of .83. Table 1 shows that all validation measures demonstrated adequate internal consistency so that estimates of validity could be made without being compromised by differential reliability among the measures. The LOF measure demonstrated both concurrent and discriminant validity (see Table 2). As predicted, face loss correlated positively with other-directedness, private self-consciousness, public self-consciousness, and negatively with extraversion, acting (the desire to perform before others), and White cultural identity. Face loss was only correlated moderately with social anxiety and social desirability. However, it was not significantly related to response acquiescence, and more importantly, it was not related to maladjustment. Similar results were found when Asians and Whites were analyzed separately. Factor analysis of the LOF measure yielded one factor that accounted for 26 percent of the variance. These results suggest that the measure is unidimensional. Table 3 shows

132   NOLAN ZANE AND MAY YEH

the item loadings by ethnic group and total sample. An inspection of these loadings indicates that the LOF factor structure is similar for both Asians and Whites.

The only discrepant finding involved the non-significant relationship between Asian cultural identification and face loss. This may have been due to technical problems with the Asian identity measure, itself. Unlike the White cultural identification measure in which respondents simply respond to standard items, the Asian identity measure requires respondents to fill in their specific Asian ethnicity so that the item can reflect adherence to a specific ethnic Asian culture. Many respondents either did not comply with the instructions or reportedly found them to be somewhat confusing.

Table 2. Correlations of Loss of Face with Each Validation Measure for Asian Americans and Whites

Measures	Asians	Caucasians	Total
Acting	.01	- .24*	- .18**
Other-directedness	.44***	.33**	.37***
Extraversion	- .28**	- .23*	- .32***
Private Self-Consciousness	.22*	.15	.20**
Public Self-Consciousness	.42***	.56***	.51***
Social Anxiety	.54***	.54***	.58***
White-American Cultural Identity	- .10	- .03	- .13*
Asian Ethnic Cultural Identity	.16	- .28**	- .03
Social Desirability	- .49***	- .35**	- .47***
Response Acquiescence	.03	.11	.08
Maladjustment	.10	.13	.11

*p<.05   **p<.01   ***p<.001

Finally, a critical question is whether face loss can account for ethnic variance in addition to what has been accounted for by personality variables already established in Western psychology. Asians ($M = 91.8$, $SD = 16.9$) scored significantly higher on face loss than Whites ($M = 80.4$, $SD = 16.3$), t (156) = 4.32, $p < .001$. Consistent with previous studies, ethnic differences between Asians and Whites were also found on social anxiety, acting, other-directedness, and White cultural identification (see Table 4). However, the Asian–White difference on face loss persisted even after controlling for ethnic differences on these other personality variables, F (1, 150) = 7.42, $p < .01$, (adjusted means of 89.7 and 82.7 for Asians and Whites, respectively). An effect size analysis provides another way of examining the sensitivity of the LOF measure to ethnic differences. The effect sizes associated with the ethnic comparisons include the following: acting = .31, other-directedness = .27, social anxiety = .38, Asian cultural identity = .83, and face loss = .64. The effect sizes associated with ethnic differences on most of the other personality variables are somewhat larger than what Cohen (1992) considers to be a small effect size, whereas the effect size associated with ethnic differences on face loss is somewhat larger

THE USE OF CULTURALLY-BASED VARIABLES IN ASSESSMENT: STUDIES ON 133
LOSS OF FACE

than a moderate effect size. These results strongly suggest that face loss was an important ethnic discriminator. In fact, the only effect size larger than the face loss effect size is the one involving Asian cultural identity that is a large effect size, according to Cohen. However, this would be expected since little overlap would be expected in the cultural identities of Whites and Asian Americans on Asian cultural identity.

Table 3. Means, Standard Deviations, and t-values of Measures by Ethnic Group

Measure	Ethnic Group		t-value
	Asian	White	
Acting			
M	2.0	2.5	- 2.16*
SD	1.6	1.6	
Other-directedness			
M	5.4	4.8	1.90*
SD	2.0	2.2	
Extraversion			
M	3.0	3.4	- 1.44
SD	1.4	1.5	
Loss of Face			
M	91.8	80.4	4.32***
SD	16.9	16.3	
Private Self Consciousness			
M	21.0	20.4	0.82
SD	4.7	4.6	
Public Self Consciousness			
M	20.4	19.5	1.39
SD	4.1	4.1	
Social Anxiety			
M	10.0	8.6	2.28*
SD	3.7	3.6	
Acculturation (White)			
M	12.2	14.2	- 5.35***
SD	2.3	2.4	
Acculturation (Ethnic)	12.5	9.9	5.62***
M	2.2	3.6	
SD			
Response Acquiescence			
M	15.0	14.5	0.79
SD	3.9	3.9	

*$p<.05$ **$p<.01$ ***$p<.001$

The results support the reliability and construct validity of the LOF measure. Moreover, they also strongly suggest that the measure is especially sensitive to ethnic/cultural differences involving Asian Americans and Whites.

5. CONCLUSION AND IMPLICATIONS

Mental health practitioners and researchers continue to be perplexed by the problem of how to increase the effectiveness of mental health services to culturally diverse groups. A major but often overlooked difficulty that hinders progress in this area is the lack of appropriate "conceptual tools" to understand the interpersonal relationships of people from different cultures. In other words, cultures often differ in the extent to which certain interpersonal dynamics such as autonomy, dependence, loss of face, etc. govern or affect social interactions. Given that therapy tends to focus on the amelioration of interpersonal problems and that change in therapy is mediated through the client-therapist relationship, it is important that *assessment practices incorporate certain interpersonal constructs that may be relatively more culturally salient for different ethnic groups.*

The study presented demonstrates the potential utility of expanding the domain of assessment constructs to include loss of face issues. It appears that, consistent with accounts of Asian American clinicians, face loss is an important interpersonal issue that may hold the key to better understanding the dynamics involved in interpersonal problems of Asian American clients, as well as the treatment process and problems in establishing the working alliance between therapists and these clients. The assessment of face loss concerns opens up a number of potentially useful avenues for clinicians and researchers to pursue. First, knowing that face loss concerns may be paramount from the client's perspective may suggest the need to do "face work" in one's relationship or in treatment itself. Goffman (1955) has delineated the strategies that people often take to avoid loss of face and the usual steps that are necessary to conduct face work once face loss has actually occurred. These steps are necessary for a person who has lost face to re-claim it. By not knowing the essentials of face work, clinicians may be inadvertently impeding progress in therapy for clients who are more shame-oriented.

Second, attention to face issues may assist in understanding why Asian American clients tend to have the highest premature termination rates and shortest treatment stays in mental health systems (Sue, Zane, & Young, 1994). Therapists are often trained to elicit extensive self-disclosure and cathartic release especially in the early stages of therapy. Murase (1977) views this procedural tendency as reflecting the confessional nature of psychotherapy that reflects its Judeo-Christian roots as a healing practice. This process, while often effective, may also generate great face loss for certain clients, especially those who are unfamiliar with sharing their most private thoughts and feelings with a stranger, albeit a professional one. It is possible that by allowing such disclosures and catharses to go unabated, great face loss may be experienced as a client realizes, following these initial sessions, that she has caused face loss to not only herself but to those with whom she is closest. Such experiences would be expected to be more poignant for clients from shame-based, collectivistic cultures. These predicaments may become exacerbated when clinicians unaware of face issues and dynamics perceive such disclosures as signs of therapeutic progress and fail to engage in face work. It is unclear if these problems actually occur and contribute to the early termination of Asian American clients. However, a face analysis strongly suggests that these should be investigated both empirically and clinically. Lastly, the assessment of face loss concerns provides clinicians with a tangible outcropping of that fuzzy construct of culture (Triandis, 1996). In this case, cultural variations map onto a specific psychological element that may affect social behavior. Moreover, since face loss issues may be intertwined with a client's interpersonal problems as well as with the process between client and therapist, this culturally-based construct is proximal to psychotherapy processes and outcomes (cf. Sue & Zane, 1987).

From a pan-cultural perspective, the results suggest that assessment research on loss of face issues can enrich the general study of interpersonal processes. Loss of face was found to be a valid individual difference variable for Whites as well as Asian Americans such that the Loss of Face measure showed similar psychometric properties for both ethnic groups. This lends empirical support to the notion that face concerns are universal but may be more salient in certain cultures (Ho, 1976). Needless to say, face loss concern is but one of many relation-oriented personality constructs that may be important for clinical assessment purposes. For example, constructs such as *personalisimo* in Latino culture, *amae* in Japanese culture, and *jen* in Chinese culture constitute some of these alternative "conceptual tools" that may greatly facilitate the development of more culturally-responsive assessment and treatment approaches for ethnic minority clients.

What distinguishes these constructs from other personality variables often used in assessment is their greater emphasis on the relational aspects of social behavior among individuals in contrast to the person-centered characteristics of individuals (Ho, 1982). Historically, assessment research and practices have tended to focus on variables that characterize individually oriented dispositions. Constructs such as self-esteem, locus of control, dependence, extraversion-introversion, and anxiety tend to refer to dispositions and attitudes that reflect how the individual perceives and experiences the world from his or her own personal perspective. While such constructs may at times point to or have implications with respect to the individual's relations with others, the major orientation is toward the person's experience and consciousness as an autonomous, independent functioning entity. In contrast, constructs often emphasized in Asian social sciences tend to be more relation-centered in that they more directly map onto the relational and reciprocal aspects of the social dynamics between people. For constructs such as face, *amae*, and *jen*, the focus is on the social relationship or the social behavior as the major unit of analysis, thereby, directly situating the person's experience within a more social rather than more person-oriented matrix.

As aptly noted by Ho (1982), the difference between relation-centered constructs and individual-centered constructs is relative in nature reflecting the frame of analysis that tends to be more salient. However, since the constructs employed affect

136   NOLAN ZANE AND MAY YEH

the way in which practitioners and clinicians organize and interpret the experiences of clients, the predominant application of Western, person-centered constructs may be a major contributor to error and/or bias involved in the assessment of individuals from collectivistic cultures and societies. Relation-centered constructs tend to be more salient for individuals who have been socialized from a more collectivistic cultural milieu. Consequently, the use of such constructs may make assessment practices and measures more effective in capturing the life circumstances and worldviews of these clients. Equally important, the inclusion of relation-centered constructs simply provides psychology, in general, and the assessment field, in particular, with a more comprehensive array of conceptual tools that can be used to account for human behavior.

6. REFERENCES

Abe, J. S., & Zane, N. W. S. (1990). Psychological maladjustment among Asian and White American college students: Controlling for confounds. *Journal of Counseling Psychology, 37* (4), 437-444.

Betancourt, H., & López, S. R. (1993). The study of culture, ethnicity, and race in American psychology. *American Psychologist, 48* (6), 629-637.

Briggs, S. R., Cheek, J. M., & Buss, A. H. (1980). An analysis of the Self-Monitoring Scale. *Journal of Personality and Social Psychology, 38* (4), 679-686.

Brislin, R. W., Lonner, W. J., & Thorndike, R. M. (1973). *Cross-cultural research methods*. New York: Wiley.

Carver, C. S., & Glass, D. C. (1976). The Self-Consciousness Scale: A discriminant validity study. *Journal of Personality Assessment, 40* (2), 169-172.

Carver, C. S., & Scheier, M. F. (1978). Self-focusing effects of dispositional self-consciousness, mirror presence, and audience presence. *Journal of Personality and Social Psychology, 36* (3), 324-332.

Chen-Louie, T. T. (1981). Bilingual families: A Chinese-American example. In C. Getty & W. Humphreys (Eds.), *Understanding the family: Status and change in American family life* (pp. 232-249). New York: Appleton, Century, & Croft.

Cohen, J. (1992). A power primer. *Psychological Bulletin, 112*(1), 155-159

Edwards, A. L. (1957). *The social desirability variable in personality assessment and research*. New York: Dryden Press.

Fenigstein, A., Scheier, M. F., & Buss, A. H. (1975). Public and private self-consciousness: Assessment and theory. *Journal of Consulting and Clinical Psychology, 43* (4), 522-527.

Goffman, E. (1955). On face-work: An analysis of ritual elements in social interaction. *Psychiatry: Journal for the Study of Interpersonal Processes, 18*, 213-231.

Ho, D. (1974). Face, social expectations, and conflict avoidance. In J. L. M. Dawson & W. J. Lonner (Eds.), *Readings in cross-cultural psychology: Proceedings of the inaugural meeting of the International Association for Cross-cultural Psychology held in Hong Kong, August, 1972* (pp. 240-251). Hong Kong: Hong Kong University Press.

Ho, D. (1991). The concept of "face" in Chinese-American interaction. In W.-C. Hu & C. L. Grove (Eds.), *Encountering the Chinese: A guide for Americans* (pp. 111-124). Yarmouth, ME: Intercultural Press.

Ho, D. Y. F. (1982). Asian concepts in the behavioral sciences. *Psychologia, 25*, 228-235.

Ho, D. Y. F. (1976). On the concept of face. *American Journal of Sociology, 81*(4), 867-884.

Horowitz, L. M. (1979). On the cognitive structure of interpersonal problems treated in psychotherapy. *Journal of Consulting and Clinical Psychology, 47*(1), 5-15.

Hu, H. C. (1944). The Chinese concepts of "face". *American Anthropologist, 46*, 45-64.

Hwang, K. K. (1987). Face and favor: The Chinese power game. *American Journal of Sociology, 92*(4), 944-974.

Kleinman, A. M. (1977). Depression, somatization and the new cross-cultural psychiatry. *Social Science and Medicine, 11*(1), 3-10.

THE USE OF CULTURALLY-BASED VARIABLES IN ASSESSMENT: STUDIES ON LOSS OF FACE

López, S. R. (1989). Patient variable biases in clinical judgment: Conceptual overview and methodological considerations. *Psychological Bulletin, 106*(2), 184-203.

Lynch, E. W., & Hanson, M. J. (1992). *Developing cross-cultural competence: A guide for working with young children and their families.* Baltimore: P.H. Brookes.

Marcos, L. R., Urcuyo, L., Kesselman, M., & Alpert, M. (1973). The language barrier in evaluating Spanish-American patients. *Archives of General Psychiatry, 29*(5), 655-659.

Murase, K. (1977). Delivery of social services to Asian Americans. In National Association of Social Workers (Ed.), *The encyclopedia of social work* (pp. 953-960). New York: Author.

Nunnally, J. (1978). *Psychometric theory* (2nd ed.). New York: McGraw Hill.

Oetting, E. R., & Beauvais, F. (1991). Orthogonal cultural identification theory: The cultural identification of minority adolescents. *International Journal of the Addictions, 25*(5A-6A), 655-685.

Shon, S. P., & Ja, D. Y. (1982). Asian families. In M. McGoldrick, J. K. Pearce, & J. Giordano (Eds.), *Ethnicity and family therapy* (pp. 208-228). New York: Guilford.

Snyder, M. (1974). Self-monitoring of expressive behavior. *Journal of Personality and Social Psychology, 30*(4), 526-537.

Sue, S., & Morishima, J. K. (1982). *The mental health of Asian Americans* (1st ed.). San Francisco: Jossey-Bass.

Sue, S., & Zane, N. (1987). The role of culture and cultural techniques in psychotherapy: A critique and reformulation. *American Psychologist, 42*(1), 37-45.

Sue, S., Zane, N. W. S., & Young, K. (1994). Research on psychotherapy with culturally diverse populations. In A. E. Bergin & S. L. Garfield (Eds.), *Handbook of psychotherapy and behavior change* (4th ed., pp. 783-817). New York: Wiley.

Triandis, H. C. (1996). The psychological measurement of cultural syndromes. *American Psychologist, 51*(4), 407-415.

Turner, R. G., Scheier, M. F., Carver, C. S., & Ickes, W. (1978). Correlates of self-consciousness. *Journal of Personality Assessment, 42*(3), 285-289.

Uba, L. (1994). *Asian Americans: Personality patterns, identity, and mental health.* New York: Guilford.

Welsh, G. S., & Dahlstrom, W. G. (1956). *Basic readings on the MMPI in psychology and medicine.* Minneapolis, MN: University of Minnesota Press.

Yang, M.-C. U. (1945). *A Chinese village: Taitou, Shantung province.* New York: Columbia University Press.

Zane, N. W. S., Enomoto, K., & Chun, C.-A. (1994). Treatment outcomes of Asian- and White-American clients in outpatient therapy. *Journal of Community Psychology, 22*, 177-191.

Appendix A. *Loss of Face Questionnaire*

Developed by Nolan Zane, University of California, Santa Barbara

Instructions: Use the scale below to indicate the extent to which you agree with each statement as it applies to you.

1 = Strongly Disagree
2 = Moderately Disagree
3 = Mildly Disagree
4 = Neither Agree or Disagree
5 = Mildly Agree
6 = Moderately Agree
7 = Strongly Agree

_____ 1. I am more affected when someone criticizes me in public than when someone criticizes me in private.

_____ 2. During a discussion, I try not to ask questions because I may appear ignorant to others.

_____ 3. I maintain a low profile because I do not want to make mistakes in front of other people.

_____ 4. Before I make comments in the presence of other people, I qualify my remarks.

_____ 5. I downplay my abilities and achievements so that others do not have unrealistically high expectations of me.

_____ 6. I carefully plan what I am going to say or do to minimize mistakes.

_____ 7. I say I may be in error before commenting on something.

_____ 8. When I meet other people, I am concerned about their expectations of me.

_____ 9. I hesitate asking for help because I think my request will be an inconvenience to others.

_____ 10. I try not to do things which call attention to myself.

_____ 11. I do not criticize others because this may embarrass them.

_____ 12. I carefully watch others' actions before I do anything.

_____ 13. I will not complain publicly even when I have been treated unfairly.

_____ 14. I try to act like others to be consistent with social norms.

_____ 15. Before I do anything in public, I prepare myself for any possible consequence.

_____ 16. I prefer to use a third party to help resolve our differences between another person and me.

_____ 17. When discussing a problem, I make an effort to let the person know that I am not blaming him or her.

_____ 18. When someone criticizes me, I try to avoid that person.

_____ 19. When I make a mistake in front of others, I try to prevent them from noticing it.

_____ 20. Even when I know another person is at fault, I am careful not to criticize that person.

_____ 21. When someone embarrasses me, I try to forget it.

SECTION III: ISSUES OF PSYCHOMETRIC EQUIVALENCE ACROSS CULTURES

10. **Universal and Indigenous Dimensions of Chinese Personality**
    Fanny M. Cheung

11. **Interpreting Cultural Variations in Cognitive Profiles**
    Lisa A. Suzuki
    Tamiko Mogami
    Ellen S. Kim

12. **The Conception of Depression in Chinese Americans**
    Yu-Wen Ying

13. **Assessing Asian and Asian American Parenting: A Review of the Literature**
    Su Yeong Kim
    Vivian Y. Wong

FANNY M. CHEUNG

CHAPTER 10

UNIVERSAL AND INDIGENOUS DIMENSIONS OF CHINESE PERSONALITY

1. USE OF TRANSLATED PERSONALITY TESTS WITH THE CHINESE

One of the early cross-cultural studies on the Minnesota Multiphasic Personality Inventory (MMPI) (S. Sue & D. W. Sue, 1974) showed that Asian American students using a psychiatric clinic had higher scale elevations on the MMPI than non-Asian students. Twenty years later, similar findings were obtained. The MMPI-2 profiles of Asian American students showed more somatic complaints, depression, anxiety, and isolation than their Caucasian counterparts (S. Sue, K. Keefe, Enomoto, Durvasula, & Chao, 1996). There may be different interpretations of this finding. First, Asian American students were more prone to psychopathology. Alternatively, the elevated scores on the MMPI scales may be less a reflection of the problems of the students than those of the MMPI itself.

A typical question for international psychologists after their training in the U.S. is: Would an empirically derived Western instrument be applicable to their own people and would they be using these instruments when they return to their home countries? As they go through the items of the MMPI, they might wonder, "What would be the relevance of a question like 'I liked *Alice in Wonderland*' back home?" Studies and applications of the Chinese MMPI in Hong Kong and in the People's Republic of China in the past 20 years confirmed that it was a practical tool for clinical psychologists (Cheung, 1985, 1995; Cheung & Ho, 1997; Cheung & Song, 1989; Cheung, Song, & J. X. Zhang, 1996). Based on studies with psychiatric patients, students and workers, it was found that the average profiles of normal Chinese persons had similar elevations on the Depression and Schizophrenia scales as in S. Sue and D. W. Sue's earlier study with Asian American students. However, Chinese patients with depressive disorders and schizophrenic disorders had significantly higher scores on these scales beyond the already elevated scores obtained by the normal respondents.

Borrowing or adapting psychological tests cross-culturally serves the practical purpose of providing useably assessment techniques within a short time frame for international psychologists. The advantage lies in the wealth of evidence accumulated to support the conceptual and psychometric properties of these measures that could also be borrowed. For example, the MMPI and the MMPI-2

141

142 FANNY M. CHEUNG

have been translated and found to have generality and applicability in many countries in Asia and Southeast Asia (Butcher, 1996; Butcher & Pancheri, 1976). In Hong Kong, the MMPI is a useful objective tool for psychologists in the young profession of clinical psychology to assess their clients' psychopathology. Even before there was a standardized translation in the 1970s, clinical psychologists there were using their own instantaneous translations as they were administering the MMPI. The need for a standardized translation was apparent.

Retaining the use of a common and equivalent test also allows for cross-cultural comparisons on the construct domains measured by that test. The MMPI profiles of Chinese psychiatric patients were found to bear many similarities with their counterparts in the U.S. as well as with those in other parts of the world using translated versions of the MMPI. However, with the Chinese normative samples obtaining different mean scores on some of the scales of the MMPI from those of the American norms, caution should be exercised in clinical interpretation. If interpreted directly according to the original American norms, the profiles of many Chinese respondents may be misjudged as pathological.

To solve the problem of using an imported test for applied purposes, local norms may be established for the translated test to reflect the score distribution of the local population. This requires large-scale data collection on a local sample that is comparable to the original normative sample. National norms have been collected in China for the Chinese MMPI. With the Chinese norms, however, the T scores are more restricted in range even among psychiatric patients. The mean T scores for psychiatric patients on the clinical scales often fall below 70. The joint use of the American and Chinese norms in clinical interpretation is recommended for the Chinese MMPI (Cheung, 1995).

What about items like "I liked *Alice in Wonderland*"? In the case of the Chinese MMPI, it was substituted with a Chinese novel *Journey to the West*, a story about the Tang dynasty monk and the Monkey King, which contained similar satirical contents. The item later turned out to be endorsed by more males than females, and so did not really provide the functional equivalence for the Masculinity-Femininity scale. Checking for functional equivalence of items is particularly pertinent when the test is empirically derived, like the MMPI.

From the cross-cultural differences at the item and scale levels, international psychologists may begin to question the sufficiency of the personality or clinical constructs included in borrowed instruments. In cross-cultural testing, it is often assumed that the underlying constructs of the translated instruments are universal or etic. This approach has been labeled as *imposed etic* (Berry, 1969; Yik & Bond, 1993). While there are advantages of using tests with imposed etic constructs which are cross-culturally valid, are there important emic (culture-specific) constructs that are indigenous to the Chinese culture but are not covered by these imported tests? These are the considerations behind the development of an indigenous personality inventory for the Chinese people.

The research team on the Chinese MMPI project in the People's Republic of China and Hong Kong (Fanny Cheung and Weizhen Song) decided to develop a comprehensive personality inventory for the Chinese culture in 1989. The aim was to develop an inventory that covered personality characteristics for normal as well as diagnostic assessment. Adopting the test construction methodology used in Western psychology, the researchers started from an empirical approach in developing the Chinese Personality Assessment Inventory (CPAI). The aim was to construct an inventory suited to the local needs while retaining the standards of validity and reliability expected of established assessment instruments.

2. DEVELOPMENT OF THE CPAI

The development of the CPAI (Cheung et al., 1996) involved a series of stages based on the methodology used in test construction in Western psychology:

2.1 Determination of culturally relevant personality constructs

The first step in the construction of the CPAI was to determine culturally relevant constructs by tapping a wide range of daily life experiences where personality descriptions were commonly used. The sources included contemporary Chinese novels, books on Chinese proverbs, statements of self-descriptions collected in an informal street survey, other-descriptions by professionals (teachers, nurses, social workers, psychiatrists, psychologists, and business managers) of their colleagues, students or clients, and studies of Chinese personality in the psychological literature.

A total of 150 distinct personality characteristics were consolidated to represent common and broad personality constructs. Using an expert committee approach, these characteristics were examined and re-grouped. Consensus was reached on 26 normal personality constructs and 12 clinical constructs, which were regarded by members of the research team to be important aspects of personality and psychopathology among the Chinese people, including those constructs that were not covered in Western inventories.

2.2 Generation of scale items

Items were written or selected from existing databases by the researchers for each of the 38 scales to be used in the preliminary trial version of the CPAI. Chinese language teachers in junior high schools were asked to review the items to ensure that the language difficulty level of each of the 900 items was appropriate for the general public. A pilot study was conducted in which 130 respondents from different walks of life in China and Hong Kong were asked to rate the items in terms of comprehension, fluency and cultural relevance. Items were modified or deleted based on their responses.

2.3 Statistical verification of the initial CPAI scales

About 1,700 adults from different backgrounds in China and Hong Kong took the 1991 trial version of the CPAI. Item analysis on each CPAI scale was conducted

144 FANNY M. CHEUNG

separately for the two samples. Items were selected if they met a common set of statistical criteria for both samples. The pattern of inter-scale correlations was used to modify or delete scales with overlapping constructs.

Table 1. Scales of the CPAI

Personality Scales		Clinical Scales		Validity Scales	
EMO	Emotionality	I-S	Inferiority vs. Self-Acceptance*	INF	Infrequency
RES	Responsibility	SOM	Somatization	GIM	Good Impression
I-S*	Inferiority vs. Self-Acceptance*	DEP	Depression	RCI	Response Consistency Index
G-M	Graciousness vs. Meanness	PHY	Physical Symptoms		
V-S	Veraciousness vs. Slickness	ANT	Antisocial Behavior		
O-P	Optimism vs. Pessimism	ANX	Anxiety		
MET	Meticulousness	SEX	Sexual Maladjustment		
E-I	External vs. Internal Locus of Control	DIS	Distortion of Reality		
FAM	Family Orientation	PAR	Paranoia		
REN	*Ren Qing*	NEE	Need for Attention		
HAR	Harmony	HYP	Hypomania		
FAC	Face	PAT	Pathological Dependence		
FLE	Flexibility				
MOD	Modernization				
T-E	Thrift vs. Extravagance				
I-E	Introversion vs. Extraversion				
LEA	Leadership				
ADV	Adventurousness				
S-S	Self vs. Social Orientation				
L-A	Logical vs. Affective Orientation				
DEF	Ah-Q Mentality/Defensiveness				

2.4 Standardization of the CPAI

The 1992 version of the CPAI was standardized on a representative sample of 1,998 respondents from China and 446 respondents from Hong Kong between the age of 18 to 65. Further refinement of a number of scales was made. The final form of the CPAI consisted of 22 personality scales, 12 clinical scales (including one that

UNIVERSAL AND INDIGENOUS DIMENSIONS OF CHINESE PERSONALITY 145

is also listed as a personality scale) and three validity scales or indices. The names of the scales are listed in Table 1.

3. UNDERLYING STRUCTURE OF THE CPAI

Four factors were extracted from the personality scales and two factors were extracted from the clinical scales for both the Chinese and Hong Kong samples. The four personality factors were Dependability, Chinese Tradition, Social Potency, and Individualism, which together explained 59.9% of the total variance. The two clinical factors were Emotional Problems and Behavioral Problems, accounting for 61.2% of the total variance (Tables 2 and 3).

Among the four personality factors, the Chinese Tradition factor is of particular interest to the study of Chinese personality. It is characterized by high positive loading on scales which were deemed to be important to the Chinese culture but were not covered in most of the translated personality inventories. These scales include: Harmony (one's inner peace of mind, contentment and interpersonal harmony); *Ren Qing* (social favors that are exchanged in the form of money, goods, information, status, service and affection according to an implicit set of social rules); Thrift vs. Extravagance (the virtuous tendency to save rather than to waste and prudence in spending); and Face (the concern for maintaining face and social behaviors that enhance others' respect toward oneself and that avoid losing one's face). This factor is also characterized by negative loadings on Flexibility, Modernization, and Adventurousness. An alternative label for this factor is Interpersonal Relatedness as the factor taps the instrumental interpersonal relationships emphasized in the Chinese culture. This factor explains 16.5% of the total variance.

As an indigenously derived personality inventory, the CPAI provides an opportunity to examine how its factor structure compares with the Five Factor Model (FFM) of personality that is purported to be universal (McCrae & Costa, 1997). According to the FFM, the Big Five personality dimensions, i.e. Neuroticism vs. Emotional Stability (N), Extraversion or Surgency (E), Openness to Experience (O), Agreeableness vs. Antagonism (A), and Conscientiousness (C) can subsume most personality traits across cultures as tapped by the current personality tests. However, McCrae and Costa admitted that "because no indigenous or emic measures of personality were included in these studies, the possibility remains that there are culturally unique factors of personality beyond N, E, O, A, and C" (pp. 514-515). The Big Five personality dimensions can be compared to the CPAI factors to see if the former could subsume the latter in explaining Chinese personality.

Table 2. Factor Structure of the CPAI Personality Scales for the Chinese Standardization Sample (N=2,444)

Personality Scales	Factor			
	1 Dependability	2 Chinese Tradition	3 Social Potency	4 Individualism
Practical Mindedness	**.75**	.14	-.30	-.11
Emotionality	**-.73**	.00	-.17	.00
Responsibility	**.73**	.28	.00	.23
Inferiority vs. Self-Acceptance	**-.66**	.36	-.39	.00
Graciousness-Meanness	**.65**	-.21	.00	**-.44**
Veraciousness-Slickness	**.61**	.00	-.18	-.31
Optimism	**.59**	-.20	**.51**	.00
Meticulousness	**.57**	.32	.00	.25
External vs. Internal Locus of Control	**-.57**	.20	-.19	.00
Family Orientation	**.54**	.21	.19	**-.42**
Ren Qing (Relationship) Orientation	-.11	**.73**	.12	.00
Harmony	.26	**.71**	.00	.00
Flexibility	.00	**-.60**	.00	**-.47**
Modernization	.00	**-.57**	.16	.00
Face	**-.54**	**.55**	.00	.17
Thrift-Extravagance	.27	**.49**	-.36	.17
Introversion-Extroversion	.00	.00	**-.73**	.17
Leadership	.00	.15	**.73**	.40
Adventurousness	.26	**-.41**	**.67**	.10
Self vs. Social Orientation	-.15	.00	.00	**.81**
Logical vs. Affective Orientation	.24	.38	.31	**.53**
Defensiveness (Ah-Q Attitude)	-.38	**.44**	.18	**.45**
Eigenvalue	4.87	3.31	2.55	2.22
Variance Explained	22.11%	15.06%	11.59%	10.10%

Note: Extraction Method was Principal Component Analysis.
Rotation Method was Varimax with Kaiser Normalization.

UNIVERSAL AND INDIGENOUS DIMENSIONS OF CHINESE PERSONALITY   147

Table 3. Factor Structure of the CPAI Clinical Scales for the Chinese
Standardization Sample (N=2,444)

	Factor	
	1	2
Clinical Scales	Emotional Problems	Behavioral Problems
Depression	**.83**	.20
Physical Symptoms	**.78**	-.11
Anxiety	**.75**	**.44**
Inferiority vs. Self-Acceptance	**.74**	.36
Somatization	**.69**	.30
Hypomania	.21	**.79**
Antisocial Behavior	.36	**.73**
Need for Attention	**.48**	**.64**
Pathological Dependence	-.18	**.63**
Distortion of Reality	**.54**	**.59**
Paranoia	**.52**	**.58**
Sexual Maladjustment	.35	**.48**
Eigenvalue	4.00	3.35
Variance Explained	33.31%	27.93%

Note: Extraction Method was Principal Component Analysis.
Rotation Method was Varimax with Kaiser Normalization.

4. JOINT FACTOR ANALYSIS OF THE CPAI AND THE BIG FIVE

In a series of studies in which the CPAI and measures of the Big Five were submitted to a joint factor analysis, the common and unique domains of the CPAI were identified (Cheung et al., 2001).

The first study involved 279 Chinese students from Beijing and Guangzhou who took both the personality scales of the CPAI and the Chinese version of the NEO-PI-R (Costa & McCrae, 1992). Based on principal components analysis with varimax rotation, a six-factor model instead of a five-factor model was found to provide the best solution. The six-factor model encompasses the Big Five and the unique CPAI Chinese Tradition or Interpersonal Relatedness factor (Table 4).

The CPAI scales loaded on four of the Big Five factors, corresponding to Neuroticism, Conscientiousness, Agreeableness, and Extraversion. None of the CPAI scales loaded on the Openness domain of the Big Five. On the other hand, none of the NEO-PI-R facets loaded on Factor Five, the Interpersonal Relatedness factor. This factor has high loadings on only CPAI scales, including positive loadings on *Ren Qing*, Defensiveness, Harmony, Face, and Logical vs. Affective Orientation, and negative loadings on Optimism vs. Pessimism and Flexibility.

To replicate the six-factor model, a joint analysis of the Big Five factors and the CPAI Interpersonal Relatedness factor was conducted in a second study with a non-student sample in China. In the second study, 372 Chinese managers from

148 FANNY M. CHEUNG

Guangzhou took a short version of the Big Five measure, the NEO-FFI (Costa & McCrae, 1992) together with selected scales from the CPAI. Four CPAI scales which formed the core of the Interpersonal Relatedness factor from both the standardization study and the first joint factors analysis were used in this joint analysis: Harmony, *Ren Qing*, Face and Flexibility.

Table 4. Six Factor Solution of Joint Factor Analysis of CPAI Personality Scales and NEO-PI-R Facets for a Chinese College Student Sample (N=279)

Scales / Facets	Factor					
	1 Neuro-ticism	2 Conscien-tiousness	3 Agree-ableness	4 Extra-version	5 Inter-personal Related-ness	6 Open-ness
Adventurousness	**-.76**	-.02	-.03	.24	-.11	.11
Inferiority vs. Self-Acceptance	**.69**	-.13	-.12	-.10	.35	-.06
N1: Anxiety*	**.63**	-.11	-.17	-.16	.04	.13
N3: Depression*	**.62**	-.25	-.13	-.17	.16	.08
N6: Vulnerability*	**.60**	**-.46**	.03	-.19	.03	-.08
N4: Self-Consciousness*	**.59**	-.12	.05	-.34	.21	.08
Ext. vs. Int. Locus of Control	**.58**	-.11	-.33	.00	-.02	.05
Leadership	**-.51**	.08	-.34	.32	**.40**	.01
Emotionality	**.48**	**-.42**	-.34	.07	-.01	.22
O5: Ideas*	**-.41**	.07	-.19	.00	.14	.36
C5: Self-Discipline*	-.20	**.72**	-.06	.15	-.06	.18
C6: Deliberation*	**-.04**	**.71**	-.03	-.08	.08	.06
C2: Order*	.01	**.68**	.03	-.03	-.03	.10
Responsibility	-.20	**.66**	.10	-.02	.16	-.19
C4: Achievement Striving*	-.16	**.62**	-.26	.27	.04	.09
Meticulousness	.03	**.59**	.09	-.16	.21	-.02
C3: Dutifulness*	-.06	**.59**	.25	.15	.14	.22
N5: Impulsiveness*	.29	**-.57**	-.22	.07	.12	.25
C1: Competence*	-.24	**.52**	-.09	.30	.18	.19
Practical Mindedness	-.22	**.45**	**.41**	-.10	-.06	-.12
Graciousness-Meanness	-.29	.09	**.65**	.02	**-.40**	.12
A4: Compliance*	.21	.14	**.63**	-.00	.01	-.11
Veraciousness-Slickness	-.09	.02	**.61**	-.07	-.17	.11
A2: Straightforwardness*	.10	-.10	**.58**	-.18	.00	-.02
A1: Trust*	-.09	-.02	**.58**	.27	.15	.19

UNIVERSAL AND INDIGENOUS DIMENSIONS OF CHINESE PERSONALITY

Scales / Facets	Factor					
	1 Neuroticism	2 Conscientiousness	3 Agreeableness	4 Extraversion	5 Interpersonal Relatedness	6 Openness
Family Orientation	.22	-.05	**.50**	-.11	-.04	-.08
N2: Angry Hostility*	.34	-.28	**-.47**	-.15	.00	.21
A3: Altruism*	.06	.34	**.44**	.33	.18	**.43**
E2: Gregariousness*	-.04	-.04	.15	**.72**	-.04	-.18
Introversion-Extroversion	.36	.11	.10	**-.66**	-.09	.01
E1: Warmth*	-.09	.06	.27	**.60**	.04	.36
E4: Activity*	-.28	.29	-.15	**.57**	-.04	.10
E3: Assertiveness*	-.35	-.03	-.32	**.53**	.08	-.01
E6: Positive Emotions*	-.16	-.08	.11	**.51**	-.04	.32
Self vs. Social Orientation	-.37	.04	**-.41**	**-.41**	.30	.11
Optimism-Pessimism	-.15	-.02	.05	-.14	**-.63**	-.07
Ren Qing (Relationship) Orientation	.00	.06	.27	-.08	**.59**	.28
Flexibility	-.11	-.28	.24	.05	**-.58**	.15
Defensiveness (Ah-Q Attitude)	.10	-.03	-.51	-.04	**.57**	-.08
Harmony	.15	.35	.39	-.02	**.57**	-.05
Face	**.41**	-.03	-.25	.09	**.56**	-.03
Logical vs. Affective Orientation	-.35	.35	-.08	-.16	**.53**	.08
O3: Feelings*	.15	.15	-.04	.16	.03	**.74**
O2: Aesthetics*	-.07	.11	.02	-.06	-.06	**.69**
O1: Fantasy*	.12	-.39	.03	-.14	.03	**.54**
A6: Tender-mindedness*	.13	.02	.22	.24	.21	**.41**
A5: Modesty*	.37	-.02	.30	-.26	-.02	-.28
O4: Actions*	-.26	-.24	-.22	.10	-.14	-.02
Thrift-Extravagance	.16	.34	.11	-.28	.22	-.08
Modernization	-.32	-.10	.35	-.05	-.19	.33
E5: Excitement-seeking*	-.08	-.28	-.31	.27	.16	.25
O6: Values*	-.16	.09	.34	.14	-.14	.35
Eigenvalue	8.35	5.06	4.92	3.66	2.16	1.82
Variance Explained	16.1%	9.7%	9.5%	7.0%	4.2%	3.5%

Note. Scales marked with * are personality facets from NEO-PI-R; unmarked scales are from CPAI.

150 FANNY M. CHEUNG

In a confirmatory factor analysis used to test the goodness of fit of the six-factor model, the statistics indicated a good fit to the data. In contrast, a principal components analysis which tried to fit the data into a five-factor model showed that the original five-factor structure was not retained. The uniqueness of the Interpersonal Relatedness factor was confirmed with an independent sample of Chinese mamagers.

4.1 Common Domains Among the CPAI and the Big Five Factors

Are there commonalities between the CPAI factors and the Big Five? In the first study, four of the Big Five domains obtained from the NEO-PI-R shared a large overlap with the CPAI factors in the six-factor solution (i.e., Neuroticism, Conscientiousness, Agreeableness, and Extraversion). These four factors represent the core domains that are shared by the NEO-PI-R and the CPAI. These results were replicated by confirmatory factor analysis in the second study.

How do these four NEO factors compare with the CPAI factors? The Emotionality-related scales of the CPAI Dependability factor are comparable to the NEO-PI Neuroticism domain. The Dependability factor of the CPAI is broader in scope and encompasses both the Conscientiousness and the Agreeableness domains of the NEO-PI. The CPAI Social Potency factor is positively related to the Extraversion domain, as well as negatively related to some of the facets in the Neuroticism domain of the NEO-PI.

In the joint factor analysis of both studies, none of the CPAI scales loaded on the Openness factor. There are several possible reasons for this absence. One possibility is that openness as defined in the five-factor model is not a culturally relevant personality dimension in the person-perception of the Chinese people. Alternatively, openness-related constructs may not have stood out prominently in the person-description method used in the development of the CPAI, or may have been deemed less important by the test developers when the constructs were selected for inclusion in the CPAI.

The relevance of the Openness factor among the Chinese people may be examined by looking at other studies of the Big Five involving Chinese respondents. The factor structure of the NEO-PI-R itself for the same group of Chinese students participating in Study One has been analyzed separately in another study using confirmatory factor analysis (Leung, Cheung, J. X. Zhang, Song, & Xie, 1997). The Big Five was basically identifiable among these Chinese students. Similarly, studies with the NEO-PI in Hong Kong (Bond, 1994) also supported the five-factor model. Even when other indigenous instruments were used with the NEO-PI, they could be "coaxed to reveal a five-factor solution that bears plausible functional similarity to the Big Five" (p.116). In a U.S. study comparing the five-factor structure of Chinese and American undergraduates in the U.S. (Trull & Geary, 1997), a high degree of congruency was also found in the pattern of factor loadings across the two samples.

The Openness domain, however, has not been consistently extracted in cross-cultural studies of the Big Five (Bond, 1994). It was found in a number of studies (Yik & Bond, 1993) and was shown to predict mutual friendship in a Chinese sample (Lee & Bond, 1998). Openness to Experience is conceptualized as a broad construct that encompasses tender-mindedness, imaginativeness, liberal thinking, receptivity to many varieties of experience, and a fluid and permeable structure of consciousness. McCrae (1990) admitted that this factor seemed to be poorly represented in natural languages especially for the less observable traits characterizing the structure of consciousness. In the Leung et al. (1997) study, two facets from the Openness domain (Actions and Values) were considered as non-equivalent across the Chinese and the American structures. These two facets also showed low variable congruence in other Hong Kong data (McCrae, Costa & Yik, 1996).

5. THE INTERPERSONAL RELATEDNESS FACTOR

Even though the five-factor model is recoverable, it does not prove that the model is adequate and sufficient in providing a comprehensive description of the Chinese personality. The results from the joint factor analyses of the CPAI and Big Five measures support a six-factor model, with one unique factor loaded entirely by CPAI scales. These scales from the Interpersonal Relatedness factor include *Ren Qing*, Harmony, Face, and Flexibility. The first three scales were developed specifically for the CPAI.

5.1 Ren Qing (Relationship Orientation)

Ren Qing is a complicated social relationship concept in the Chinese culture in which social favors are exchanged in the form of money, goods, information, status, service, and affection according to the category of social ties between the individuals involved in the interaction. The forms of interaction include courteous rituals, exchange of resources, reciprocity, maintaining and utilizing useful ties, and nepotism. This scale is designed to assess adherence to the cultural norms of interaction based on reciprocity, exchange of social favors, and exchange of affection according to the implicit social rules (Bond & Hwang, 1986; Gabrenya & Hwang, 1996).

5.2 Harmony

Harmony assesses one's inner peace of mind, contentment, interpersonal harmony, avoidance of conflict, and maintenance of equilibrium, which are considered to be virtues in the Chinese culture (Gabrenya & Hwang, 1996; Gao, Ting-Toomey, & Gudykunst, 1996).

5.3 Face

Face is a dominant concept in interpreting and regulating social behavior in the Chinese culture. This scale taps the Chinese concept of face in an interpersonal and

152 FANNY M. CHEUNG

hierarchical connection, and social behaviors to protect and enhance one's face, to promote others' respect toward oneself, and to avoid losing one's face (Bond & Hwang, 1986; Gabrenya & Hwang, 1996).

5.4 Value of the Interpersonal Relatedness Factor

The characteristics associated with these personality scales reflect a strong orientation toward instrumental relationships, avoidance of internal, external and interpersonal conflict, and adherence to norms and tradition. Is the Interpersonal Relatedness factor useful to the study of the Chinese personality? The personality characteristics associated with the Interpersonal Relatedness factor have been drawn from the works of Chinese social psychologists who have advocated for the development of an indigenous psychology of the Chinese people (Hwang, 1987; Yang, 1986). These constructs have been found to be related to conflict avoidance, conflict resolution, self-esteem, as well as life satisfaction (Kwan, Bond, & Singelis, 1997; Leung, 1997).

The original Chinese Tradition factor scales of the CPAI have been used in a number of studies on social relationships in the Chinese culture. The results support the utility of the Chinese Tradition factor in predicting Chinese social behavior. For example, J. X. Zhang (1997) found that the Chinese Tradition factor as a whole predicted the general trust trait across different situations. Specific CPAI scales were related to target-based trust. Trust of intimate persons in one's in-group was positively related to the Harmony scale, whereas trust of strangers in the out-group was negatively related to the *Ren Qing* scale. In another study with Chinese students in Hong Kong and Beijing, the Harmony and *Ren Qing* scales were also found to add predictive value beyond those contributed by the Big Five dimensions in predicting filial piety (J. X. Zhang & Bond, 1998). In a study with Chinese managers in Guangzhou, the Chinese Tradition items associated with the Face, Harmony and Flexibility scales contributed additional variance beyond that of the NEO-FFI facets in predicting the use of interpersonal persuasion tactics (Sun, 1997).

The Interpersonal Relatedness scales have been found to predict life satisfaction and psychopathology (Gan & Cheung, 1996). The Interpersonal Relatedness factor consisting of four CPAI scales (positive loadings on Harmony and *Ren Qing*, negative loadings on Modernization and Flexibility) predicted greater life satisfaction and somatization and less antisocial behavior for both males and females in the CPAI standardization sample. However, the Interpersonal Relatedness factor predicted depression only for the Chinese female respondents.

This pattern of relationships was replicated in another study which examined the interrelations between personality, coping and mental health among Hong Kong and Hawaiian college students (Gan, 1998). The Chinese Tradition/Interpersonal Relatedness factor was associated with active coping especially related to support-seeking behavior for the Hong Kong sample. In addition to the Interpersonal Relatedness factor, a Dominance factor consisting of four CPAI scales (Logical vs. affective orientation, Leadership, Self vs. social orientation, and Introversion) was included in a number of discriminant analysis models to explore the pattern of

UNIVERSAL AND INDIGENOUS DIMENSIONS OF CHINESE PERSONALITY   153

relationships between personality and psychopathology. In the discriminant analysis models, high Chinese Tradition and Dominance scores were associated with life satisfaction for the Hong Kong students. Specifically, high Chinese Tradition and low Dominance scores were associated with high scores on somatization and low scores on antisocial behavior among the Hong Kong male students; this score pattern was associated with high somatization and low depression among the Hong Kong female students.

It is evident that the Interpersonal Relatedness factor is relevant and useful to the study of Chinese psychology. It is not simply a measure of collectivism vs. individualism that is usually ascribed to the Chinese or other Asian culture. This factor is independent of the Big Five and untapped by all the translated personality measures. Studies on Chinese people using translated personality tests would have left out an important dimension of the Chinese personality.

6.   THE CULTURE-SPECIFIC V. CROSS-CULTURAL NATURE OF THE INTERPERSONAL RELATEDNESS FACTOR

Is the Interpersonal Relatedness factor unique to the Chinese culture, or is it also relevant to non-Chinese cultures as well? The Interpersonal Relatedness factor is derived from scales that are indigenous to the study of Chinese personality. They assess the interpersonal aspects of personality that are important to person-perception in the Chinese culture. These aspects of personality are associated with complex instrumental relationships that have not been covered in Western personality measures. The major Western theories of personality have focused on the intrapsychic aspects of the person, and neglected these aspects of the interpersonal domains. If the Interpersonal Relatedness factor is also identified in non-Chinese samples, it may point to this blind spot in Western theories and assessment tools.

Preliminary findings from one study support the cross-cultural relevance of the Interpersonal Relatedness or Chinese Tradition factor. In Gan's (1998) dcctoral thesis on the coping behavior and mental health of college students in Hong Kong and Hawai'i, the NEO-FFI and scales from the English version of the CPAI were administered to both groups. Data from the NEO-FFI and the Interpersonal Relatedness factor scales for the Hawaiian sample were submitted to a confirmatory factor analysis as in the study with Chinese managers (Cheung et al., 2001). The 6-factor model was still retained in the mixed ethnic group of American students consisting of Caucasian, Hispanic and Asian ethnicities. The goodness of fit of the model, however, was not as high as that found in the study of Chinese managers. If a 6-factor model is used in exploratory factor analysis, a distinct Interpersonal Relatedness factor was also obtained. However, if the facets were forced into a 5-factor model in exploratory factor analysis, then the original NEO facets retained their structure whereas the Interpersonal Relatedness scales were dispersed among three of the dimensions: Neuroticism, Openness, and Agreeableness. Cross-cultural differences were also found in terms of the mean score on the Interpersonal Relatedness factor scales in Gan's study. Hong Kong students scored significantly higher than their Hawaiian counterparts on the *Ren Qing* and Harmony scales.

154 FANNY M. CHEUNG

Gan's study further explored the predictive value of personality traits on mental health indicators including life satisfaction, depression, and somatization. She conducted discriminant factor analyses by gender and by culture. The Chinese Tradition or Interpersonal Relatedness factor was found to be associated with the life satisfaction root and the somatization root in both the Hong Kong and the Hawaiian samples. For both males and females in the two samples, a high Chinese Tradition and high Dominance profile is associated with life satisfaction. A high Chinese Tradition and low Dominance profile is associated with somatization.

Although the results from the exploratory factor analyses from Gan's study show that the original Big Five Model may have a better fit among multi-ethnic respondents from Hawai'i than among Chinese in the People's Republic of China, the Interpersonal Relatedness factor may still have functional utility in a non-Chinese group. This finding suggests that this factor is not only important to the Chinese people, but may also have relevance outside of the Chinese culture. In this sense, it would be more appropriate to label the factor as Interpersonal Relatedness rather than the label of Chinese Tradition to represent the personality characteristics associated with instrumental interpersonal relationships.

One may argue that Hawaiian culture is not typical of Western culture given its strong Asian presence, and would not be a good test for the cross-cultural relevance of the Interpersonal Relatedness factor. The next step is to try out the CPAI in a more typical Western culture in continental America, as well as in other multicultural contexts. In Singapore, the English version of the CPAI has been tested in a sample of 536 ethnic Chinese respondents (Cheung, Kwonk, J. X. Zhang, & Ward, 2001). The structure of the personality scales closely matched that of the Chinese samples in the CPAI standardization sample. In a joint factor analysis of the CPAI and the NEO-FFI, the Interpersonal Relatedness factor again stood out as the sixth factor, as in the case of the Chinese studies. Colleagues are now collecting data from Asian American and Caucasian American samples in continental USA.

7. IMPLICATIONS FOR ASIAN AMERICANS

Clinical and counseling psychologists have found cross-cultural differences in the assessment of Asian Americans (Okazaki & S. Sue, 1995). The pattern of the relationship between personality and attitudes or behaviors was also shown to vary between Asian Americans and Caucasian Americans (Dunbar, 1995). The importance of cultural considerations in psychological assessment has been highlighted since the 1980s. Leong (1986) pointed to the problems with the use of clinical and personality tests among Asian Americans. Mokuau and Matsuoka (1992) queried the appropriateness of Western personality theories when working with Asian Americans. D. Sue and S. Sue (1987) critically evaluated the role of cultural factors in the clinical assessment of Asian Americans. They suggested that cultural factors should be considered not only in test interpretations, but also in the conceptual and methodological strategies of test development.

Research with the CPAI provides the link in cross-cultural personality assessment for Asian Americans. Psychological studies of Asians and Asian

UNIVERSAL AND INDIGENOUS DIMENSIONS OF CHINESE PERSONALITY   155

Americans show common patterns of cross-cultural differences. On the standard Western personality tests, similar patterns of scale elevations were found among overseas Chinese and Chinese Americans. In clinical research and practice, similar patterns of distress phenomenology and attitudes toward psychological treatment were also found (Okazaki, in press). The continuity of cultural roots of ethnic groups is often maintained through parental socialization, even after generations of acculturation. The CPAI factor structure has been found to be consistent across samples in China, Hong Kong as well as Singapore. These societies differ in terms of modernization, western influence, and socioeconomic conditions. It is expected that the "interpersonal relatedness" dimension tapped by the Interpersonal Relatedness factor of the CPAI will be relevant to the personality structure of Asian Americans as well.

One should note, however, that the size and ethnic composition of Asian American populations in the US have changed dramatically (Okazaki, 1998). With different waves of immigration, there is an increase in diversity and shifts in the make-up of the Asian American populations. Asian Americans as a group is not a homogenous ethnic minority. They vary in terms of socioeconomic background as well as degree of acculturation. For example, S. Sue et al. (1996) found significant differences in the MMPI-2 profiles among the less acculturated and the more acculturated Asian American students. Study of the personality structure of the ethnic populations in their original cultural contexts as well as in the acculturated contexts will enhance our sensitivity in assessment. Research on the CPAI with Asian Americans will promote the development of culturally relevant personality theories and assessment.

8. CONCLUSION

Research with the CPAI provides an opportunity to explore the universal and unique dimensions of Chinese personality. Our original aim was to provide Chinese psychologists with an instrument that is culturally relevant to their applied needs. We were able to develop an instrument that captured important dimensions of personality of the Chinese people. Our research findings have led us down a more theoretical path to look at how the cultural reality that is cut by this indigenous instrument reflects upon the imposed reality that we used to know, based on borrowed instruments and borrowed theories.

9. REFERENCES

Berry, J. W. (1969). On cross-cultural comparability. *International Journal of Psychology, 4,* 119-128.
Bond, M. H. (1994). Trait theory and cross-cultural studies of person perception. *Psychological Enquiry, 5,* 114-117.
Bond, M. H., & Hwang, K. K. (1986). The social psychology of the Chinese people. In M. H. Bond (Ed.), *The psychology of the Chinese people* (pp. 213-266). Hong Kong: Oxford University Press.
Butcher, J. N. (Ed.) (1996). *International adaptations of the MMPI-2: Research and clinical applications.* Minneapolis: University of Minnesota Press.
Butcher, J. N., & Pancheri, P. (1976). *A handbook of cross-national MMPI research.* Minneapolis: University of Minnesota Press.

156 FANNY M. CHEUNG

Cheung, F. M. (1985). Cross-cultural considerations for the translation and adaptation of the Chinese MMPI in Hong Kong. In J. N. Butcher & C. D. Spielberger (Eds.), *Advances in personality assessment* (Vol. 4; pp. 131-158). Hillsdale, NF: Erlbaum.

Cheung, F. M. (1995). *Administration manual of the Minnesota Multiphasic Personality Inventory (MMPI), Chinese edition.* Hong Kong: The Chinese University Press.

Cheung, F. M., & Ho, R. M. (1997). Standardization of the Chinese MMPI-A in Hong Kong: A preliminary study. *Psychological Assessment, 9,* 499-502.

Cheung, F. M., Leung, K., Fan, F. M., Song, W. Z., Zhang, J. X., & Zhang, J. P. (1996). Development of the Chinese Personality Assessment Inventory. *Journal of Cross-Cultural Psychology, 27,* 181-199.

Cheung, F. M., Leung, K., Zhang, J. X., Sun, H. F., Gan, Y. Q., Song, W. Z., & Xie, D. (2001). Indigenous Chinese personality constructs: Is the Five Factor Model complete? *Journal of Cross-Cultural Psychology, 32,* 407-433.

Cheung, F. M., & Leung, K., Zhang, J.X., & Ward, C. (2001). *Factor structure of the Chinese Personality Assessment Inventory (CPAI).* Paper presented a the Symposium of "Chinese Personality Assessment Inventory: Factor structure and cross-cultural relevance" at the 109th Annual Convention of the American Psychological Association, August 24-28, 2001, San Francisco, CA.

Cheung, F. M., & Song, W. Z. (1989). A review of the clinical applications of the Chinese MMPI. *Psychological Assessment: A Journal of Consulting and Clinical Psychology, 1,* 230-237.

Cheung, F. M., Song, W. Z., & Zhang, J. X. (1996). In J. N. Butcher (Ed.), *International adaptations of MMPI-2: A handbook of research and clinical applications* (pp. 137-161). Minneapolis: University of Minnesota Press.

Costa, P. T., Jr., & McCrae, R. R. (1992). *Revised NEO Personality Inventory (NEO-PI-R) and NEO Five Factor Inventory (NEO-FFI) professional manual.* Odessa, FL: Psychological Assessment Resources, Inc.

Dunbar, E. (1995). The prejudiced personality, racism, and anti-Semitism: The PR scale forty years later. *Journal of Personality Assessment, 65,* 270-277.

Gabrenya, W., Jr., & Hwang, K. K. (1996) Chinese social interaction: Harmony and hierarchy on the good earth. In M. H. Bond (Ed.), *The handbook of Chinese psychology* (pp. 309-321). Hong Kong: Oxford University Press.

Gan, Y. Q. (1998). *Healthy personality traits and unique pathways to psychological adjustment: Cultural and gender perspectives.* Unpublished doctoral dissertation, Chinese University of Hong Kong, Hong Kong.

Gan, Y. Q., & Cheung, F. M. (1996, August). *Personality traits as predictors of mental health in Chinese: Cultural and gender issues.* Paper presented in the 13th International Congress of the International Association of Cross-Cultural Psychology, Montreal, Canada.

Gao, G., Ting-Toomey, S., & Gudykunst, W. B. (1996). Chinese communication processes. In Bond, M. H. (Ed.), *The handbook of Chinese psychology* (pp. 280-293). Hong Kong: Oxford University Press.

Hwang, K. K. (1987). Face and favor: The Chinese power game. *American Journal of Sociology, 81,* 867-884.

Kwan, V. S. Y., Bond, M. H., & Singelis, T. M. (1997). Pancultural explanations for life satisfaction: Adding relationship harmony to self-esteem. *Journal of Personality and Social Psychology, 73,* 1038-1051.

Lee, R. Y. P. & Bond, M. H. (1998). Personality and roommate friendship in Chinese culture. *Asian Journal of Social Psychology, 1,* 179-190.

Leong, F. T. L. (1986). Counseling and psychotherapy with Asian-Americans: Review of the literature. *Journal of Counseling Psychology, 33,* 196-206.

Leung, K. (1997). Negotiation and reward allocations across cultures. In P. C. Earley & M. Erez (Eds.), *New perspectives on international industrial/organizational psychology.* San Francisco: Jossey-Bass.

Leung, K., Cheung, F. M., Zhang, J. X., Song, W. Z., & Xie, D. (1997). The five factor model of personality in China. In K. Leung, Y. Kashima, U. Kim, & S. Yamaguchi (Eds.), *Progress in Asian social psychology* (Vol. 1) (pp. 231-244).

McCrae, R. R. (1990). Traits and trait names: How well is Openness represented in natural languages? *European Journal of Personality, 4,* 119-129.

McCrae, R. R. & Costa, P. T., Jr. (1997). Personality trait structure as a human universal. *American Psychologist, 52,* 509-516.

UNIVERSAL AND INDIGENOUS DIMENSIONS OF CHINESE PERSONALITY   157

McCrae, R. R., Costa, P. T., Jr., & Yik, M. S. M. (1996). Universal aspects of Chinese personality structure. In M. H. Bond (Ed.), *The handbook of Chinese psychology* (pp. 189-207). Hong Kong: Oxford University Press.

Mokuau, N., & Matsuoka, J. (1992). The appropriateness of personality theories for social work with Asian Americans. In S. M. Furuto et al. (Eds.), *Social work practice with Asian Americans* (pp. 67-84). Newbury Park, CA: Sage.

Okazaki, S. (1998). Psychological assessment of Asian Americans: Research agenda for cultural competency. *Journal of Personality Assessment, 70,* 54-70.

Okazaki, S. (2000). Assessing and treating Asian Americans: Recent advances. In I. Cuéllar & F. A. Paniagua (Eds.), *Handbook of multicultural mental health: Assessment and treatment of diverse populations* (pp. 171-193). New York: Academic Press.

Okazaki, S., & Sue, S. (1995). Cultural considerations in psychological assessment of Asian Americans. In J. N. Butcher (Ed.), *Clinical personality assessment: Practical approaches* (pp. 107-119). New York: Oxford University Press.

Sue, D., & Sue, S. (1987). Cultural factors in the clinical assessment of Asian Americans. *Journal of Consulting and Clinical Psychology, 55,* 479-487.

Sun, H. F. (1997). *Choice of influence tactics in Chinese organizations: The effect of the interactants' personality and status.* Unpublished doctoral dissertation, Chinese University of Hong Kong.

Sue, S., Keefe, K., Enomoto, K., Durvasula, R. S., & Chao, R. (1996). Asian American and White college students' performance on the MMPI-2. In J. N. Butcher (Ed.). *International adaptations of the MMPI-2: Research and clinical applications* (pp. 206-218). Minneapolis: University of Minnesota Press.

Sue, S., & Sue, D. W. (1974). MMPI comparisons between Asian-American and Non-Asian students utilizing a student health psychiatric clinic. *Journal of Counseling Psychology, 21,* 423-427.

Trull, T. J., & Geary, D. C. (1997). Comparison of the Big-Five Factor structure across samples of Chinese and American adults. *Journal of Personality Assessment, 69,* 324-341.

Yang, K.-S. (1986). Chinese personality and its change. In M. H. Bond (Ed.), *The psychology of the Chinese people* (pp. 106-170). Hong Kong: Oxford University Press.

Yik, M. S. M. & Bond, M. B. (1993). Exploring the dimensions of Chinese person perception with indigenous and imported constructs: Creating a culturally balanced scale. *International Journal of Psychology, 28,* 75-95.

Zhang, J. X. (1997). *Distinction between general trust and specific trust: Their unique patterns with personality trait domains, distinct roles in interpersonal situations, and different functions in path models of trusting behavior.* Unpublished doctoral dissertation, Chinese University of Hong Kong, Hong Kong.

Zhang, J. X., & Bond, M. H. (1998). Personality and filial piety among college students in two Chinese societies: The added value of indigenous constructs. *Journal of Cross-Cultural Psychology, 29,* 402-417.

LISA A. SUZUKI, TAMIKO MOGAMI, AND ELLEN S. KIM

CHAPTER 11

INTERPRETING CULTURAL VARIATIONS IN COGNITIVE PROFILES

1. INTRODUCTION

The prevailing view that Asian Americans are a "model minority" and a homogeneous group often obscures the reality of complex cultural variations in cognitive profiles of Asian Americans. In general, the research conducted on abilities primarily focuses on only a few Asian American subgroups (e.g., Japanese and Chinese) to the exclusion of other subgroups. While studies indicate that Asian Americans as a group tend to score higher on quantitative measures in comparison to verbal measures on aptitude tests, there is also evidence that significant subgroup differences in performance exist (e.g., Hsia & Peng, 1998). Issues of standardization, test validity and reliability also impact the interpretation of test performance of Asian Americans given diversity in language, level of acculturation, and other culturally relevant variables.

The purpose of this chapter is to highlight more specifically the cognitive profiles of Asian Americans while attending to subgroup differences whenever possible. The following areas will be discussed: a) Asian American cognitive profiles on standardized measures (i.e., achievement tests, aptitude measures), b) issues of standardization, test reliability and validity, c) factors impacting performance on ability tests, d) interpretive strategies for understanding profile differences, and e) future directions in testing research and test development practices.

2. ASIAN AMERICAN COGNITIVE PROFILES ON STANDARDIZED MEASURES

In this section, Asian American cognitive profiles based upon scores obtained on standardized achievement and aptitude measures will be highlighted. It should be noted that the distinction between achievement tests and aptitude tests is often blurred and researchers may discuss both concepts in reference to the same test. In this discussion we have attempted to differentiate these measures as much as possible. Specific trends in the literature on Asian Americans and related subgroups will be considered.

2.1 Standardized Achievement Tests

Standardized achievement tests are based upon knowledge of curriculum areas (e.g., reading, language, mathematics) that all students are expected to have had the opportunity to learn at various grade levels. Test developers provide normative information to understand the meaning of derived scores related to a nationally representative standardization sample. Studies indicate that Asian Americans demonstrate strengths on tests in the area of math achievement (e.g., Hsia & Peng, 1998). However, Hsia and Peng (1998) cite recent data obtained on the American College Test Assessment which indicate that Asian American students earned comparable scores to White high school graduates on English, Mathematics, Reading, Science and Reasoning, and the overall Composite score.

Intragroup variations exist across Asian ethnic groups in the U.S. with regard to performance on achievement tests. For example, studies utilizing the National Educational Longitudinal Study (NELS) of 1998 suggest that South Asians, as represented by persons of Asian Indian and Pakistani origin, score higher in comparison to other Asian American subgroups in both the verbal and quantitative domains, followed by the Korean American, Chinese American, and other Asian American groups (e.g., Hsia & Peng, 1998). Kao (1995) reports that the South Asians were higher than the other Asian American subgroups in parental SES, educational aspirations, educational resources, outside classes, and other family variables. Kao also notes that Chinese American, Korean American, and Southeast Asian (i.e., Vietnamese American, Cambodian American, Laotian American, Hmong American) students obtain higher math scores in comparison to their White peer group. Pacific Islander Americans, however, obtained lower math and reading scores. Subgroup differences in educational and economic resources may contribute to intragroup variations in performance, which in turn challenge the model minority myth. Furthermore, research by Fuligni (1997) suggests that high achievement may be associated with the emphasis placed upon education shared by students of Asian descent, their parents, and their peer group.

2.2 Aptitude Tests

Aptitude tests assess an individual's performance on particular tasks that are used to predict future performance in a given setting (e.g., school, occupation) utilizing estimates of general ability areas. Some of the most popular aptitude measures are intelligence tests.

Studies in this area often focus on Asian Americans as one group, neglecting potential subgroup differences. The literature indicates that Asian Americans attain relatively higher quantitative skills in comparison to their verbal abilities (Fuertes, Sedlacek & Liu, 1994; Hsia & Peng, 1998; Reglin & Adams, 1990; Sue, 1985; Sue & Okazaki, 1990). For example, it is well documented that Asian American students demonstrate this quantitative greater than verbal profile on the Scholastic Aptitude Test. Hsia and Peng (1998) report findings from the College Board (1990-1991) on average SAT scores of Asian American college bound seniors. The following averages are noted: Asian Americans (n=76,500) Verbal 410 (SD=131), Math 528 (SD=132) in comparison to White students (n=729,245) Verbal 442 (SD=104), Math 491 (SD=117). Reglin and Adams (1990) identified average quantitative SAT scores for Asian Americans 535.5 and average verbal scores of 407.3. This achievement profile in the Reglin and Adams study was in contrast to students of non-Asian heritage, whose average scores were lower quantitative (431.7) and higher verbal (459.9) test scores.

Similar quantitative greater than verbal ability profiles are also reported on the Graduate Record Examination (Wah & Robinson, 1990 as cited in Hsia & Peng, 1998). Asian American U.S. citizen examinees (n=6,133) obtained the following averages: Verbal 480 (SD=127), Quantitative 612 (SD=131) and Analytic 539 (SD=134) in comparison to their White counterparts, Verbal 520 (SD=108), Quantitative 546 (SD=128) and Analytic 557 (SD=118). These profiles are consistent with other literature (e.g., Sue & Okazaki, 1990).

A consistent profile of higher quantitative and visual-spatial abilities in comparison to verbal abilities has also been noted in the intelligence test literature on Asians and Asian Americans (Jensen & Inouye, 1980; Lynn & Hampson, 1985-1986; Vernon, 1982). Studies examining the abilities of Asian children on the Wechsler scales reflect this profile (e.g., Suzuki & Gutkin, 1992). In a study comparing Japanese children to White American children on the WISC-R, Japanese children were found to score lower on verbal comprehension and perceptual speed and higher on memory span, numerical, and spatial abilities (Lynn & Hampson, 1985-1986). Most studies located in our search reflect performance of Asian international students and not Asian Americans on these scales. While Asian Americans are included in the standardization samples of all Wechsler scales, information regarding their specific cognitive profiles is not provided in the test manuals.

In addition, on the Stanford-Binet Intelligence Scale (4th Edition) (Thorndike, Hagen, & Sattler, 1986), the Asian sample included in the standardization obtained the following scores based upon a mean of 100 (SD=16) for the standardization sample: Abstract/Visual Reasoning 102.6; Quantitative Reasoning 103.3; and Verbal Reasoning 96.5. These scores were derived from the 12 to 23 year age grouping.

On measures of nonverbal reasoning, Asians tend to score much higher than average. For example, on the Universal Nonverbal Intelligence Test (UNIT) (Bracken & McCallum, 1998) Standard Battery, Asian Americans/Pacific Islanders (n=49) were compared with a demographically matched White sample (n = 49). Asian Americans/Pacific Islanders obtained a mean of 112.69 (SD=11.81) in comparison to the White sample that obtained an average of 103.29 (SD=14.31).

162   LISA A. SUZUKI, TAMIKO MOGAMI, AND ELLEN S. KIM

3. ISSUES OF STANDARDIZATION, RELIABILITY AND VALIDITY

In considering the meaning of the profiles obtained on achievement and aptitude tests with Asian Americans, it is important to examine the test development process—specifically, the standardization and the establishment of reliability and validity for these measures. The most popular ability tests are often standardized on a nationally representative sample. Stratification variables include gender, parental education, parental occupation, race/ethnicity, socioeconomic status, etc. The standardization sample often represents the most well-formulated and largest research sample obtained on a particular measure. In order for a test to be reliable and valid, the score derivation sample (i.e., standardization sample) must be representative of the population of people for which the test was designed. It should be noted that "nationally representative" often refers to proportional representation based upon U.S. census data. The proportion of Asians in the U.S. is very low relative to other groups; therefore, the number of Asian Americans in standardization samples is often quite small. For example, the Leiter-R (Roid & Miller, 1997) includes only 55 Asian Americans in comparison to 1,138 Caucasian. On some measures (e.g., Kaufman Brief Intelligence Test spanning ages 4–90) persons of Asian ancestry are allocated to the "other" minority category (that includes Native Americans) in terms of racial/ethnic composition of the standardization sample.

Another concern that is often mentioned in the Asian American literature has to do with the issue of language. Most of the tests described in this chapter were developed for native English speakers. Few verbal ability tests have been translated and renormed for other non-native speakers of English. The lack of non-English based measures has proven problematic for clinicians and educators working with clients with limited English proficiency. A few exceptions do exist with translated versions of the Wechsler scales (e.g., Japanese Wechsler Intelligence Scale for Children – III, Nihonban WISC-III Kanko- Inkai, 1998) currently available and new measures like the Bilingual Verbal Abilities Test (BVAT) (Munoz-Sandoval, Cummins, Alvarado, & Ruef, 1998). The BVAT is derived from three subtests adapted from the language proficiency battery of the Woodcock-Johnson Tests of Cognitive Ability Revised (Woodcock & Johnson, 1989), namely Picture Vocabulary, Oral Vocabulary, and Verbal Analogies. According to the instructions, the BVAT "… can provide a more accurate estimate of academic potential than assessments administered nonverbally, only in English, only in the student's first language, or through separate measures of the student's abilities in English and first language" (Munoz-Sandoval et al., 1998, p. 12).

In the case of achievement and aptitude tests, reliability is often established through test-retest, item-total correlations, alternative forms, and split half techniques. Often these procedures are conducted as part of the test development process and involve the entire standardization sample without examining particular racial/ethnic subgroups in separate analyses. Validity of achievement and aptitude measures is often established by examination of content (e.g., achievement tests based upon curriculum content appropriate for age range) and correlations with other popular instruments (e.g., concurrent, predictive validity) such as the Wechsler scales. In the test construction process validity and reliability procedures are often not conducted on subsamples of Asian Americans but instead on the entire standardization sample. Thus, the reliability and validity of these tests with Asian Americans is questionable unless other studies were conducted after the test development process was completed.

4. FACTORS IMPACTING PERFORMANCE ON ABILITY TESTS

Researchers have identified a number of factors that may influence and mediate the performance of Asian Americans on achievement and cognitive ability measures. The focus has been not only on test scores but also on other indicators of educational achievement (e.g., grades, graduation from high school, college enrollment, etc.). It is beyond the scope of this chapter to provide in depth information regarding these different variables. Therefore, only highlights of this literature base with regard to educational achievement are noted in Table 1.

Table 1. Factors Impacting Asian American Performance on Ability Tests

Variable	Definition	Findings
Achievement Motivation	Attitudes toward achievement	Achievement of Asian-American and East Asian students linked to: "... having parents and peers who hold high standards, believing that the road to success through effort, having positive attitudes about achievement, studying diligently, and facing less interference with their schoolwork from jobs and informal peer interactions" (Chen & Stevenson, 1995, p. 1215). Asian American students revealed lower levels of self-efficacy beliefs but outperformed their non-Asian peers on a novel achievement task. Fear of failure explained achievement motivation better than self-efficacy beliefs (Eaton & Dembo, 1997).
Acculturation	Level of acculturation	Inconclusive findings (i.e., presents no significant impact on academic performance for South Asians, Lese & Robbins, 1994).
Brain Size	Magnetic Resonance Imaging	At birth, 4 months, 1 year, and 7 years an Asian sample (n=100) "averaged a higher

Variable	Definition	Findings
		cranial capacity than did the whites or blacks despite being smaller in stature and lighter in weight" (p. 7). Asian intelligence test scores averaged 110 at age 7 compared to 102 for Whites and 90 for Blacks (Rushton, 1997).
Educational Resources	Availability of outside school educational resources (e.g., after school lessons)	Inconclusive findings (i.e., presence of a home computer and books has a positive impact on some ethnic groups like the Chinese and Filipino but not on others such as Korean or Southeast Asian and afterschool lessons were positively associated with academic achievement, Blair & Qian, 1998; Peng & Wright, 1994).
Effort Attribution	Academic success and failure attributed to ability or effort	Effort attribution was positively associated with achievement for Indo-Chinese students (Bempechat, Graham, & Jimenez, 1999) and for Chinese, Filipino, Japanese, Korean, Vietnamese, and other Southeast Asians (Mizokawa & Ryckman, 1998).
Ethnic Identity Salience	e.g., language spoken at home, generational status	High achieving Asian American female undergraduates performed better on a mathematics test when their ethnic identity was made salient, but worse when their gender identity was activated. (Shih, Pittinsky, & Ambady, 1999).
Gender and Math Achievement	Math achievement	Asian males scored higher on math achievement than Asian females at the higher score levels (Fan, Chen, & Matsumoto, 1997)
Generation	Generational status (e.g., immigrant, native-born)	Asian American students from immigrant families of primarily Chinese and Filipino backgrounds had higher grades in both math and English compared to native borns (Fuligni, 1997). Hsia and Peng (1998) found that U.S.-born Asian Americans of various ethnic backgrounds

INTEPRETING CULTURAL VARIATIONS IN COGNITIVE PROFILES 165

Variable	Definition	Findings
		(i.e., Chinese, Filipino, Japanese, Korean, Southeast Asian, Pacific Islander, South Asian, and West Asian) had higher reading scores than overseas-born Asian students.
Home Environment	Home environmental factors pertinent to education (e.g., monitoring children's free time, intact family)	Two parent households were positively correlated with achievement for Korean, Chinese, Filipino, and Southeast Asian Americans (Blair &Qian, 1998; Peng & Wright, 1994). Monitoring free time was positively associated with achievement (Bempechat, Graham, & Jimenez, 1999).
Language	Bilingualism and usage of native language vs. English at home	Speaking a language other than English was positively related to course grades but negatively related to standardized test scores in reading for Asian Americans of Chinese, Filipino, Japanese, Korean, and Southeast descent (Kennedy & Park, 1994). Native language use in the home was positively related to academic achievement for Vietnamese youth (Bankston & Zhou, 1995). Comparison of Chinese American children (ages 9-12) indicated that an overall mean IQ of bilinguals was higher than that of monolinguals (Hsieh & Tori, 1993). The benefits of bilingualism are moderated by factors such as parental proficiency in English (Mouw & Xie, 1999). Use of a native language at home was positively correlated with educational performance among Chinese and Southeast Asian students (Blair & Qian, 1998).
Math Coursework	Number and difficulty of math courses	Higher math achievement was related to completing more coursework and taking more demanding courses in mathematics

Variable	Definition	Findings
		for Chinese, Filipino,Japanese, Korean, Southeast Asian, South Asian, West Asian, and Pacific Islanders (Hsia & Peng, 1998).
Neuropsychological Bilateral Function	Cerebral dominance based upon language	Asian American groups show neuropsychological phenomena (i.e., right to left language orientation) found among Jews of Ashkenazic descent, which may have implications for bilateral cerebral dominance (Fox, 1991).
Parental Education	Years of parental formal education	Parental education level was positively associated with academic achievement for Chinese, Korean, Filipino, and Southeast Asian Americans (Blair & Qian, 1998; Peng & Wright, 1994).
Parental Expectation	Parents' expectation for the children's academic achievement (e.g., years of education to be completed, grades in classes)	Asian American students, including Chinese, Korean, Filipino, and Southeast Asians, had higher parental expectations, which were positively associated with higher performance in math and English (Blair & Qian, 1998; Fuligni, 1997). Years of education expected were positively associated with academic achievement (Slaughter-Defoe, Nakagawa, Takanishi, & Johnson, 1990). Agreement between parents and children on educational expectations enhanced children's academic achievement for Chinese, Filipino, and Korean-Americans (Hao & Bonstead-Bruns, 1998).
Parental Investment	Cultural Financial Social Capital	East Asian (i.e., Chinese, Japanese, and Korean) families of 8th grade students were found to invest more "aggressively in financial, human, and within-family social capital than families from other racial groups (Sun, 1998, p. 432)." Some investment measures indicated more educational return for East Asian students than those from other racial groups.

Variable	Definition	Findings
Parental Involvement	Involvement with schoolwork (e.g., help with homework); two parent vs. single parent involvement	Indo-Chinese (5th and 6th grade, low SES) students' perception of relatively "... frequent parental emphasis on the value of effort" was associated with lower math scores (Bempechat, Graham, & Jimenez, 1999). Negative relationships between parental involvement and academic achievement for Asian immigrants and Asian-Americans were noted (Mau, 1997). [See also home environment]
Peer Relationships	Peer Relationships	The support of peers who share a strong emphasis on achievement has been linked to high academic achievement among Asian American students of Chinese and Filipino descent (Fuligni, 1997; Steinberg, Dornbusch, & Brown, 1992).
Reaction Time	Reaction time of a response to a nonverbal ability task	Inconclusive findings with regard to relationship between reaction time and intelligence. Asians scored higher than Caucasians on the Ravens Progressive Matrices test. Chinese Americans had a longer reaction time and movement time than Caucasians (Jensen & Whang, 1993).
Religion	Catholicism	Catholicism was correlated significantly with educational performance among Filipino and Southeast Asian students (Blair & Qian, 1998).
Socioeconomic Status	Parental occupation, educational level, finances	Higher SES indicators are positively correlated with achievement and intelligence for Chinese and Korean Americans (e.g., Blair & Qian, 1998).

Note: Variables are presented in alphabetical order.

It is evident that there is great complexity in understanding the multitude of variables that may impact the development of particular cognitive abilities for Asian Americans. These range from issues regarding achievement motivation (Chen & Stevenson, 1995) to controversial factors such as biological aspects of brain size (Rushton, 1997). However, a major focus of this literature base has been on language and family variables (e.g., home environment, language use in the home, parental expectations, parental education, and parental involvement). For example, while usage of native language at home has been positively correlated with educational performance for Vietnamese-, Chinese-, and Southeast Asian American students (Bankston & Zhou, 1995; Blair & Qian, 1998), there is also evidence that presents a more complex relationship between language and cognitive functioning of Asian Americans. One study found that speaking a language other than English in the home was positively related to course grades but negatively related to standardized test scores in reading (Kennedy & Park, 1994). At the same time, the potential benefits of bilingualism may be moderated by factors such as parental proficiency in the English language (Mouw & Xie, 1999). Mouw and Xie (1999) suggest that native language use has a positive effect on achievement only when the parents are not English proficient. Thus, bilingualism may serve a functional purpose in enhancing communication with parents.

Many studies yield inconsistent findings related to variables impacting Asian American performance. Inconclusive and contradictory results may be due to different methods of measurement, Asian subgroup differences, or a combination of both .factors. In addition, even national studies (e.g., NELS) have not examined critical variables such as acculturation in relation to educational achievement. Students with limited English proficiency were excluded from the NELS study involving reading assessment tests. This likely resulted in elevated mean score reports for Asian Americans (Hsia & Peng, 1998), which can contribute to the perception that Asians as a group are performing at a high academic level and thus are not in need of educational interventions.

5. INTERPRETIVE STRATEGIES FOR UNDERSTANDING PROFILE DIFFERENCES

There are numerous interpretations that have been put forth in the literature to account for the profiles of abilities noted on standardized tests. The quantitative/nonverbal greater than verbal abilities discrepancy may be explained by the finding that Asian Americans tend to spend more time in mathematics classes (e.g., Hsia & Peng, 1998). In addition, relative lower verbal scores may be attributed to limited English proficiency in home language use and enrollment in English as a Second Language courses (Hsia & Peng, 1998). Hsia and Peng also raise questions regarding the validity of current assessment instruments in evaluating the communication (i.e., verbal) skills of Asian Americans.

The number of variables that may impact performance on achievement and aptitude tests underscores the need to merge quantitative and qualitative methods of assessment in order to obtain a more comprehensive understanding of an individual's abilities. Given that ability tests tend to assess what a person has learned, it is imperative to have information about the examinees' educational background and other historical information (Armour-Thomas & GoPaul-McNicol, 1998).

In addition, the literature has cited differences in the ways in which various cultures view intelligence and ability. Sternberg and Kaufman (1998) provide an excellent review of cultural variations in defining cognitive abilities. With regard to Asian conceptions of ability, Chen and Chen (1988) note that the term *chih li* is equated with intelligence. They found that Chinese undergraduates at two Hong Kong universities indicated that *chih li* was comprised of verbal and nonverbal abilities. However, the study indicated that nonverbal reasoning was the most highly valued skill. Chen and Chen concluded that their findings may be due to the emphasis in Chinese schooling on "... silent mental activities, whereas that of the English schools stressed more group discussion and verbal inquisitiveness" (p. 485). Similarly, Azuma and Kashiwagi (1987) noted the Japanese term for highly intelligent is *atama ga yoi*. People viewed as being *atama ga yoi* were found to be socially competent, task efficient and original. These studies indicate that cultural differences in the value placed upon particular ability areas may also impact performance on cognitive ability tests. Thus, understanding the historical and educational background of Asian American group members is critical in order to interpret the meaning of cognitive profiles.

6. FUTURE DIRECTIONS IN TESTING RESEARCH AND TEST DEVELOPMENT STRATEGIES

Our understanding of Asian American cognitive abilities remains limited given the issues mentioned in the preceding sections of this chapter (e.g., lack of attention to subgroup differences). More research is needed on newer immigrant groups, such as Southeast Asians, Koreans, and Filipinos, given the indications of subgroup differences in achievement. Clearly, the model minority myth misrepresents the educational experiences and achievement of different Asian American subgroups. The educational needs of certain Asian American subgroups are overlooked when stereotyped over-generalizations of high ability and achievement are perpetuated.

There are limitations in both assessment practices and cognitive instruments. A need exists to have more ability measures that are standardized on Asian American samples (i.e., oversampling of minority groups beyond census proportions). In the absence of measures developed for non-native speakers of English, translators and interpreters must participate in the testing procedure. In addition, factors impacting test performance should be addressed in evaluation reports.

Armour-Thomas and GoPaul-McNicol (1998) suggest important future directions needed for the appropriate assessment of all minority group members. These are applicable to Asian Americans and highlight the findings noted in this chapter.

They note that multiple forms of assessment must be developed (p. 17) that:

- Sample a broad range of cognitive processes
- Sample content that is functionally equivalent for the groups targeted for assessment

170 LISA A. SUZUKI, TAMIKO MOGAMI, AND ELLEN S. KIM

- Are sufficiently diagnostic so as to uncover strengths and weaknesses of manifest cognitions as well as emerging cognitive potentials
- Are sensitive to the sociolinguistic patterns that children bring to the assessment environment
- Assess the manifestation of these processes in more real-world environments

Understanding the cognitive profiles and abilities of Asian Americans involves better assessment practices, examination of subgroup differences, broadening of variables studied in research, and development of a model incorporating the complexity of variables which impact the assessment of the abilities of members of the Asian American group.

7. REFERENCES

Armour-Thomas, E., & Gopaul-McNicol, S. (1998). *Assessing intelligence: Applying a bio-cultural model.* Thousand Oaks, CA: Sage Publications.

Azuma, H., & Kashiwagi, K. (1987). Descriptors for an intelligent person: A Japanese study. *Japanese Psychological Research, 29,* 17-26.

Bankston, C. L., & Zhou, M. (1995). Effects of minority-language literacy on the academic achievement of Vietnamese youths in New Orleans. *Sociology of Education, 68,* 1-17.

Bempechat, J., Graham, S. E., & Jimenez, N. V. (1999). The socialization achievement in poor and minority students: A comparative study. *Journal of Cross-Cultural Psychology, 30,* 139-158.

Blair, S. L., & Qian, Z. (1998). Family and Asian students' educational performance: A consideration of diversity. *Journal of Family Issues, 19,* 355-374.

Bracken, B. A., & McCallum, R. S. (1998). *Universal Nonverbal Intelligence Test.* Itasca, IL: Riverside Publishing.

Chen, M. J., & Chen, H. C. (1988). Concepts of intelligence: A comparison of Chinese graduates from Chinese and English schools in Hong Kong. *International Journal of Psychology, 23,* 471-487.

Chen, C., & Stevenson, H. W. (1995). Motivation and mathematics achievement: A comparative study of Asian-American, Caucasian-American, and East Asian high school students. *Child Development, 66,* 1215-1234.

Eaton, M. J., & Dembo, M. H. (1997). Differences in the motivational beliefs of Asian American and Non-Asian students. *Journal of Educational Psychology, 89,* 433-440.

Fan, X., Chen, M., & Matsumoto, A. R. (1997). Gender differences in mathematics achievement: Findings from the National Education Longitudinal Study of 1998. *The Journal of Experimental Education, 65,* 229-242.

Fox, D. (1991). Neuropsychology, achievement, and Asian American culture: Is relative functionalism oriented times three. *American Psychologist, 46,* 877-878.

Fuertes, J. N., Sedlacek, W. E., & Liu, W. M. (1994). Using the SAT and noncognitive variables to predict the grades and retention of Asian American university students. *Measurement and Evaluation in Counseling and Development, 27,* 74-84.

Fuligni, A. J. (1997). The academic achievement of adolescents from immigrant families: The roles of family background, attitudes, and behavior. *Child Development, 68,* 351-363.

Hao, L., & Bonstead-Bruns, M. (1998). Parent-child differences in educational expectations and the academic achievement of immigrant and native students. *Sociology of Education, 71,* 175-198.

Hsia, J., & Peng, S. S. (1998). Academic achievement and performance. In L. C. Lee & N. W. S. Zane (Eds.), *Handbook of Asian American Psychology* (pp. 325-357). Thousand Oaks: Sage.

Hsieh, S. J. & Tori, C. D. (1993). Neuropsychological and cognitive effects of Chinese language instruction. *Perceptual and Motor Skills, 77,* 1071-1081.

Jensen, A. R., & Inouye, A. R. (1980). Level I and Level II abilities in Asian, White, and Black children. *Intelligence, 4,* 41-49.

Jensen, A. R., & Whang, P. A. (1993). Reaction time and intelligence: A comparison of Chinese American and Anglo-American children. *Journal of Biosocial Science, 25*, 397-410.

Kao, G. (1995). Asian Americans as model minorities? A look at their academic performance. *American Journal of Education, 103*, 121-159.

Kennedy, E., & Park, H. S. (1994). Home language as a predictor of academic achievement: A comparative study of Mexican- and Asian-American youth. *Journal of Research and Development in Education, 27*(3), 188-194.

Lese, K. P., & Robbins, S. B. (1994). Relationship between goal attributes and the academic achievement of Southeast Asian adolescent refugees. *Journal of Counseling Psychology, 41*, 45-52.

Lynn, R., & Hampson, S. (1985-86). The structure of Japanese abilities: An analysis in terms of the hierarchical model of intelligence. *Current Psychological Research and Reviews, 4*, 309-322.

Mau, W. C. (1997). Parental influences on the high school students' academic achievement: A comparison of Asian immigrants, Asian Americans, and White Americans. *Psychology in the Schools, 34*, 267-277.

Mouw, T., & Xie, Y. (1999). Bilingualism and the academic achievement of first-and second-generation Asian Americans: Accommodation with or without assimilation? *American Sociological Review, 64*, 232-252.

Munoz-Sandoval, A. F., Cummins, J., Alvarado, C. G., & Ruef, M. L. (1998). *Bilingual verbal ability tests.* Itasca, IL; Riverside.

Nihonban WISC-III Kanko- Inkai. (1998). *Japanese WISC-III Intelligence Test.* Tokyo: Nihon Bunka Kagakusha.

Peng, S. S., & Wright, D. (1994). Explanation of academic achievement of Asian American students. *Journal of Educational Research, 87*, 346-352.

Reglin, G. L., & Adams, D. R. (1990). Why Asian-American high school students have higher grade point averages and SAT scores than other high school students. *High School Journal, 73*, 143-149.

Roid, G. H., & Miller, L. J. (1997). *Leiter International Performance Scale- Revised.* Wood Dale, IL: Stoelting.

Rushton, J. P. (1997). Cranial size and IQ in Asian Americans from birth to age seven. *Intelligence, 25*, 7-20.

Shih, M., Pittinsky, T. L., & Ambady, N. (1999). Stereotype susceptibility: Identity salience and shifts in quantitative performance. *Psychological Science, 10*, 80-83.

Slaughter-Defoe, D. T., Nakagawa, K., Takanishi, R., & Johnson, D. J. (1990). Toward cultural/ecological perspectives on schooling and achievement in African and Asian-American children. *Child Development, 61*, 363-383.

Steinberg, L., Dornbusch, S. M., & Brown, B. B. (1992). Ethnic differences in adolescent achievement: An ecological perspective. *American Psychologist, 47*, 723-729.

Sternberg, R. J., & Kaufman, J. C. (1998). Human abilities. *Annual Review of Psychology, 49*, 479-502.

Sue, S. (1985). Asian Americans and educational pursuits: Are the doors beginning to close? *Asian American Psychological Association Journal*, 16-19.

Sue, S., & Okazaki, S. (1990). Asian American educational achievements: A phenomenon in search of an explanation. *American Psychologist, 45*, 913-920.

Sun, Y. (1998). The academic success of East-Asian-American students – An investment model. *Social Science Research, 27*, 432-456.

Suzuki, L. A., & Gutkin, T. G. (1993, August). *Ethnic ability patterns on the WISC-R and theories of intelligence.* Paper presented at the American Psychological Association Convention, Toronto, Canada.

Thorndike, R. L., Hagen, E. P., & Sattler, J. M. (1986). *Technical manual for the Stanford-Binet Intelligence Scale* (4th ed.). Chicago: Riverside.

Vernon, P. E. (1982). *The abilities and achievements of Orientals in North America.* San Diego, CA: Academic Press.

Woodcock, R. W., & Johnson, M. B. (1989). *Woodcock-Johnson Tests of Cognitive Ability - Revised.* Chicago: Riverside.

YU-WEN YING

CHAPTER 12

THE CONCEPTION OF DEPRESSION IN CHINESE AMERICANS

1. INTRODUCTION

The conception of depression has been demonstrated to vary across cultures (Kleinman & Good, 1985). In particular, research has focused on monocultural individuals (see Cheung, 1985; Kleinman, 1986 for a discussion on the conception of depression in Chinese people). Relatively little research has assessed the conception of depression in individuals exposed to more than one culture secondary to cross-cultural living. The chapter reviews the literature on the conception of depression of ethnic Chinese people living in the United States.

The conception of depression in individuals living in a cross-cultural context is of interest due to increased worldwide migration. In the United States, close to 10% of its population consists of immigrants, the majority of whom originated from culturally-different, non-European countries, mostly Latin America and Asia (U.S. Bureau of the Census, 1997). In the case of Chinese Americans, two-thirds are overseas-born and the majority of the remainder consists of children of immigrants (U.S. Bureau of the Census, 1990). Thus, understanding how the conception of depression changes secondary to cross-cultural living is particularly salient for this group. This chapter compares and contrasts major differences between Chinese and American cultures that inform the conception of depression, followed by a review of empirical research on the conception of depression in Chinese Americans and potential variation secondary to differential exposures to Chinese and American cultures.

2. VARIATION BETWEEN CHINESE AND AMERICAN CULTURES

Chinese and American cultures vary significantly. Differences most germane to the conception of depression are highlighted here: the body-mind relationship, self-other relationship, and the view of positive self-concept and affect.

173

174 YU-WEN YING

2.1 Body-Mind Relationship

The body and mind are viewed as dualistic, dichotomous entities in mainstream American culture. Thus, physical and psychological illness are clearly differentiated (Lutz, 1985). The DSM classification of depression as a mood disorder accompanied by somatic symptoms further reflects this division (Jenkins, 1994). In fact, the term "somatization" which describes the concurrent occurrence of psychological and physical symptoms, is believed to result from a transformation of psychological distress into physical illness, rather than the two concurrently and mutually influencing each other (Cheung, 1985).

In contrast, the mind and body are viewed as integrated with each other in Chinese culture and medicine (Kaptchuk, 1983; Wu, 1982). In writing about Traditional Chinese Medicine, Kaptchuk (1983) states, "In the West, the final concern is always the creator or cause...for the Chinese, the web has no weaver...the desire [is] to understand the interrelationships" (p.15). While Western medicine focuses on specific and discrete organs, Traditional Chinese Medicine views the human body as connected by an extensive network of meridians, which link these organs and serve as pathways for the circulation of *chi* (or energy) throughout the body (Kaptchuk, 1983; Wu, 1982). Thus, the functioning of each organ cannot be separated from that of the rest of the body. Illness of the soma also cannot be separated from illness of the psyche, and vice versa. In this context, the diagnosis of neurasthenia or "nerve weakness" is strongly preferred by professionals and lay people alike over the diagnosis of major depression as it acknowledges the significant contribution of a physical process and incorporates more physical symptoms in its criteria (Kleinman, 1986). Western-trained mental health professionals have interpreted this presentation as somatization, but from a Chinese point of view, such a designation fails to acknowledge the significant intertwining of physical and psychological etiologies and manifestations (Cheung, 1995, Tung, 1994).

2.2 The Self-Other Relationship

Francis Hsu (1985) has observed that, whereas in the West, a person is defined by her uniqueness and separateness from others, in the East, a person (or *jen,* written with two strokes, each representing one person, see Kagawa-Singer & Chung, this volume) is defined by her relationships. As such, the Chinese conception of self is a social one. The interdependence of the self and other is reflected in the use of body parts to describe intimate relationships in the Chinese language. For example, biological children are referred to as bone and flesh, and siblings are referred to as hand and foot.

Thus, a fundamental concern of Confucian philosophy, a major source of Chinese culture, is self-cultivation, which serves as the basis for family harmony, national prosperity, and world peace. The primary objective of socialization is *tsuo jen* (which literally means to make/become human), that is, to teach a child the proper social rules of conduct and submission of personal desires to that of others in order to avoid interpersonal conflict and social disapproval (Russell & Yik, 1996; Yang, 1995).

Confucian teaching is reinforced by Mahayana Buddhism, another major influence on Chinese culture. The development of compassion is founded on the realization that any self-other distinction is illusionary (Thich, 1987). In addition, the Buddhist concept of *yuan* shows the value that Chinese people accord to social relationships. The concept of *yuan* has no equivalence in English. It suggests current social relationships occur because of attachments from previous lives, and as such, are to be treasured (Chang & Holt, 1991; Yang, 1995). Thus, a Chinese saying states: When people have *yuan*, they will travel thousands of miles to meet. When people have no *yuan*, they will come to face-to-face without meeting.

In contrast, mainstream Americans define themselves by how they differ from others. The American identity may be characterized as individualistic and autonomous (Lutz, 1985; Markus & Kitayama, 1991). Americans guard their privacy, value being in control and free from other people's interference (Bellah, Madsen, Sullivan, Swidler, & Tipton, 1985). This emphasis on the individual is reflected in the capitalization of "I" but no other personal pronoun. Indeed, empirical research has demonstrated that Americans score significantly higher on individualism than Chinese people (Hofstede, 1980).

2.3 Positive Self Concept and Affect

Modesty and self-effacement are highly valued characteristics in Chinese culture and are believed to reflect personal cultivation and wisdom, and enhance social harmony (Russell & Yik, 1996). Thus, Chinese students have been found to report a poorer self-concept than American students (Bond & Cheung, 1983). Moderation of affect, especially positive ones, is highly valued (Russell & Yik, 1996). The Chinese saying *le chi sheng pei* warns that too much happiness results in sorrow (e.g., consider a man who wins the lottery and suffers a fatal heart attack in his ecstasy). In contrast, in American culture, self-enhancing views of the self and positive emotion are believed to reflect individual uniqueness and self-worth (Heine & Lehman, 1995; Markus & Kitayama, 1991). Thus, when given a compliment, the proper Chinese response is to express embarrassment (at being singled out), to modestly deny the compliment, and to diminish or disavow responsibility for the good deed being praised. In contrast, the proper American response is to express pleasure and gratitude, to accept the recognition, and to take credit for one's actions. Americans would misinterpret the Chinese response as lack of confidence and poor self-esteem. The Chinese people would interpret the American response as shameless immodesty and poor social upbringing.

In summary, significant differences exist between Chinese and American cultures with regard to the sense of self and depression. The Chinese conception is likely to integrate the body, psyche, and social relationship, while the American conception is likely to differentiate these. In addition, Chinese people tend to minimize positive self-concept and positive affect, while Americans admire a positive sense of self and open expression of positive emotion. Next, empirical

176 YU-WEN YING

evidence for the American conception of depression is presented, against which the research findings of Chinese American conceptions of depression may be compared. Due to limited space, the discussion will focus on research using the same instrument, the Center for Epidemiologic Studies-Depression Scale (CES-D).

3. THE CONCEPTION OF DEPRESSION IN WHITE AMERICANS

Using the CES-D, Lenore Radloff (1977) examined the conception of depression in large samples of White American adults (sample size ranged from 1,060 to 2,514). The CES-D is a self-report measure that consists of 20 items assessing the presence and extent of depression symptoms in the last week, four of which are presented in the positive direction (thus, reverse coded when calculating a sum score). Employing principal components factor analysis with varimax rotation, Radloff (1977) identified four conceptually distinct factors of depression: depressed affect, positive affect, somatic and retarded activity, and interpersonal relationship (see WA in Table 1 for factor loading, adapted from Ying, Lee, Tsai, Yeh, & Huang, 2000). The loading of psychological, physical, and social items on separate factors supports the earlier discussion of main American culture's body-mind duality and self-other distinction.

4. THE CONCEPTION OF DEPRESSION IN CHINESE AMERICANS

4.1 The General Chinese American Community

Two community-based investigations published in the 1980's examined the conception of depression in Chinese Americans (Ying, 1988) and Asian Americans (Kuo, 1984), using the previously mentioned CES-D (Radloff, 1977). Unfortunately, neither study explicitly assessed acculturation. Kuo (1984) provided less demographic information (from which degree of acculturation may be inferred) than Ying (1988), and his sample also included non-Chinese Americans), (i.e., Korean, Japanese, and Filipinos Americans). Of these, the Filipino Americans are significantly and culturally different from the other Asian American groups under study as they do not share a Confucian and Buddhist heritage. As the chapter focuses exclusively on Chinese Americans, Ying's (1988) study will be presented in fuller detail here.

Recruited through a random selection of Chinese-surnamed households in the San Francisco Public Telephone Directory, Ying's (1988) sample of 360 Chinese Americans was quite heterogeneous. With roughly equal representation of men and women, the participants' mean age was 41 (with a range from 19 to 91). Their educational level was quite varied as well: 26% did not graduate from high school, 16% were high school graduated, 21% had some college education, and 37% were college graduated. In addition, the sample included a large number of immigrants (76%), and recent arrivals (25% for less than 5 years, 19% for 5 - 9 years, and 13%

THE CONCEPTION OF DEPRESSION IN CHINESE AMERICANS 177

for 10-14 years, 8% for 15-19 years, and only 11% for 20 years or more). Although acculturation level was not directly assessed, these characteristics suggest the sample, as a whole, may be somewhat limited on acculturation as 44% had lived in the United States for less than ten years. Also, their high educational level does not necessarily reflect Westernization as immigrants were likely to have been schooled outside of the United States.

Using the same method as Radloff (1977), Ying identified three CES-D factors in this Chinese American community sample: depressed affect/vegetative signs, positive affect, and interpersonal/vegetative/depressed (see CO in Table 1 for factor loading). Notably, two of these factors were conceptually mixed, suggesting that Chinese Americans, on the whole, may continue to hold a body-mind and self-other integrated conception of depression, consistent with Chinese cultural views and values. Recent findings from the Chinese American Psychiatric Epidemiological Study based on interviews with 1,747 Chinese Americans (Zheng et al., 1997) also support the persistence of a body-mind integrated conception of depression in Chinese Americans. Zheng et al. (1997) found that 6.4% of their participants met diagnostic criteria for neurasthenia, a condition that entails the experience of significant psychological and physical symptoms. In addition, over half of those diagnosed with neurasthenia (58.3%) did not meet criteria for any other current and lifetime DSM-III-R diagnoses (Zheng et al., 1997). In conclusion, these researchers argued for the inclusion of neurasthenia as a distinct diagnosis in psychiatric classification schemes used with Chinese Americans.

Returning to Ying's (1988) CES-D study, although her participants had a choice of being interviewed in English, Cantonese or Mandarin Chinese, a significant number (21%) were unable to complete the CES-D in spite of the interviewer's encouragement. The non-completers were further examined in a later study (Ying, 1989). Compared to completers, the demographic characteristics of the non-completers (i.e., being older, more likely to be immigrants, more recently arrived, and less well-educated than the completers) reflected a lower acculturation level. Radloff (1977) suggested four missed items as the cut-off for rendering a questionnaire invalid. Among those who missed more than four items, no clear pattern emerged as to which type of item was more likely to be missed. However, among those who missed between one to four items, the most commonly missed CES-D items were those that assessed positive self-concept and positive affect, that is, "4) I felt I was as good as other people," "8) I felt hopeful about the future," "12) I was happy," and "16) I enjoyed things." These items may be difficult for minimally acculturated Chinese Americans to respond to, as Chinese culture de-emphasizes positive self-concept and minimizes positive affect.

178 YU-WEN YING

Table 1. A Comparison of CES-D Factor Loading of White Americans (WA, Radloff, 1977), Chinese American College Student (ST, Ying et al., 2000), and Chinese Americans in the Community (CO, Ying, 1988)

	Factors				
White Americans (WA):	Depressed Affect	Positive Affect	Somatic/ Retarded	Interpersonal	
College Students (ST):	Depressed Affect	Positive Affect	Somatic/ Retarded	Interpersonal	Somatic
Community (CO):	Depressed Affect/ Vegetative Signs	Positive Affect		Interpersonal/ Vegetative/ Depressed	
1) Bothered	ST		WA		
2) Poor Appetite	CO		WA		ST
3) Have the Blues	WA ST CO				
4) Good as Others		WA ST CO			
5) Keep mind on things	CO		ST		
6) Depressed	WA ST				
7) Everything is an effort			WA		
8) Hopeful		WA ST CO			
9) Life is a failure	CO		ST		
10) Fearful	ST				
11) Restless Sleep			WA ST	CO	ST
12) Happy		WA ST CO			
13) Talk Less	CO				ST
14) Lonely	WA ST CO				
15) Unfriendly				WA ST CO	
16) Enjoy Life		WA ST CO			
17) Crying	WA ST			CO	
18) Sad	WA ST				
19) People dislike me				WA ST CO	
20) Can't get going	CO		WA ST		

Note: From "The conception of depression in Chinese American college students" by Y. Ying, P. A. Lee, J. L. Tsai, Y. Yeh, & Huang, J. S., 2000, *Cultural Diversity and Ethnic Minority Psychology, 6*(2), 183-195.
© 2000 Educational Publishing Foundation. Reprinted with permission.

THE CONCEPTION OF DEPRESSION IN CHINESE AMERICANS

This postulation was empirically tested (Ying, 1987). The CES-D was administered (in Cantonese) to a handful of recently migrated, monolingual Chinese American women. They, too, stumbled on the positive items. When asked about their difficulty in answering these, some comments they gave were "I don't think about being good/hopeful/happy/enjoying things," and "I can't say I am as good as other people, that would mean that there is no room for improvement" or "to think I am as good as other people is rather conceited." These remarks indicate that positive self-concept and affect are indeed viewed as irrelevant, frivolous, and immodest Chinese Americans with limited contact with mainstream American culture. Taken together then, these findings raise serious questions about the appropriateness of using the CES-D to assess depression in primarily monocultural Chinese American individuals.

4.2 Recently Immigrated Chinese American Women

To better understand the conception of depression in minimally acculturated Chinese Americans, Ying (1990) also utilized a qualitative method, and recruited 40 recently immigrated Chinese American women at a Chinatown public health center, where they were receiving postnatal care for their infants or young children. The women were all originally from China and had lived in the United States on average for only 2.7 years (SD=1.6). Their mean age was 29.5 (SD=4.7). They had an average of 8.9 years of education (SD=1.7). About one-third worked in sewing factories and the remainder were housewives. These characteristics suggest very limited contact and engagement with mainstream American culture. All were interviewed in Cantonese Chinese, their preferred language.

The women were presented with a vignette describing a woman with a similar background as themselves, but met DSM-III criteria for major depression. The vignette is reproduced here in its entirety:

> Mrs. Wong is 35 years old. Three years ago, she and her husband emigrated from China to the U.S. They have a two-year old son. During the last two months, Mrs. Wong has lost interest in many things she usually enjoys, such as chatting with her neighbors, taking her son to the playground and watching Chinese television programs. During this time, she lost her appetite, feels tired but has trouble falling asleep. She has difficulty concentrating in the sewing factory. She is worried about her problem, and thinks she ought to find someone to help her with them (Ying, 1990, p. 395).

The women were then asked to provide an explanatory model (Kleinman, 1980) for the case, that is, the name for the problem, its cause, impact, chief complaint, severity, and most feared aspect. Of the participants, 57% described Mrs. Wong's problem as primarily psychological (i.e., unstable mood, worry, anxiety, melancholia, and psychiatric disorder), 30% described it as physical (i.e.,

180   YU-WEN YING

neurasthenia, heart disorder, common cold, or pregnancy), and the rest did not know (Ying, 1990). However, regardless of what they named the problem, a significant intermingling of psychological, physical and social elements was evident when the complete explanatory model was considered (Ying, 1990). For example, a psychological problem could have a social cause, a physical impact and chief complaint. Notably, while the vignette did not identify an interpersonal conflict, the majority of the respondents cited it as a cause, a chief problem, or the most feared aspect of the problem. The projection of participants' own experiences onto Mrs. Wong was evidenced by several women referring to themselves rather than Mrs. Wong in providing their responses (Ying, 1990). Thus, using a qualitative method, the findings also support a highly integrated view of depression in Chinese Americans who have limited exposure to mainstream American culture.

4.3 Bicultural Chinese American College Students

However, the Chinese American population is a heterogeneous one. Although Ying's (1988, 1990) findings reflected an integrated conception of depression among Chinese Americans discussed thus far, it is plausible that there is a segment of the Chinese American population who is more acculturated and therefore holds a more differentiated conception of depression, approximating that of mainstream White Americans. Ying et al. (2000) postulated that Chinese American college students who have been educated in the American educational system are likely to represent such a group, and assessed their conception of depression.

A total of 353 Chinese American students at a prestigious public university on the West Coast were recruited. Of the sample, 34.56% were American-born and the rest were immigrants, with a mean age of migration of 11.71 (SD=5.60). Their mean age was 20.23 (SD=1.77). The study was conducted in English. The students' cultural orientation was empirically examined, and found to be bicultural, as they scored above the midpoint on 9 out of 12 subscales that assessed degree of endorsement of American and Chinese cultures (Tsai, Ying, & Lee, 2000). Their conception of depression was assessed with the CES-D (Radloff, 1977). In contrast to Ying's community sample (1989), there were no missing responses. A principal component factor analysis with varimax rotation revealed five conceptually pure factors of depression: depressed affect, positive affect, somatic/retarded, interpersonal, and somatic (see ST in Table 1 for factor loading). Table 1 shows that the Chinese American college students' factor loadings (ST) were more similar to that of White American adults (WA, Radloff, 1977) than those of the Chinese American community sample (CO, Ying, 1988). Two confirmatory factor analyses further showed that the Chinese Americans students had a better fit with the White Americans' differentiated conception than the Chinese American general community sample's integrated view (Ying, et al., 2000). Thus, there appears to be a significant shift in Chinese American college students' conception of depression from body-mind and self-other integration to body-mind and self-other differentiation, secondary to significant engagement with American culture.

5. DIRECTIONS FOR FUTURE RESEARCH

In summary, the empirical studies reviewed here suggest heterogeneity in the conception of depression in Chinese Americans. More research is clearly needed. In particular, it would be of interest to empirically assess the association of self-concept and the conception of depression (Okazaki, 1997), that is, whether a more individualistic self-concept predicts a differentiated conception of depression, and whether a collectivistic self-concept predicts an integrated conception of depression in Chinese Americans.

Finally, while a Western-conceptualized measurement such as the CES-D is often favored in the study of depression in ethnic minority Americans because of its ease of administration, it falls short of capturing the experience of depression among individuals who do not fully or solely embrace mainstream American culture. This was demonstrated with the problem of non-response in Chinese Americans who have limited contact with American culture (Ying, 1989). Also, the approximation of the Chinese American college students' conception to that of White Americans on the CES-D does not necessarily imply that variation would not be uncovered if an open-ended qualitative method was used.

6. IMPLICATIONS

As Chinese Americans vary in their conception of depression, careful assessment of the client's problem conceptualization prior to embarking on psychological intervention is recommended (Sue & Zane, 1987). Clients with an integrated conception may prefer an intervention that concurrently addresses psychological, physical, and interpersonal distress. This may include problem-solving oriented and supportive psychotherapy, the practice of *chi-gong* and *tai-chi*, and consultation with practitioners of Traditional Chinese Medicine (Ying, 1997). In contrast, clients with a differentiated conception of depression may require less modification of traditional psychotherapy techniques. Still, Tung (1991) has noted that even acculturated Chinese American clients (e.g., those with American college and post-graduate education) in insight-oriented psychotherapy attend to their social relationships significantly more than White Americans, suggesting the persistence of a collectivistic sense of self. Clearly more research is needed to identify means for increasing therapy effectiveness with even acculturated Chinese Americans.

7. REFERENCES

Bellah, R. N., Madsen, R., Sullivan, W. M., Swidler, A., & Tipton, S. M. (1985). *Habits of the heart: Individualism and commitment in American life*. Berkeley, CA: University of California Press.

Bond, M. H., & Cheung, T. S. (1983). College students' spontaneous positive self-concept: The effect of culture among respondents in Hong Kong, Japan, and the United States. *Journal of Cross-Cultural Psychology, 14*(2), 153-171.

Chang, H., & Holt, R. (1991). The concept of *yuan* and Chinese interpersonal relationships. In S. Ting-Toomey & F. Korzenny (Eds.), *Cross-cultural interpersonal communication* (pp. 28-57). Newbury Park, CA: Sage Publications.

Cheung, F. M. (1985). An overview of psychopathology in Hong Kong with special reference for somatic presentation. In. W. S. Tseng & D. Y. H. Wu (Eds.), *Chinese culture and mental health* (pp. 287-304). Orlando, FL: Academic Press.

Cheung, F. M. (1995). Facts and myths about somatization among the Chinese. In T. Y. Lin, W. S. Tseng, & E. K. Yeh (Eds.), *Chinese society and mental health* (pp. 156-166). Hong Kong: Oxford University Press.

Heine, S. J., & Lehman, D. R. (1995). Cultural variation in unrealistic optimism: Does the West feel more vulnerable than the East? *Journal of Personality and Social Psychology, 68*(4), 595-607.

Hofstede, G. H. (1980). *Culture's consequences: International differences in work-related values.* Beverly Hills, CA: Sage.

Hsu, F. L. K. (1985). The self in cross-cultural perspective. In A. Marsella, G. DeVos, & F. L. K. Hsu (Eds.), *Culture and self: Asian and Western perspectives* (pp.24-55). New York: Tavistock.

Jenkins, J. H. (1994). Culture, emotion, and psychopathology. In S. Kitayama & H. Markus (Eds.), *Emotion and culture: Empirical studies of mutual influence* (pp. 307-335). Washington, DC: The American Psychological Association.

Kaptchuk, T. J. (1983). *The web that has no weaver: Understanding Chinese medicine.* Chicago: Congdon and Weed.

Kleinman, A. M. (1980). *Patient and healers in the context of culture: An exploration of the borderland between anthropology, medicine and psychiatry.* Berkeley, CA: University of California Press.

Kleinman, A. M. (1986). *Social origins of distress and disease: Depression, neurasthenia, and pain in modern China.* New Haven, CT: Yale University Press.

Kleinman, A. M., & Good, B. (1985). *Culture and depression: Studies in the anthropology and cross-cultural psychiatry of affect and disorder.* Berkeley, CA: University of California Press.

Kuo, W. H., (1984). Prevalence of depression among Asian Americans. *Journal of Nervous and Mental Disease, 172,* 449-457.

Lutz, C. (1985). Depression and the translation of emotional worlds. In A. Kleinman & B. Good (Eds.), *Culture and depression* (pp.63-100). Berkeley, CA: University of California Press.

Markus, H., & Kitayama, S. (1991). Culture and self: Implications for cognition, emotion, and motivation. *Psychological Review, 98,* 224-253.

Okazaki, S. (1997). Sources of ethnic differences between Asian American and White American college students on measures of depression and social anxiety. *Journal of Abnormal Psychology, 106*(1), 52-60.

Radloff, L. (1977). The CES-D Scale: A self-report depression scale for research in the general population. *Applied Psychological Measurement, 1,* 385-401.

Russell, J. A, & Yik, M. S. M. (1996). Emotion among the Chinese. In M. H. Bond (Ed.), *The handbook of Chinese psychology* (pp. 166-188). Hong Kong: Oxford University Press.

Sue, S., & Zane, N. (1987). The role of culture and cultural techniques in psychotherapy: A critique and reformulation. *American Psychologist, 42*(1), 37-45.

Thich, N. H. (1987). *Being peace.* Berkeley, CA: Parallax Press.

Tsai, J. L., Ying, Y., & Lee, P. A. (2000). The meaning of "being Chinese" and "being American": Variation among Chinese American young adults. *Journal of Cross-Cultural Psychology, 31*(3), 302-322.

Tung, M. (1991). Insight-oriented psychotherapy and the Chinese patient. *American Journal of Orthopsychiatry, 61*(2), 186-194.

Tung, M. (1994). Symbolic meanings of the body in Chinese culture and "somatization." *Culture, Medicine and Psychiatry, 18,* 483-492.

U.S. Bureau of the Census (September, 1997). *CPS publication - Country of origin and year of entry into the U.S. of the foreign-born: March 1997* [WWW Document]. URL: http://www.bls.census.gov/cps/pub/1997/forborn.htm

Wu, D. Y. H. (1982). Psychotherapy and emotion in Traditional Chinese Medicine. In A. J. Marsella & G. M. White (Eds.), *Cultural conceptions of mental health and therapy* (pp. 285-301). Dordrecht, the Netherlands: D. Reidel.

Yang, K.-S. (1995). Chinese social orientation: An integrative analysis. In T. Y. Lin, W. S. Tseng, & E. K. Yeh (Eds.), *Chinese society and mental health* (pp. 19-39). Hong Kong: Oxford University Press.

Ying, Y. (1987). *Depression in Cantonese Chinese American immigrant women.* Unpublished study.

Ying, Y. (1988). Depressive symptomatology among Chinese Americans as measured by the CES-D. *Journal of Clinical Psychology, 44,* 739-746.

Ying, Y. (1989). Nonresponse on the Center for Epidemiologic Studies - Depression Scale in Chinese Americans. *International Journal of Social Psychiatry, 35*(2), 156-163.

Ying, Y. (1990). Explanatory models of major depression and implications for help-seeking among immigrant Chinese-American women. *Culture, Medicine, and Psychiatry, 14*, 393-408.

Ying, Y. (1997). Psychotherapy for East Asian Americans with major depression. In E. Lee (Ed.), *Working with Asian Americans: A guide for clinicians* (pp.252-264). New York: Guilford Press.

Ying, Y., Lee, P. A., Tsai, J. L., Yeh, Y., & Huang, J. S. (2000). The conception of depression in Chinese American college students. *Cultural Diversity and Ethnic Minority Psychology, 6*(2), 183-195.

Zheng, Y.-P., Lin, K.-M., Takeuchi, D., Kurasaki, K. S., Wang, Y., & Cheung, F. M. (1997). An epidemiological study of neurasthenia in Chinese Americans of Los Angeles. *Comprehensive Psychiatry, 38*(5), 249-259.

SU YEONG KIM AND VIVIAN Y. WONG[1]

CHAPTER 13

ASSESSING ASIAN AND ASIAN AMERICAN PARENTING: A REVIEW OF THE LITERATURE

1. INTRODUCTION

Parenting is the primary method for socializing children (Darling & Steinberg, 1993). Culture is a critical force in this socialization process. Cultural values shape socialization goals to influence parenting style and practices, which in turn relate to child outcomes (Chao, 2000; Darling & Steinberg, 1993). Chao's (1995) study demonstrates these relationships by comparing the cultural values and parenting practices of mothers from European American and Asian American backgrounds. She found that socialization goals of Asian American mothers were consistent with an interdependent and collectivistic orientation of Asian culture (Markus & Kitayama, 1991; Triandis, 1995). Asian American mothers emphasized interdependence by encouraging children toward high academic achievement to bring honor to the family. This contrasted with the European American socialization goal of emphasizing an independent and individualistic orientation (Markus & Kitayama, 1991; Triandis, 1995). European American mothers emphasized a sense of self-esteem in their children, stressing the personal well-being of the individual.

Chao's (1995) study underscores the role of culture in parenting. Yet, today's parenting literature is dominated by concepts and measures based on Western cultures even though Asian cultures constitute approximately 60% of the world's population ("Six Billion and Counting," 1999). These numbers demonstrate the need to understand parenting practices and their outcomes as they apply to more than half of the world's population.

Two methods of inquiry have been used to examine Asian and Asian American parenting. One line of research evaluates parenting practices based on mainstream or Western parenting concepts and measures. Another line of research examines

---

[1] We thank Xiaojia Ge for our discussions on many of the topics presented in this chapter. Support for the writing of this chapter was provided through the Jewell L. Taylor and Ellen H. Richards Fellowships from the American Association of Family and Consumer Sciences to the first author and the Cota-Robles Fellowship from the University of California, Davis, to the second author.

indigenous parenting concepts as it applies to child-rearing practices among Asians or Asian Americans. We report here on research findings from both types of inquiry. In order to provide a basis for developing culturally appropriate Asian American parenting measures, we extensively discuss how parenting values, goals, and practices are expressed among Asians/Asian Americans.

2. PARENTING CONCEPTS IN WESTERN MEASURES

The use of Baumrind's (1967) parenting typology is most pervasive in studies of Asian and Asian American parenting. The most commonly studied are the authoritarian and authoritative styles. Authoritative parents are warm, democratic, and firm with their children. Authoritarian parents control their children through a set of standards, emphasize respect for authority and order, and discourage democratic exchanges between the parent and child.

Investigators vary in how they operationalize the authoritarian and authoritative parenting styles. For example, Chao (1994) derived her authoritative style from Kochanska's (1990) earlier work. Chao's authoritative construct consists of the following concepts: encouragement of independence, expression of affection, and rational guidance. Research by Dornbusch and colleagues (1987), on the other hand, conceptualized authoritative parenting as follows: examining both sides of an issue, admitting that the youth sometimes know more, and insisting that everyone should help with decisions in the family. Still, another approach by Maccoby and Martin (1983) was to combine the parenting dimensions derived from the early work of Schaefer (1959) and Becker (1964) to construct the authoritative and authoritarian styles. Maccoby and Martin focused on two parenting dimensions, parental control and parental responsiveness/warmth. Parenting with high levels of responsiveness and high levels of control were identified as authoritative in style, while parenting with high levels of control but low levels of responsiveness were identified as authoritarian in style. Clearly, despite the universality of the typology used, researchers did not agree on how to operationalize the construct.

While Maccoby and Martin (1983) combined the study of parenting dimensions with parenting styles, other researchers focus soley on the various parenting dimensions. The most commonly studied parenting dimensions are parental control and parental warmth. Examples of such investigations include research by Berndt and his colleagues and Rosenthal and her colleagues (Berndt, Cheung, Lau, & Hau, 1993; Lau, Lew, Hau, Cheung, & Berndt, 1990). Both the parental control and parental warmth dimensions have shown perplexing and inconsistent findings across studies involving Asian/Asian Americans. Researchers have been puzzled that Asian Americans show more parental control, while also encouraging more independence in their children than European Americans (Lin & Fu, 1990; Wang & Phinney, 1998). This contradictory evidence may be due to the lack of attention paid by researchers in distinguishing the various types of parental control. Darling and Steinberg (1993, p.492) note that parental control can range from restrictive control, to firm control, to coercive control. While firm control is likely to be associated with positive developmental outcomes in children, restrictive and coercive control are likely to be associated with unfavorable developmental outcomes in children. Researchers must distinguish among the various types of parental control to better understand its role in Asian American parenting. Parental warmth also shows contradictory findings. Overseas Chinese adolescents report more parental warmth than adolescents in the United States (Greenberger, Chen, Tally, & Dong, 2000). Within the United States, however, Asian American adolescents report less parental warmth than European American adolescents (Greenberger & Chen, 1996). More comparative studies are needed to better understand how parental warmth is conceived by Asians living in an Asian country and abroad. One way to resolve this discrepancy may be through Chao's (2000) recommendation of examining an aspect of Asian/Asian American parents' devotion and sacrifice for their children, particularly in the area of children's education, as an alternative to assessing parental warmth in a Western derived manner.

Another common parenting dimension is monitoring (Patterson, DeBaryshe, & Ramsey, 1989). Monitoring assesses how often parents track and know the whereabouts of their children and is generally associated with positive developmental outcomes for children. Researchers using the monitoring dimension include Feldman and colleagues (Feldman, Rosenthal, Mont-Reynaud, & Leung, 1991) and Mantzicopoulor and Oh-Hwang (1998).

Other aspects of parenting have also emerged, such as parents' use of induction or reasoning when disciplining their children (Kim & Ge, 2000). In Maccoby and Martin's influential review, they note that the use of induction is not captured in their conceptualization of parenting styles, but is nonetheless important as a dimension of effective parent-child communication.

2.1 Most Commonly Used Western Developed Parenting Measures

2.1.1 Parent-child measures

As discussed thus far, parenting measures employ either the typological or the dimensional approach. This pattern holds for two of the most commonly used measures to assess Asian/Asian American parenting, which are the Child Rearing Practices Report (CRPR) by Block (1986) and the parenting measure developed by Steinberg and his colleagues (Dornbusch et al., 1987; Steinberg, Elmen, & Mounts, 1989).

The CRPR has been used primarily by researchers studying young children (preschoolers and toddlers) while the Steinberg measure has been used primarily by researchers studying adolescents (junior high and high school). The CRPR is a 91-item scale to assess child-rearing attitudes, goals, values, and behaviors. Researchers have used a variety of factors from this scale in their studies, ranging from encouragement of expressivity and psychological discipline (Zahn-Waxler, Friedman, Cole, & Mizuta, 1996) to expression of affection and emphasis on achievement (Lin & Fu, 1990). While the CRPR measure is typically used by investigators as a dimensional measure of parenting, the Steinberg measures can be used as a typological or a dimensional measure. For example, Steinberg, Mounts, Lamborn, and Dornbusch (1991) used a composite of their warm, firm, and democratic parenting dimensions to construct an authoritative parenting style. Yet, a study by Chiu, Feldman, and Rosenthal (1992) examined each of these dimensions separately, rather than as a composite of the authoritative style.

The popularity of the CRPR can be attributed to its use by Lin and Fu (1990), whose paper appeared in *Child Development*. This was one of the first studies on Asian parenting to appear in a top developmental journal. The popularity of the Steinberg scale can be attributed to the notable findings by Dornbusch, Ritter, Leiderman, Roberts, and Fraleigh (1987). They found that Asian Americans and European Americans show differential relationships between parenting and academic achievement. Since then, numerous studies have been devoted to understanding this discrepant relationship (e.g., Chao, 1994; Leung, Lau, & Lam, 1998). Researchers who followed Lin and Fu (1990) and Dornbusch et al. (1987) were likely to use the CRPR or Steinberg measures for replicability of research findings and for comparative purposes.

2.1.2 Family measures

Also commonly used are global measures of the family, including the Family Environment Scale (FES) (Moos & Moos, 1974) and the Family Adaptability and Cohesion Evaluation Scale (FACES) (Olson, Sprenkle, & Russell, 1979). The FES is a 90-item scale for assessing levels of family cohesion, expressiveness, conflict, independence, achievement orientation, intellectual-cultural orientation, active recreational orientation, moral-religious emphasis, organization, and control. Most researchers elect to use several dimensions from this scale, rather than administering the entire scale to their study participants. The most commonly used factors include cohesion, control, and conflict (e.g., Chiu et al., 1992; Greenberger & Chen, 1996). Moos and Moos' factors may be reconceptualized when other researchers use their scale. For example, Chiu et al. subsumed the cohesion subscale of FES as part of the parental warmth construct in their study. In general, Asian/Asian American parenting is characterized by less cohesion, more conflict, and more control when compared to European American parenting.

Another global measure is the FACES, a 30-item scale assessing two areas of family functioning, including family cohesion and family adaptability. Family cohesion refers to the emotional bonding among family members, while family adaptability refers to how well the family can change and adjust to environmental stressors. Scholars using this scale on Asian Americans have elected to administer the cohesion subscale only (e.g., Fuligni, 1998; Tseng & Fuligni, 2000). Fuligni (1998) found that levels of cohesion are similar among children of various ethnicities and generations. In his study, Asian Americans were represented by Chinese and Filipino adolescents.

ASSESSING ASIAN AND ASIAN AMERICAN PARENTING: A REVIEW OF THE LITERATURE

2.2 Limitations of Assessing Asian Parenting Using Western Based Measures

One of the consequences of using Western based measures to assess Asian/Asian American parenting has been that Asian/Asian American parenting is depicted unfavorably when compared to European American parenting. In general, Asian American parents are described as stricter in discipline and more restrictive (Chao, 1994; Kelley & Tseng, 1992; Wang & Phinney, 1998) than their European American counterparts. Consistent with these findings, Honig and Chung (1989) report Korean mothers to be the most punitive of the ethnic groups (Indian was the only other Asian group) they examined. Further, Bornstein and colleagues (1998) showed that Japanese mothers self-rate themselves to be the least competent and satisfied with their parenting compared to any of the other non-Asian ethnic groups they examined. Bornstein and colleagues argue that due to the high value placed on modesty in Japanese culture, it may be culturally inappropriate for the Japanese to assert their competence and satisfaction in parenting. It is therefore critical to interpret research findings by considering the appropriate expression of behaviors within a particular culture.

It is also unfortunate that empirical research on Asian versus European American parenting practices has paid little attention to the role of socioeconomic status. Researchers have noted the difficulty of having a comparable sample of Chinese and European Americans in terms of socioeconomic status, with the Chinese typically showing lower SES than European Americans (e.g., Leung et al., 1998). This has dire consequences, since the negative relationship between SES and parenting has depicted Asian parenting as less favorable than European American parenting.

Unfortunately, the bulk of the research on Asian/Asian American parenting have blindly applied Western parenting concepts to Asian/Asian Americans. Some have proceeded with great care in translating questionnaires to an Asian language and are sensitive to idioms and measurement equivalence across cultures. Despite such efforts, there is an appalling lack of indigenous and culture-specific Asian parenting concepts in the studies examined. This may be due to the large number of Western investigators initiating research studies on Asian/Asian Americans. For many, the goal is to apply measures that they have normed and validated on a Western sample to a non-Western sample. Another reason may be that quantitative researchers have overlooked the qualitative research, which has focused on culture-specific concepts of Asian/Asian American parenting. This is due to the difficulty of crossing disciplinary lines between quantitative and qualitative research. The work of qualitative researchers (most notably anthropologists) typically does not involve developing items for scales and measures. Therefore, psychologists who rely on scales have generally overlooked the qualitative research. As psychologists are acknowledging the need to integrate qualitative and quantitative research methodologies, we foresee newly developed parenting scales incorporating culture-specific parenting items. It is critical that researchers continuously re-evaluate the validity and reliability of their measures, as culture is not stagnant but changing over time.

3. ASIAN PARENTING CONCEPTS DERIVED FROM QUALITATIVE INVESTIGATIONS

Qualitative research provides insight into important indigenous concepts of Asian parenting. Most of the qualitative information about parenting has come from anthropological fieldwork. Researchers stayed in various villages in Asia for a period of time and made observations within the cultural context of the society. The anthropologists generally did not use standardized measures to collect information. Instead, they learned about the villagers' parenting beliefs and practices through observations and through informal interviews and discussions with the village people. As a result of the qualitative approach, several parenting themes have emerged. These themes include parenting responsibility, filial piety and family structure, parental affect, discipline, and autonomy and control.

3.1 Parenting Responsibility

For Asian parents, especially for Chinese parents, Confucius' teachings formed the basis of the cultural model of childcare and education (Wu, 1996). Confucius taught that a person does not become a competent human being unless educated through deliberate efforts. It was the parents' responsibility to teach and the child's responsibility to learn. Teaching by example and modeling was an important way through which parents and teachers could socialize the child.

3.2 Filial Piety and Family Structure

Confucian philosophy was the basis for one of the most important concepts in Asian families, filial piety. This ideal, the devotion of children to the parents, not only involves supporting one's parents, but also includes showing respect and warmth (Lang, 1946). Filial piety also consists of total and unconditional obedience, an unquestioned compliance of parents' wishes, and ancestral worship after the death of the parents (Harrell, 1982). A related concept, that has also originated from Confucian thought, was the tradition of a hierarchical, authoritarian, patriarchal family based on "deference, submission, and respect" (Anderson, 1998). The familial hierarchy followed the status of one's generation, age, and sex (Lang, 1946). Those who were older in generation and in age were superior over those younger in generation and in age. Males were superior to females. In patriarchal families, the father held the most power and authority in the household. In most of the fieldwork involving Chinese families, this tradition was observed.

3.3 Parental Affect

Parents' attitudes towards expression of emotions and warmth are another recurring theme in qualitative research. In general, infants and young children received much affection from parents. On the other hand, relationships with older children were devoid of nurturance. Lang (1946) and Wolf (1972) found that parents believed that if they showed the children affection, they would spoil the children, and the children would not respect or fear the parents anymore. The parents also felt that they should not praise older children while they were present. They believed that praise would cause the child to think that they were good enough and not improve him or herself. These parents felt that this was the only way they could teach their children.

3.4 Discipline

Parental discipline is another main issue in the qualitative literature. As seen throughout the literature, traditional Asian families placed great emphasis on training children to behave properly and to be obedient. Wolf (1972) discovered that a basic philosophy of socialization for Taiwanese families was that if you wanted to train a child, the child must fear you. "The only way to encourage desired behavior is to punish undesired behavior severely" (p. 68). This belief was related to the parent practices of not showing affection and not praising the children, so that the children would not be spoiled, and that they would obey.

3.5 Autonomy and Control

A final recurring theme found in the qualitative literature is the amount of autonomy and control the parent exerts over the child. This area includes the practices of monitoring, impulse control, and control of aggression. Confucian philosophy stressed composed, reverential behavior in children. As a result, Asian parents exercised high impulse control over their children, who were trained to behave properly and discouraged from showing their emotions. Children were to behave solemnly and with self-control. Mothers constantly stayed close to their young children out of protectiveness and physical caring rather than out of consideration for their emotional needs. Although children had their physical needs met, they were not allowed to be active or explore. Prohibitive training in the areas of sex and aggression were the most severe. In general, traditional Chinese parents did not encourage their children to be independent or participate in active or exploratory activities, especially if there was a risk of physical injury (Ho, 1986). These restrictions on physical activity were based on the Confucian principle of filial piety, which greatly emphasized discipline and proper behavior. It was also possible that parents did not want children to injure themselves because they were the ones who would care for aged parents in the future. From the literature, it appears that children were allowed minimal amount of freedom and autonomy.

192   SU YEONG KIM AND VIVIAN Y. WONG

4. ASIAN/ASIAN AMERICAN PARENTING MEASURES AND RESEARCH DESIGN

4.1 Parenting Measures Using Culturally Derived Concepts

In recent years, several psychologists have begun to address the need for culture-specific parenting scales. The first well-known scale was developed by Chao (1994), to assess the degree to which Chinese parents endorse *guan*, or "training" as their parenting goal. This "training" concept expects children to follow a standard of conduct, stresses the role of parents as teachers of appropriate behavior for children, and emphasizes academic success from children to reflect positively on the family. These goals are accomplished through parental involvement, especially through parents' devotion and sacrifice for the child. This 13-item scale addresses parenting goals as they apply to "ideologies on child development and learning" and "ideologies on the mother-child relationship" (Chao, 1994, p.1115). Chao finds that this culturally derived concept of "training" or teaching is endorsed more often by Asian American parents than European American parents. Further work on this scale has extended beyond parenting goals to include parenting practices, or behavioral indicators of *guan* (Stewart et al., 1998).

Family obligation is another concept that has recently emerged in the Asian American parenting literature (Fuligni, Tseng, & Lam, 1999; Phinney, Ong, & Madden, 2000). The measures developed by Fuligni et al. and Phinney et al. were developed on immigrant populations, including Asian immigrants. Fuligni et al.'s measure includes three subscales of current assistance (11-items), respect for family (7-items), and future support (6-items). Adolescents rate how often they are expected to contribute to the household, how important it is to show respect for the family, and also how much they expect to support their parents when they are older. A similar scale was also developed by Phinney et al. as an 8-item measure. Items assess how much children should obey their parents and how important it is to follow parents' wishes and desires.

There is also a family conflict measure for use with Asian Americans (Lee, Choe, Kim, & Ngo, 2000). This 10-item scale assess common intergenerational conflicts in Asian immigrant families, such as adolescent's personal sacrifices for the sake of the family, or parents demanding more respect than adolescents want to display to elders. This scale has conceptual overlap with the family obligation measures developed by Phinney et al. (2000) and Fuligni et al. (1999), in that it emphasizes the importance of meeting familial and parental expectations.

4.2 Parenting Assessment Research Designs

There are some consistencies in research design for quantitative studies of Asian/Asian American parenting. In research with preschoolers, a parent, typically the mother, is asked to complete questionnaires regarding the child's behavior and her parenting practices. In research with adolescents, studies are typically conducted

ASSESSING ASIAN AND ASIAN AMERICAN PARENTING: A REVIEW OF THE LITERATURE

in schools where adolescents self-report their perceptions of parenting practices in the home. These study designs are limiting since they are based on single informant, single method, and single level assessments. Researchers have advocated the need for multimethod, multi-informant, and multilevel assessment of the family (Bank, Dishion, Skinner, & Patterson, 1990; Cook & Goldstein, 1993; Hayden et al., 1998; Jacob & Windle, 1999). This use of multimethods is recommended to reduce method variance. Multiple informants can include self-report, clinical ratings, and observer ratings. This insures that both the "insider" and "outsider" view of family relationships are assessed (Carlson, 1995). Carlson notes that the correspondence between the "insider" and "outsider' view of the family is not always high, but that both are needed to capture a more objective view of the family. Multilevel assessments can include the dyadic as well as family level ratings (Hayden et al., 1998). For example, Jacob and Windle (1999) use the same measure and ask informants to assess family functioning several times, between parent-child, between the spouses, and the family. A recent study by X. Chen and colleagues (X. Chen et al., 2000a) appears promising, where multiple methods including mothers' self-ratings and observation ratings were used to assess parenting relations.

5. ASIAN/ASIAN AMERICAN PARENTING RESEARCH

5.1 Migration, Acculturation, and Parenting

Although there has been a large influx of immigrants from Asia to the United States since 1965, only a few studies have examined the role of migration and acculturation on parenting practices. Chiu, Feldman, and Rosenthal (1992) showed that immigration can change parental control and involvement, while parental warmth does not change. Also, Lin and Fu (1990) showed that immigrant Chinese fall between the Chinese in Taiwan and European Americans on measures of parental control, suggesting that immigrant Chinese are more Western in their parenting practices than the Chinese in Taiwan. Another study by Jain and Belsky (1997) suggested that with acculturation, Asian American fathers become more engaged and involved in parenting their children. These researchers have been concerned with how migration and acculturation may change Asian parenting practices to become more Westernized. Gorman (1998), however, has argued that Asian immigrants' parenting should be examined as its own entity, as qualitatively distinct and dissimilar from either Asian or European American parenting.

One shortcoming of the migration/acculturation literature is that none of the studies we reviewed followed the same families before and after migration to understand how parenting practices are influenced by acculturation. The existing studies attempting to untangle this question have used indirect measures of acculturation, such as immigrant status. For example, Lin and Fu's (1990) study included Chinese in Taiwan, Chinese immigrants, and European Americans. They infer the role of acculturation on parenting practices by comparing the parenting scores of Chinese in Taiwan versus Chinese immigrants in the U.S. While researchers typically use immigrant status as a proxy for acculturation, Rogler, Cortes, & Malgady (1991) advocate for a direct measure of acculturation. The assumption that parenting practices of immigrant Chinese in the U.S. are always more Western than parenting practices in Taiwan ignores the variability and range of parenting practices within each of these groups.

5.2 Parenting Across Age

Qualitative research on Chinese child rearing supports the ideas that patterns of socialization change as a function of the child's age (Ho, 1986; Ho, 1989; Wu, 1996). An infant or young child (under six years old) was considered to be incapable of understanding things. At about age six, the child had reached an "age of reason" (Wolf, 1970, p.41). This view that the child could not comprehend or learn things until about age six resulted in different treatment of younger and older children. Ho noted that parents tended to be indulgent and highly lenient with infants and young children, who were viewed as passive, dependent creatures. Young children were closely monitored and received a lot of attention and affection. In most Asian families, after the child has reached the age of understanding, treatment of the child changed drastically. Parents felt that at age six or seven, the child could be considered a small-scale adult, expected to work, learn, and adhere to their sex roles (Ward, 1985). The period of leniency and indulgence ended abruptly. Instead, strict, harsh discipline was imposed on the child (Ho, 1986). Parents now expected their children to be obedient, responsible, and helpful. Otherwise, they were punished.

Due to the lack of quantitative longitudinal research on Asian parenting, it is difficult to use quantitative research to reach conclusions on how Asian parenting practices change over time. Almost all of the quantiative studies examined were cross-sectional. For a couple of studies which were longitudinal in design (e.g. Shek, 1995), data collection was typically only a year apart, making it difficult to draw inferences regarding developmental change over the course of childhood and adolescence.

5.3 Gender of Child and Parent

There is a dearth of quantitative investigations focusing on how gender of the child or parent impacts parenting practices. Due to the small sample size for many of the studies on Asian and Asian American parenting, dividing the sample even further by child gender would not provide enough statistical power to detect gender differences in parenting. A reason for the lack of investigations on the role of parent gender may be due to the heavy reliance on Asian mothers as study informants, as they are typically the primary caregivers in the home. In many cases, fathers do not participate in a research study. When adolescents are asked to report on mother's and father's parenting separately, researchers have collapsed the two reports due to a lack of significant gender difference in adolescent perception of parenting by mothers and fathers (e.g., Greenberger & Chen, 1996).

ASSESSING ASIAN AND ASIAN AMERICAN PARENTING: A REVIEW OF THE LITERATURE

In our review, we found four quantitative studies focusing on the role of parent or child gender on parenting practices (Berndt et al., 1993; X. Chen, Liu, & Li, 2000b; Lau et al., 1990; Shek, 2000). Two of the three studies were based on data collected by the same research team (Berndt et al., 1993; Lau et al., 1990). In general, adolescents viewed their relationship with mothers more favorably than with fathers (Shek, 2000). Mothers were perceived as warmer, more indulgent, and less controlling than fathers (Berndt et al., 1993; Lau et al., 1990). Fathers' parenting was perceived as harsher than mothers' parenting (Shek, 2000), possibly due to their role as the disciplinarian in the family (Ho, 1986). There was also an effect for child gender, with daughters being more likely than sons to perceive their fathers as warmer and less controlling (Berndt et al., 1993). Also, sons were more likely to report their fathers as more controlling than their mothers (Lau et al., 1990). In addition, sons were more likely to nominate their fathers as the disciplinarians (Lau et al., 1990). Parent gender also impacts child developmental outcomes. Maternal warmth predicts children's emotional adjustment, while paternal warmth predicts children's academic achievement (X. Chen et al., 2000b). A limitation of the two studies by Berndt and colleagues is that parenting was reported retrospectively, where adults in China and Hong Kong were asked to recollect their parents' parenting practices before they were 12 years of age. On the other hand, the studies by Shek (2000) and X. Chen et al. (2000b) were prospective studies.

Although there is a lack of quantitative research investigating the role of gender, both of the parent and of the child, on parenting behavior, a great deal of information on this topic can be found in qualitative research. Anthropological works show a clear differentiation of paternal and maternal roles, and that the sex of the child can affect the parent-child relationship. In Chinese societies, there was a clear separation of sex roles. These roles, which were taught in early childhood, led to the development of different parental roles in adulthood (Ho, 1989). Chinese families were patriarchal; the father was the powerful head of the family. He was regarded as the provider, the one who made the decisions, and the one with the final authority in matters. He was seen by the children as a stern disciplinarian who was to be feared (Ho, 1989). Wolf (1970) observed that fathers in Taiwan were aloof and distant with older children in order to maintain a position of authority. Fathers felt that by behaving in this way, they could command obedience and respect in order to teach their children. Fathers were the most feared in the household.

In contrast to the role of the father in the Asian family, the role of the mother was quite different. Asian mothers were traditionally characterized as being "affectionate, kind, lenient, protective, and even indulgent" (Ho, 1989, p.155). While the father was a symbol of dignity and sternness, the mother was a symbol of kindness (Lang, 1946). She was more open about her love for the children. The main function of the maternal role was to act as the primary caregiver and provide child-care duties (i.e., nurturing the children, meeting their needs, and communicating with them). Mothers monitored the emotional well-being of the family (Uba, 1994). At the same time, however, mothers also punished the children. Wolf (1972) observed that mothers were actually the most frequent and violent punishers. Another function that the mother served was to act as a mitigator or someone who could intervene between the children and the father (Lang, 1946; Yang, 1945). Mothers also helped to build the image of authority for the fathers (Wolf, 1970). From the literature, it can be seen how there is a differentiation of parental roles, and how these roles complement each other in the Asian family.

The sex of the child and its relationship with parenting is another recurring theme in qualitative research on Asian patterns of socialization. In general, with regards to parents' attitudes, there was considerable emphasis on family continuity and care for the aged. Since parents expected to be cared for in old age by their children, as part of their children's filial responsibilities, all children were welcomed and loved (Gallin, 1966). However, within many traditional East Asian cultures, the Confucian principle of patriarchal, patrilineal families still had much influence. As a result, in many families, sons were more highly valued and occupied a higher status than daughters (Ho, 1989; Shon & Ja, 1982). This differentiation in value correlated with the differentiation in sex roles. Sons were the ones who would carry on the family name and lineage. Sons married and brought women and children into the family. They were the ones who would take over the family property and had the responsibility of caring for aged parents. Usually, the eldest son in Asian families was considered to be the most important child (Uba, 1994). Daughters were raised by parents so that they could join another family when they married. Especially for poor families, girls were viewed as a burden and expense (Eastman, 1988). During desperate times, infant girls were allowed to die at birth.

The gender of the child affected the relationship that he or she had with both the father and the mother. Although fathers were generally distant, dignified, and stern with all their children, they were more so with their sons. According to Confucian philosophy, the father-son relationship was the most important relationship of all (Lang, 1946). The father-son relationship could be characterized by "dominance, submission, unity, division, solidarity or competition" (Cohen, 1976, p.193). During early childhood, fathers were allowed to be more affectionate with their sons, but as the child grew older, fathers assumed their distant role. The distance in the relationship was intended to create the position of authority, respect, and fear that the bond commanded (Wolf, 1970). Fathers wanted to ensure that their sons would care for them in their old age, but not take over as the head of the family until then. Sons had to follow in their father's footsteps and be filial and obedient. At times, if the father and son were in competition for power and resources, the relationship was filled with tension and antagonism (Lang, 1946).

The mother-son relationship differed from the father-son relation in that it was characterized by affection and love (Lang, 1946). Their bond was warm and comparatively close (Yang, 1945). Mothers spent more time with their sons and had more influence over their actions and attitudes. Wolf (1970) noted that a Chinese father wanted obedience and respect from the son, even at the price of affection, but the Chinese mother would prefer affection. It would be the affection and sentiment in their bond that would provide the basis for sons to care for their mothers in old age (Wolf, 1972). There was a mixture of warmth and harsh discipline in the relation. Mothers had to establish their authority in the family as well.

The father-daughter relationship greatly contrasted the one between father and son. Lang (1946) characterized the father-daughter bond as being respectful and one of tender love. Wolf (1970) also observed that many fathers enjoyed a "relaxed informal exchange" (p. 45) with their daughters. They would not be criticized as long as they followed the general rules of propriety. The contrast between the father-daughter relationship and the father-son relationship was due to the fact that in adulthood, the daughter's actions would be irrelevant to the father, since she would marry into another family anyway. It was the son who had the responsibility of caring for the aged father, so the father needed to establish the respect and authority early on.

The mother-daughter relationship was similar to the mother-son relation. Mothers and daughters often had a warm and intimate relationship (Wolf, 1970). Mothers also had to train the daughter to be obedient and to help around the home. The daughter's job was to follow in the footsteps of her mother. The mother's job was to raise the daughter to be a good wife and mother. Anything the daughter did or did not do reflected on her mother's training.

5.4 Parenting Outcomes

A wide range of developmental outcomes have been investigated in relation to parenting practices. The most commonly studied outcome is academic achievement, perhaps due to the academic success of many Asian children both abroad and in the United States (e.g., Leung et al., 1998; Okagaki & Frensch, 1998). Other developmental outcomes correlated with parenting practices include mental health such as depression, problem behavior such as conduct disorder, and social competence such as psychosocial maturity. In general, the results seem to parallel the relationship found between parenting practices and developmental outcomes of European Americans, where authoritative and nurturant parenting (e.g., high level of monitoring, high level of warmth) are associated with positive developmental outcomes (e.g., Kim & Ge, 2000). Such a pattern provides some support for Rowe, Vazsonyi, and Flannery's (1994) position that despite mean level differences in developmental outcomes by ethnicity, the underlying developmental processes are similar regardless of ethnicity.

Studies by Dornbusch et al. (1987) and X. Chen et al. (1998) were notable exceptions to the argument advanced by Rowe, Vazsonyi, and Flannery (1994). Dornbusch and colleagues showed that authoritative parenting is not predictive of high academic achievement for Asian American adolescents as it was for European Americans. Also, X. Chen et al. (1998) found that the relationship between child behavioral inhibition and parenting practices are dissimilar between European Americans and Asian Americans. While child behavioral inhibition is associated with parental rejection and punishment orientation for European Americans, for the Chinese it is associated with parental warmth and accepting attitudes. The researchers attribute these findings to cultural norms, where behavioral inhibition or shyness is viewed as a positive personality trait by the Chinese, although as a negative personality trait by European Americans.

6. CLOSING REMARKS

This chapter reviewed the current state of research on Asian and Asian American parenting with regards to the types of parenting measures and concepts used, role of acculturation and migration, differences and similarities across age, child gender/parent gender, and developmental outcomes. Western derived parenting concepts and measures has provided the framework for the bulk of the quantitative studies on Asian and Asian American parenting. While using a Western derived framework may be useful for comparative purposes, this has resulted in limited understanding of Asian/Asian American parenting as its own entity.

Although a few parenting measures assessing culture-specific dimensions of Asian parenting have emerged, there is a need to develop grounded theories of Asian parenting. The review provided in this chapter can offer insights into this process. First, Asian parents or more specifically, Chinese parents, draw many child-rearing beliefs from the traditional teachings of Confucius. There is great emphasis on filial piety and on proper behavior. Second, these beliefs are correlated with the differentiation of parental roles: "strict father, kind mother." Because of the hierarchy in traditional families, there is also sex role differentiation: males are more valued than females. Also, fathers and mothers have different types of relationships with their sons and daughters. Another conclusion that can be made is that parenting behaviors change with the age of the child. Young children are indulged, while older children are expected to be obedient and responsible. Affective control is another recurring theme that is based on Confucian principles. Parents and children are trained not to show their emotions and to act properly. Parents want the children to fear them so that they would be obedient.

It is notable that only a handful of investigative teams have contributed the bulk of the research on Asian parenting, using their same dataset to publish a number of papers on Asian and Asian American parenting. Other investigators have shown little follow up work on Asian parenting. Most discontinue their inquiry of Asian/Asian American parenting after testing the generalizability of their scales on a non-Western population.

We have several suggestions for future research on Asian and Asian American parenting. There is a dire need for studies sampling multiple informants using multiple methods and multiple measures to capture a more comprehensive view of the family. This needs to be incorporated in a longitudinal study design. There is also a need for more culture-specific and indigenous parenting concepts in Asian/Asian American parenting measures. Our review of both the quantitative and qualitative research provides a foundation for developing measures incorporating such culture-specific dimensions, which will allow readers to better understand Asian and Asian American parenting practices.

7. REFERENCES

Anderson, E. N. (1998). Child-raising among Hong Kong Fisherfolk: Variations on Chinese themes. *Bulletin of the Institute of Ethnology Academia Sinica, 86,* 121-155.

ASSESSING ASIAN AND ASIAN AMERICAN PARENTING: A REVIEW OF THE LITERATURE

Bank, L., Dishion, T., Skinner, M., & Patterson, G. (1990). Method variance in structural equation modeling: Living with "GLOP". In G. R. Patterson (Ed.), *Depression and aggression in family interaction* (pp. 247-249). Hillsdale, N.J.: Erlbaum.

Baumrind, D., & Black, A. E. (1967). Socialization practices associated with dimensions of competence in preschool boys and girls. *Child Development, 38*(2), 291-327.

Becker, W. C. (1964). Consequence of different kinds of parental discipline. In M. L. Hoffman & L. W. H. Hoffman (Eds.), *Review of child development research* (vol. 1, pp. 169-208). New York: Russell Sage Foundation.

Berndt, T. J., Cheung, P. C., Lau, S., & Hau, K. T. (1993). Perceptions of parenting in mainland China, Taiwan, and Hong Kong: Sex differences and societal differences. *Developmental Psychology, 29*(1), 156-164.

Block, J. (1986). *The child-rearing practices report (CRPR): A set of Q items for the description of parental socialization attitudes and values.* Berkeley: University of California.

Bornstein, M. H., Haynes, O. M., Azuma, H., Galperin, C., Maital, S., Ogino, M., Painter, K., Pascual, L., Pecheux, M.-G., Rahn, C., Toda, S., Venuti, P., Vyt, A., & Wright, B. (1998). A cross-national study of self-evaluations and attributions in parenting: Argentina, Belgium, France, Israel, Italy, Japan, and the United States. *Developmental Psychology, 34*(4), 662-676.

Carlson, C. I. (1995). Families as the focus of assessment: Theoretical and practical issues. In J. C. Conoley & E. B. Werth (Eds.), *Family assessment* (pp. 19-63). Lincoln, NE: Buros Institute of Mental Measurements University of Nebraska-Lincoln.

Chao, R. K. (1994). Beyond parental control and authoritarian parenting style: Understanding Chinese parenting through the cultural notion of training. *Child Development, 65*(4), 1111-1119.

Chao, R. K. (1995). Chinese and European American cultural models of the self reflected in mothers' child rearing beliefs. *Ethos, 23*(3), 328-354.

Chao, R. K. (2000). The parenting of immigrant Chinese and European American mothers: Relations between parenting styles, socialization goals, and parental practices. *Journal of Applied Developmental Psychology, 21*(2), 233-248.

Chen, X., Hastings, P. D., Rubin, K. H., Chen, H., Cen, G., & Stewart, S. L. (1998). Child-rearing attitudes and behavioral inhibition in Chinese and Canadian toddlers: A cross-cultural study. *Developmental Psychology, 34*(4), 677-686.

Chen, X., Liu, M., Li, B., Cen, G., Chen, H., & Wang, L. (2000a). Maternal authoritative and authoritarian attitudes and mother-child interactions and relationships in urban China. *International Journal of Behavioral Development, 24*(1), 119-126.

Chen, X., Liu, M., & Li, D. (2000b). Parental warmth, control, and indulgence and their relations to adjustment in Chinese children: A longitudinal study. *Journal of Family Psychology, 14*(3), 401-419.

Chiu, M. L., Feldman, S. S., & Rosenthal, D. A. (1992). The influence of immigration on parental behavior and adolescent distress in Chinese families residing in two western nations. *Journal of Research on Adolescence, 2*(3), 205-239.

Cohen, M. L. (1976). *House united, house divided: The Chinese family in Taiwan.* New York: Columbia University Press.

Cook, W. L., & Goldstein, M. J. (1993). Multiple perspectives on family relationships: A latent variables model. *Child Development, 64*(5), 1377-1388.

Darling, N., & Steinberg, L. (1993). Parenting style as context: An integrative model. *Psychological Bulletin, 113*(3), 487-496.

Dornbusch, S. M., Ritter, P. L., Leiderman, P. H., Roberts, D. F., & Fraleigh, M. J. (1987). The relation of parenting style to adolescent school performance. *Child Development, 58*(5), 1244-1257.

Eastman, L. E. (1988). *Family, fields, and ancestors: Constancy and change in China's social and economic history, 1550-1949.* New York: Oxford University Press.

Feldman, S. S., Rosenthal, D. A., Mont-Reynaud, R., & Leung, K. (1991). Ain't misbehavin': Adolescent values and family environments as correlates of misconduct in Australia, Hong Kong, and the United States. *Journal of Research on Adolescence, 1*(2), 109-134.

Fuligni, A. J. (1998). Authority, autonomy, and parent-adolescent conflict and cohesion: A study of adolescents from Mexican, Chinese, Filipino, and European backgrounds. *Developmental Psychology, 34*(4), 782-792.

Fuligni, A. J., Tseng, V., & Lam, M. (1999). Attitudes toward family obligations among American adolescents with Asian, Latin American, and European backgrounds. *Child Development, 70*(4), 1030-1044.

Gallin, B. (1966). *Hsin Hsing, Taiwan: A Chinese village in change.* Berkeley, CA: University of California Press.

Gorman, J. C. (1998). Parenting attitudes and practices of immigrant Chinese mothers of adolescents. *Family Relations: Interdisciplinary Journal of Applied Family Studies, 47*(1), 73-80.

Greenberger, E., & Chen, C. (1996). Perceived family relationships and depressed mood in early and late adolescence: A comparison of European and Asian Americans. *Developmental Psychology, 32*(4), 707-716.

Greenberger, E., Chen, C., Tally, S. R., & Dong, Q. (2000). Family, peer, and individual correlates of depressive symptomatology among U.S. and Chinese adolescents. *Journal of Consulting and Clinical Psychology, 68*(2), 209-219.

Harrell, S. (1982). *Ploughshare village: Culture and context in Taiwan.* Seattle, WA: University of Washington Press.

Hayden, L. C., Schiller, M., Dickstein, S., Seifer, R., Sameroff, S., Miller, I., Keitner, G., & Rasmussen, S. (1998). Levels of family assessment: I. Family, marital, and parent-child interaction. *Journal of Family Psychology, 12*(1), 7-22.

Ho, D. Y. F. (1986). Chinese patterns of socialization: A critical review. In M. H. Bond (Ed.), *The psychology of the Chinese people* (pp. 1-37). New York: Oxford University Press.

Ho, D. Y. F. (1989). Continuity and variation in Chinese patterns of socialization. *Journal of Marriage and the Family, 51*(1), 149-163.

Honig, A. S., & Chung, M. (1989). Child-rearing practices of urban poor mothers of infants and three-year-olds in five cultures. *Early Child Development and Care, 50,* 75-97.

Jacob, T., & Windle, M. (1999). Family assessment: Instrument dimensionality and correspondence across family reporters. *Journal of Family Psychology, 13*(3), 339-354.

Jain, A., & Belsky, J. (1997). Fathering and acculturation: Immigrant Indian families with young children. *Journal of Marriage & the Family, 59*(4), 873-883.

Kelley, M. L., & Tseng, H. M. (1992). Cultural differences in child rearing: A comparison of immigrant Chinese and Caucasian American mothers. *Journal of Cross-Cultural Psychology, 23*(4), 444-455.

Kim, S. Y., & Ge, X. (2000). Parenting practices and adolescent depressive symptoms in Chinese American families. *Journal of Family Psychology, 14*(3), 420-435.

Kochanska, G. (1990). Maternal beliefs as long-term predictors of mother-child interaction and report. *Child Development, 61*(6), 1934-1943.

Lang, O. (1946). *Chinese family and society.* New Haven, CT: Yale University Press.

Lau, S., Lew, W. J., Hau, K. T., Cheung, P. C., & Berndt, T. J. (1990). Relations among perceived parental control, warmth, indulgence, and family harmony of Chinese in mainland China. *Developmental Psychology, 26*(4), 674-677.

Lee, R. M., Choe, J., Kim, G., & Ngo, V. (2000). Construction of the Asian American Family Conflicts Scale. *Journal of Counseling Psychology, 47*(2), 211-222.

Leung, K., Lau, S., & Lam, W. L. (1998). Parenting styles and academic achievement: A cross-cultural study. *Merrill-Palmer Quarterly, 44*(2), 157-172.

Lin, C. C., & Fu, V. R. (1990). A comparison of child-rearing practices among Chinese, immigrant Chinese, and Caucasian-American parents. *Child Development, 61*(2), 429-433.

Maccoby, E. E., & Martin, J. A. (1983). Socialization in the context of the family: Parent-child interaction. In P. H. Mussen (Series Ed.) & E. M. Hetherington (Vol. Ed.), *Handbook of child psychology: Vol. 1. Socialization, personality, and social development* (5th ed., pp. 1-101). New York: J. Wiley.

Mantzicopoulos, P. Y., & Oh-Hwang, Y. (1998). The relationship of psychosocial maturity to parenting quality and intellectual ability for American and Korean adolescents. *Contemporary Educational Psychology, 23*(2), 195-206.

Markus, H. R., & Kitayama, S. (1991). Culture and the self: Implications for cognition, emotion, and motivation. *Psychological Review, 98*(2), 224-253.

Moos, R. H., & Moos, B. S. (1974). *Family environment scale.* Palo Alto, CA: Consulting Psychology Press.

Okagaki, L., & Frensch, P. A. (1998). Parenting and children's school achievement: A multiethnic perspective. *American Educational Research Journal, 35*(1), 123-144.

Olson, D. H., Sprenkle, D. H., & Russell, C. S. (1979). Circumplex model of marital and family systems: I. Cohesion and adaptability dimensions, family types, and clinical applications. *Family Process, 18*(1), 3-28.

Patterson, G. R., DeBaryshe, B. D., & Ramsey, E. (1989). A developmental perspective on antisocial behavior. *American Psychologist, 44*(2), 329-335.

Phinney, J. S., Ong, A., & Madden, T. (2000). Cultural values and intergenerational value discrepancies in immigrant and non-immigrant families. *Child Development, 71*(2), 528-539.

Rogler, L. H., Cortes, D. E., & Malgady, R. G. (1991). Acculturation and mental health status among Hispanics: Convergence and new directions for research. *American Psychologist, 46*(6), 585-597.

Rowe, D. C., Vazsonyi, A. T., & Flannery, D. J. (1994). No more than skin deep: Ethnic and racial similarity in developmental process. *Psychological Review, 101*(3), 396-413.

Schaefer, E. S. (1959). A circumplex model for maternal behavior. *Journal of Abnormal and Social Psychology, 59*, 226-235.

Shek, D. T. L. (1995). The relation of family environments to adolescent psychological well-being, school adjustment and problem behavior: What can we learn from the Chinese culture? *International Journal of Adolescent Medicine and Health, 8*(3), 199-218.

Shek, D. T. L. (2000). Differences between fathers and mothers in the treatment of, and relationship with, their teenage children: Perceptions of Chinese adolescents. *Adolescence, 35*(137), 135-146.

Shon, S. P., & Ja, D. Y. (1982). Asian Families. In M. McGoldrick, J. K. Pearce, & J. Giordano (Eds.), *Ethnicity and family therapy* (pp. 208-228). New York: Guilford Press.

Six billion... and counting (1999, October 18). *Time, 154*, 61.

Steinberg, L., Elmen, J. D., & Mounts, N. S. (1989). Authoritative parenting, psychosocial maturity, and academic success among adolescents. *Child Development, 60*(6), 1424-1436.

Steinberg, L., Mounts, N. S., Lamborn, S. D., & Dornbusch, S. M. (1991). Authoritative parenting and adolescent adjustment across varied ecological niches. *Journal of Research on Adolescence, 1*(1), 19-36.

Stewart, S. M., Rao, N., Bond, M. H., McBride-Chang, C., Fielding, R., & Kennard, B. D. (1998). Chinese dimensions of parenting: Broadening Western predictors and outcomes. *International Journal of Psychology, 33*(5), 345-358.

Triandis, H. C. (1995). *Individualism and collectivism.* Boulder, CO: Westview Press.

Tseng, V., & Fuligni, A. J. (2000). Parent-adolescent language use and relationships among immigrant families with East Asian, Filipino and Latin American backgrounds. *Journal of Marriage and the Family, 62*(2), 465-476.

Uba, L. (1994). *Asian Americans: Personality patterns, identity, and mental health.* New York: Guilford Press.

Wang, C. H. C., & Phinney, J. S. (1998). Differences in child rearing attitudes between immigrant Chinese mothers and Anglo-American mothers. *Early Development and Parenting, 7*(4), 181-189.

Ward, B. E. (1985). *Through other eyes: Essays in understanding 'conscious models', mostly in Hong Kong.* Hong Kong: Chinese University Press.

Wolf, M. (1970). Child training and the Chinese family. In A. L. S. Chin, and M. Freedman (Eds.), *Family and kinship in Chinese society* (pp. 37-62). Stanford, CA: Stanford University Press.

Wolf, M. (1972). *Women and the family in rural Taiwan.* Stanford, CA: Stanford University Press.

Wu, D. Y. H. (1996). Chinese childhood socialization. In M. H. Bond (Ed.), *The handbook of Chinese psychology* (pp. 143-154). New York: Oxford University Press.

Yang, M.-C. U. (1945). *A Chinese village: Taitou, Shantung province.* New York: Columbia University Press.

Zahn-Waxler, C., Friedman, R. J., Cole, P. M., & Mizuta, I. (1996). Japanese and United States preschool children's responses to conflict and distress. *Child Development, 67*(5), 2462-2477.

SECTION IV: CULTURALLY INFORMED ASSESSMENT, RESEARCH, AND PRACTICE

14. **Assessing Psychiatric Prevalence Rates Among Asian Americans**
Karen S. Kurasaki
Alan K. Koike

15. **The Place of Ethnographic Understanding in the Assessment of Asian American Mental Health**
Edwina S. Uehara
Nancy Farwell
Greg Yamashiro
Michael Smukler

16. **The Clinical Assessment of Asian American Children**
May Yeh
Joyce Wu Yeh

17. **Examining the Role of Culture in Educational Assessment**
Jonathan Sandoval

18. **A Cultural Accommodation Approach to Career Assessment with Asian Americans**
Frederick T. L. Leong
Mei Tang

19. **Theory and Method of Multicultural Counseling Competency Assessment**
Richard M. Lee
Adam J. Darnell

20. **Assessment of Cultural Competence in Mental Health Systems of Care for Asian Americans**
Jean Lau Chin

KAREN S. KURASAKI AND ALAN K. KOIKE

CHAPTER 14

ASSESSING PSYCHIATRIC PREVALENCE RATES AMONG ASIAN AMERICANS

1. INTRODUCTION

This chapter examines the challenges that researchers face when estimating prevalence rates of psychiatric disorders among Asian Americans, and provides recommendations for designing and implementing culturally valid epidemiological research. Our present understanding of psychiatric prevalence rates, pathogenesis, and correlates of mental disorders among Asian Americans is woefully inadequate. Large scale epidemiological studies of mental disorders in this country (e.g., Kessler et al., 1994; Robins & Regier, 1991) have failed to include sufficient numbers of Asian Americans, limiting our ability to make meaningful comparisons of the rates of mental illness between Asian Americans and the general United States population. The magnitude of this problem is troubling. Our knowledge base has lagged far behind the population growth of Asian Americans. The Asian American population doubled in size between 1980 and 1990, and has grown by an average of 4.5 percent annually since 1990 (Hajime-Shinagawa, 1996). At this rate, by the year 2050, it is estimated that the Asian American population will have grown to five times its size in 1995 and will make up ten percent of the nation's population (Hajime-Shinagawa, 1996). In order to improve our response to the treatment needs of this growing population of Americans, more, well-designed studies are needed to determine the rates and correlates of mental illness among Asian Americans. In this chapter, our discussion begins with an examination of the ideological and methodological challenges that have hampered prevalence research in Asian American communities. We use the Chinese American Psychiatric Epidemiological Study[1] (CAPES) as a model to present strategies for: 1) sampling small populations; 2) selecting and establishing culturally valid measures; and 3) encouraging community participation in research studies.

---

[1] The Chinese American Psychiatric Epidemiological Study (CAPES) was conducted with the support of NIMH Grant No. 47460. The principal investigator of the CAPES was David T. Takeuchi, Ph.D. Neuropsychiatric Institute (now at the Department of Sociology, Indiana University). The former Project Director of the study was Karen S. Kurasaki, Ph.D., Neuropsychiatric Institute (now at the California Endowment).

2. CHALLENGES TO ESTIMATING PREVALENCE RATES AMONG ASIAN AMERICANS

2.1 Values and the Practice of Science

One of the challenges to conducting prevalence studies among Asian Americans lies in what is valued in science, which in turn affects how science is practiced. Internal and external validity should be equal partners in science, but in practice the scientific community has favored internal over external validity (Sue, 1999). Internal validity is the ability to draw conclusions about the causal relationship between two variables. External validity is the degree to which scientific findings can be generalized to various populations of interest. Favoring internal over external validity, the field of psychology more often assumes, rather than tests, the generality of its findings based on the majority white population. As a consequence, ethnic research has suffered. Because of this bias in how science has been practiced, many psychological principles and measures have not been cross-validated with different ethnocultural populations.

2.2 Cost of Sampling a Small Population

A practical challenge is the cost of conducting prevalence studies among a small population. In epidemiological research, random sampling of the general population is conducted according to a multi-stage probability sampling design. The effort, and thus cost involved in obtaining a representative sample of rare or small populations using such a design is high, and consequently has hampered prevalence research in Asian American communities (Takeuchi et al., 1998). Obtaining a true random sample representative of the community population can be accomplished by sampling telephone directories or conducting door-to-door household sampling. Household interviewing allows researchers to ask more extensive questions than over the telephone surveys. In door-to-door household sampling, workers go from residence to residence to find households with eligible persons. In some neighborhoods in the U.S., workers may need to visit hundreds of households before finding one Asian American household. The yield is therefore quite low for such a time consuming and thus costly procedure.

Only two mental health prevalence studies have conducted systematic data collection of large numbers of Asian Americans using a random sampling frame (Takeuchi et al., 1998; Takeuchi, Kuo, Kim, & Leaf, 1989). More often, little effort is made to include adequate numbers of Asian Americans in the research design. Although several large-scale studies have been conducted to assess psychiatric prevalence rates across the U.S., Asian Americans have been poorly represented in each of these studies' samples. Asian Americans were underrepresented in the two largest national studies—the Epidemiological Catchment Area (ECA) study (Robins & Regier, 1991) and the National Comorbidity Study (NCS) (Kessler et al., 1994)—which have been touted as landmark epidemiological investigations of psychiatric disorders in the U.S. In the ECA study, which was conducted in the early 1980's, there were only 242 Asian Americans among a total sample of 18,152 (Zhang & Snowden, 1999). The NCS was conducted after the ECA study, and included no Asian American sub-sample. Instead the NCS lumped Asian Americans into category labeled "others," which represented 3% of the total sample (Zhang & Snowden, 1999).

Because sampling pools (i.e., pool of those available to be sampled) are a relatively small proportion in any given geographical area, methodological rigor is often compromised to lower the costs involved in obtaining the sample. The most typical methodological compromise is the use of a convenience sample. For example, some studies have reported findings based on clinical samples (Takeuchi & Uehara, 1996). One of the problems with using clinical samples to estimate the prevalence rates for Asian Americans is that Asian Americans have been found to be underrepresented in services with respect to their representation in the general population and in comparison to other racial groups (Snowden & Cheung, 1990; S. Sue et al., 1991). Consequently, prevalence rates yielded from clinical samples are likely to produce biased estimates. Rates based on clinical samples are more likely to reflect their patterns of mainstream service use than the actual level of psychopathology in the general community. Studies of psychopathology among Asian Americans have compromised their methodological rigor by relying on convenience samples such as college students (Abe & Zane, 1990; Marsella, Kinzie & Gordon, 1973; Okazaki, 1997; S. Sue & D. W. Sue, 1974) whose characteristics often do not reflect those of the general community. Similarly, other non-random sampling frames such as phone directory or ethnic association lists (Kuo, 1984) can produce biased samples by systematically leaving out individuals who do not have telephones or Asian surnames, or who are not members of particular ethnic organizations. Another problem is that ethnic groups (e.g., Vietnamese, Chinese, Korean, etc.) are often combined into the overarching racial category "Asian Americans" (or even worse lumped into an "other" category with dissimilar ethnic groups such as persons originating from Middle Eastern countries who are also underrepresented in most studies) in order to achieve a large enough sample. For instance, the ECA study (Robins & Regier, 1991) made no ethnic distinctions among Asian Americans. The assumption that Asian Americans fit into one homogenous category ignores the rich diversity among the many ethnic groups. Asian Americans represent more than 25 distinct ethnic groups (Uba, 1994), each with their own set of languages and dialects, culture, history, and experiences. For instance, it may not be appropriate to lump Japanese Americans with a Southeast Asian refugee group like Hmong Americans. Japanese Americans have one of the highest average household incomes in the U.S and many of them are fourth or fifth generation in this country (Yin, 2000). In contrast, many Hmong Americans are recent refugees from Laos, have experienced a number of traumas and have one of the lowest average household incomes in the country (Yin, 2000). When studies combine the different Asian American ethnic groups together, variations in prevalence rates among these ethnic groups cannot be determined from their data.

2.3 Validity of Western Diagnostic Criteria

Another problem is an over-reliance on assessment tools that follow Western diagnostic taxonomies, which may or may not have cultural validity for the different Asian American ethnic groups. The Diagnostic and Statistical Manual of Mental Disorders (DSM) (American Psychiatric Association, 1994) is a system that is widely used in the U.S. to determine psychiatric diagnoses across populations. This use of the DSM system assumes that psychiatric distress is manifested similarly across people from a variety of ethnic heritages and racial groups. However, it is unclear whether DSM criteria are valid for non-Western ethnic groups. Evidence from cross-cultural studies on depression does not unanimously support this assumption of universality. According to the NCS (Kessler et al., 1994), lifetime depression prevalence rates were 17.1% among their sample that consisted of 75.1% White, 12.5% Black, 9.1% Latino, and 3.3% Other. In contrast, the rates of depression obtained from studies conducted in China, Taiwan, and Hong Kong are strikingly lower. The Shanghai Psychiatric Epidemiological Study (Wang et al., 1992) reported less than 1% Major Depressive Disorder (MDD) in Xuhui, a metropolitan district in Shanghai. The Taiwan Psychiatric Epidemiologic Project (Hwu, Yeh, & Chang, 1989) estimated MDD in Metropolitan Taipei to be 0.9%, and the Shatin Community Mental Health Survey (Chen et al., 1993) estimated MDD at 1.9% in the Shatin community of Hong Kong. These findings raise a number of important questions. Do Asians suffer from lower rates of psychiatric disorders or is there a problem with the tools we use to assess for psychiatric disorders? Is depression a valid diagnosis for Asians? If depression is not culturally valid for Asians in Asia, then what about their counterparts in the U.S.? That is, are Asian Americans more likely to manifest psychiatric distress like their counterparts in Asia or like non-Asians in the U.S.?

Furthermore, among studies that examined symptom configuration, differences between Asian American and White American samples were found. Using the Center for Epidemiologic Studies Depression scale on a population-based sample in Seattle, Washington, Kuo (1984) found that depressed affect and somatic complaints loaded on the same factor among Asian Americans, but were separate factors among the White American comparison group. In another study (Marsella et al., 1973) a University of Hawai'i student sample who earned raw scores above 50 on the Zung Self-Rating Depression Scale (Zung, 1965) were operationally defined as depressed. Among their sample, Marsella et al. found different patterns of concomitant symptoms among Japanese Americans, Chinese Americans, and White Americans. One of their most interesting findings was that somatic symptoms were scattered across factors for both Japanese Americans and Chinese Americans, but not for White Americans. Moreover, the somatic symptoms most often endorsed were not the same as the physical symptom included in the DSM-III-R (American Psychiatric Association, 1987) Major Depressive Episode diagnostic criteria.

3. RECOMMENDATIONS

3.1 Sampling a Small Population

The basic methodology for obtaining a random sample of a specific ethnic population is no different than the procedures for performing random sampling in the general population. In epidemiological research, a multi-stage probability sampling design is used to randomly sample the general population. A multi-stage probability sampling design consists of randomly selecting individuals within households within blocks within census tracts. In other words, random sampling is performed at every selection level.

However, random sampling of a specific and small ethnic population in this same manner, although possible, can be time-consuming, and as a result quite costly. As an example, the Chinese American Epidemiological Study (CAPES) set forth in the early 1990s to estimate mental disorder prevalence rates and their correlates among the Chinese American population in Los Angeles County (Takeuchi et al., 1998). The aim was a sample size of 1,700. On the outset, it might appear that finding Chinese American households in Los Angeles County would be relatively easy to come by. After all, in 1990, the number of Chinese Americans across the entire U.S. was 1,645,472 (Asian Week, 1991), 704,850 (or 43%) of whom resided in the State of California, and more than one-third (35%) of those made their homes in Los Angeles County. However, despite the fact Chinese Americans represented the largest Asian American ethnic group in Los Angeles County and 14% of the entire Chinese American population in the United States, ultimately Chinese Americans represented fewer than three-percent of the total Los Angeles County population. With such small numbers, conducting door-to-door household sampling of the entire Los Angeles County would have produced a very low yield.

A more cost-effective solution, which would still allow the application of a sophisticated sampling technique to study a small ethnic population, is to sample geographic areas where the target population represents a larger percentage of the population. This approach is, admittedly, not without its own set of limitations. However, let us first examine its utility and how it can be applied before discussing the limitations. The CAPES (Takeuchi et al., 1998) investigators selected only those census tracts with six-percent or greater Chinese American households. This criterion increased the probability of finding the targeted 1,700 Chinese American households, and thereby was more cost-effective than sampling the entire 1,652 census tracts in the County. Following standard epidemiological procedures, the census tracts were further cross-stratified by the percent of Chinese American households within tracts (which ranged from 6% to 72.3%), median household income of Asian American households (which ranged from $3,000 to $108,000), and percent of race-ethnicity composition (which ranged from 14% to 82% born outside of the U.S.). The next two stages of the multi-stage probability sampling design consisted of randomly selecting 12 blocks within each tract, then randomly selecting 4 households in each block. A total of 16,916 households were visited and screened to locate eligible respondents. Finally, one individual per household was selected according to whomever had the most recent birth date. This final step helped to minimize a selection bias toward only the English-speaking members of the household who might be more likely to answer the door, or non-English-speaking elders in the household who might be more likely to be home during the day.

Sampling geographic areas where the target population represents a larger percentage of the population increases the feasibility of applying a sophisticated, multi-stage sampling design to the study of a small ethnic population. In the case of the CAPES, it resulted in the most extensive epidemiological investigation of a single Asian American ethnic group conducted to date. Still, in employing this approach, it is important that researchers also be aware of its potential limitations. Primarily, this approach results in an undersampling of those persons who reside in less ethnically dense areas. One can speculate that those individuals who reside in less ethnically dense areas are less likely to be immigrants, and more likely to have higher incomes than those who live in areas that are more ethnically diverse (S. Sue, Kurasaki, & Srinivasan, 1999). By undersampling these areas, researchers may miss a characteristically different segment of their targeted ethnic population and reduce the generalizability of their findings.

3.2 Selecting and Establishing Culturally Valid Measures

Selecting culturally valid measures is one of the major challenges of doing mental health research with Asian Americans. Issues include selecting and adapting mainstream measures; translating measures; and developing instruments to measure non-Western constructs.

3.2.1 Selecting and adapting mainstream measures

Recall that earlier in the chapter we questioned the universal validity of Western diagnostic categories and criteria. The findings obtained by administering mainstream instruments that are based on Western notions of mental illness are of limited value unless we know that the concepts being measured are also valid for the targeted ethnic population. The issue of concern here is known as conceptual equivalence. Conceptual equivalence refers to "whether the construct being measured exists in the thinking of the target culture and is understood in the same way" (S. Sue et al., 1999, p. 59). When selecting a mainstream instrument to study an ethnic population, it is necessary to consider whether the instrument has established reliability and validity with the intended target population in order to have confidence that the constructs being measured are conceptually equivalent. Unfortunately, more often than not, mainstream instruments have neither been validated, nor have their reliability been tested among non-mainstream populations. What do we do then? The following is an example of the steps one might take in order to overcome this measurement dilemma commonly encountered by those conducting research among Asian American populations.

One of the aims of the CAPES was to estimate the prevalence rate of the Western diagnostic category of depression among Chinese Americans. Our interest in estimating depression among our Chinese American sample was two-fold. First, we wanted to understand the patterns of psychiatric disorder prevalence among Chinese Americans, including Western-developed conditions such as depression. Do Chinese Americans suffer from depression at the same rates as other ethnic groups? Are the rates of depression similar to indigenous conditions? What is the level of comorbidity between depression and indigenous conditions? Second, we wanted to examine whether the pattern of depression prevalence among Chinese Americans changed as the population became more acculturated to U.S. societal norms.

The approach for finding a culturally appropriate instrument to measure depression required a series of steps. First, the investigators searched for an instrument that had been established to be reliable and valid for Chinese Americans. The University of Michigan version of the Composite Diagnostic Interview Schedule (UM-CIDI) (Kessler et al., 1994) is a structured interview that was derived from the Diagnostic Interview Schedule (DIS). The DIS was originally developed by the National Institute of Mental Health to assess psychiatric disorders (as per the criteria set by the DSM III) (American Psychiatric Association, 1980) among an adult sample of persons age 18 to 65. Substantive international research has been conducted with the DIS. Researchers using the DIS have reported consistently high reliability and validity, including with Chinese samples in Hong Kong, Taiwan, and China (Hwu, Yeh, & Chang, 1986; Hwu et al., 1989; Hwu, Yeh, Chang, & Y. L. Yeh, 1986). Based on the psychometric research reported on the DIS with overseas Chinese samples, the UM-CIDI (based on DSM-III-R criteria) was selected as the diagnostic instrument to be administered in the CAPES.

Although the DIS had demonstrated high reliability and validity for overseas Chinese samples, the UM-CIDI itself had not been used with a Chinese American sample. Therefore, the CAPES investigators conducted a series of focus groups with participants who were representative of the population of interest to determine whether the idioms used in the UM-CIDI to assess depression made sense. Where potentially problematic individual words and/or phrases were identified, supplemental questions were developed that were more consistent with the idioms used by Chinese Americans to describe depressive symptoms. For example, in attempting to translate the item "In your lifetime, have you ever had two weeks or more when nearly every day you felt sad, blue, or depressed?" to assess a primary symptom of depression, the CAPES investigators learned that the color idiom "blue" was not one that Chinese Americans used to describe depressive symptoms. Rather, the focus group informants indicated that the descriptors "down in the dumps, low, or gloomy" were words that made more sense when translated. In order to avoid significant deviation from the standardized administration of the UM-CIDI (so as to remain comparable to other studies that administered the UM-CIDI), the standard items were administered first, followed by supplemental questions that included the alternative wording.

3.2.2 Translating measures and language equivalence

When conducting prevalence research in Asian American communities, it is frequently necessary to administer the measures in more than one language in order to obtain a more representative sample. Collecting data in only one language (e.g., English) will bias the sample toward the subset of those who are fluent enough to be interviewed in English. Most likely, English-speaking samples will be comprised of more acculturated persons; that is, mostly non-immigrants, or persons who have been in the U.S. for a longer period of time, and possibly also a more highly educated sector of the target population. Likewise, collecting data in only Korean, for example, may bias the sample toward more recent immigrants whose language of preference, or perhaps the only language, may be Korean. In either case, the findings may not be generalizable to a substantial subset of the ethnic group you are studying.

Translating instruments involve more than simply translating each item word-for-word. Translating instruments requires that there is language equivalence between the two translated versions of an instrument. Language equivalence exists "when the descriptors and measures of psychological concepts can be translated well across languages" (S. Sue et al., 1999, p. 59). Often, language equivalence does not exist for even common words (e.g., there is no exact equivalent for the word parent in the Hmong language), but especially for psychological terms. When language equivalence cannot be achieved, conceptual equivalence should be the goal. Conceptual equivalence refers to "whether the construct being measured exists in the thinking of the target culture and is understood in the same way" (Sue et al., 1999, p. 59).

Translating instruments also requires that the level of understanding match that of the target population. Specifically, translated instruments should match the cultural, socioeconomic, and reading level of the target population. For example, an instrument that is translated into the Cambodian language using idioms understandable to more educated, urban persons may not necessarily be understandable to those who are less educated and came from one of the rural villages.

Cross-cultural researchers recommend following a three-step method for ensuring reliable and valid instrument translations (e.g., Herrera, Delcampo, & Ames, 1993; Sue et al., 1999). These three steps include: 1) translation into the second language; 2) back-translation to the original language; and 3) field testing the measures for reliability. When translating, it is beneficial to employ more than two translators who complete their translations independently. Once the independent translations are completed, the team of translators along with linguistic experts should convene to discuss and resolve discrepancies among the independent translations. Back-translating refers to a step where the translated instrument is translated back into the original language. Back-translation is valuable to ensure that the translation in the second language is accurate, thus it should be completed by more than two persons working independently. At the end of the back-translation step, once again, it is advisable to have linguistic experts examine for and correct any discrepancies between the independent back-translations.

ASSESSING PSYCHIATRIC PREVALENCE RATES AMONG ASIAN AMERICANS 213

In both these steps – translation and back-translation – it is important to provide clear instructions for the translators because the research standards may not be the same as the translation work they may have performed for others in different professional fields. For instance, it is important to clearly instruct the translators to translate the measures using words that are relevant to the cultural, socioeconomic, and reading level characteristics of the target population. Optimally, researchers should use translators with comparable background to the target population. However, there may be times when the low educational level of the target population does not permit one to do so. In such a case, it is important to make certain that the translators use words that are understandable to the target population. It is also advisable to hire linguistic experts to check that the vocabulary level is not too high. Also, it is very important that the back-translators do not make inferences as they back-translate. If they do, errors and sloppiness in the original translation cannot be identified.

Finally, pilot testing the instruments should be done on a sample that is truly linguistically representative of the intended target population. It is important to note that if the intended population is monolingual, than a bilingual sample is not an equivalent group (e.g., Diaz, 1988). Correctly interpreting the field trial data is critical to knowing whether or not there are problems with your translated measure that require correction. Good test-retest reliability in the English version of a measure and poor test-retest reliability in the translated version indicates problems in the translated version. By contrast, poor test-retest reliability in the English version (the original version) of the measure indicates problems with the original instrument. Establishing the reliability of an instrument that is intended for administration to a bilingual sample is slightly more complex. Field data from two bilingual samples should be obtained. The order of administration of the two language versions to the same group of individuals (i.e., English-second language vs. second language-English) should differ between the two groups in order to control for administration order effects. Low test-retest reliability for the two language versions across multiple bilingual samples most likely indicates problems with the translation.

3.2.3 Developing instruments to measure indigenous conditions

How people experience and express mental illness is inextricably related to what Kleinman (1980) has termed their social reality. Social reality is comprised of the surrounding value systems and behavioral norms in a cultural setting that favor certain behaviors over others. In Chinese culture, for example, the social reality surrounding individuals looks unfavorably upon the outward display of dysphoric affect. This social reality is internalized by individuals at such a degree that Chinese individuals are known to manage their dysphoric affect and manifest distress through physical symptoms. Because mental illness is culturally laden in this manner, assessing for only Western-derived diagnoses among an Asian American population may not fully capture the level of psychiatric need in that population. Depending on the level of acculturation, Asian Americans may continue to be influenced by a social reality that is different from the normative social reality in the

214 KAREN S. KURASAKI AND ALAN K. KOIKE

U.S. It is therefore important that prevalence studies among Asian American populations also assess for disorders indigenous to Asia.

In the CAPES, the investigators included questions about neurasthenia as a candidate condition that may be prevalent among Chinese Americans but not classified by the DSM nomenclature. Neurasthenia is a mental disorder that is characterized by more physical than affective manifestations of distress. Originally coined by George Beard, neurasthenia has fallen out of favor among mental health professionals in the West and was omitted from the third and fourth editions of the DSM. In contrast, neurasthenia is routinely diagnosed and treated in China (Zheng et al., 1997). Neurasthenia is an indigenous syndrome characterized as a persistent and distressing complaint of fatigue after mental effort, or persistent and distressing complaint of bodily weakness and exhaustion after minimal effort. The mental fatigability is typically described as unpleasant intrusion of distracting associations or recollections, difficulty in concentrating, and general ineffective thinking. The bodily complaints are accompanied by muscular aches and pains and an inability to relax. In both cases, there are a variety of accompanying physical complaints (e.g., dizziness, tension headaches, sleep disturbance, and dyspepsia) along with irritability and anhedonia. While not included in the DSM system, neurasthenia is however recognized by and included in the International Classification of Diseases (ICD) (World Health Organization, 1992). Following the ICD criteria, one of the CAPES researchers[2] developed a structured interview schedule to assess the presence of neurasthenia. This neurasthenia module was administered as a supplement to the UM-CIDI in order to obtain a more accurate estimate of psychiatric need than if the UM-CIDI was administered alone.

When diagnostic criteria for conditions indigenous to the target Asian American population are not known to the extent that was known for neurasthenia, researchers may consider employing qualitative methods of inquiry. Qualitative methods encompass a number of different methodological techniques (e.g., interview, focus group, observation) for collecting in-depth data. A primary feature of such methods is that they elicit open-ended and information-rich data that allow the researcher to discover new or indigenous concepts. Qualitative methods are especially useful for cross-cultural clinical research in which the aim is to better understand emic or culture-specific patterns and concepts related to mental illness.

3.3 Encouraging Community Participation in Research Studies

A major challenge in conducting epidemiological research with Asian Americans is gaining cooperation from the research participants in order to have an adequate response rate. CAPES made specific efforts to encourage maximum community participation in the study, and in this section we review the recruitment and sampling procedures used. Data was collected in the three most common languages among Chinese Americans who reside in Los Angeles County – Mandarin, Cantonese, and English – to try to include as much of the Chinese American

---

[2] Keh-Ming Lin, M.D., MPH, of Harbor-UCLA Medical Center

population as possible. Bilingual interviewers were recruited for the data collection, and as much as possible, they were recruited from the census tract areas where sampling was being conducted, which helped to maximize their interviewer rapport and familiarity with the neighborhood, as well as efficiency in travel time and mileage. In using the UM-CIDI and other instruments that could be administered by lay interviewers, CAPES was able to recruit persons who did not necessarily have any clinical training. Instead, individuals were screened for their reading and writing abilities in both languages, access to transportation, and style of presentation. Although it was not a requirement, it turns out that most of the interviewers had at least some college education.

When a Chinese American household was identified, the screening for eligibility was performed by the interviewers in the potential respondent's preferred language. In cases when the interviewer did not speak the language of the potential respondent, a different interviewer with the language abilities in the appropriate language was sent to the site to complete the screening process. Eligible respondents were immediately identified through the screening process. The investigation's purpose, procedures, potential benefits to the community, and their rights as participants of a research study were explained fully, and written informed consent was obtained in their preferred language.

The interviews were conducted in Mandarin, Cantonese, or English, depending on the respondent's language preference. On average, each interview lasted approximately 90 minutes. Data was collected at two time points from the same respondents, 15 months apart, which allowed us to examine changes in level of functioning that occurred over time. The interviews opened with demographic information, such as age, marital status, education level, age of immigration, etc., and an assessment of behaviors that served as an indication of their acculturation level. When interviewers came to this point in the interviews, using a standard format, they let the respondents know that they were moving into a section that covered emotional functioning, and asked whether the respondents were still certain that they wanted to continue with the interview. Of the total eligible respondents screened, 1,747 interviews were completed, which resulted in an 82% response rate at Time 1. Respondents from Time 1 were asked to provide contact information for a close relative or friend for the purpose of tracking them for the second round of data collection. At Time 2, 1,503 interviews were completed for a response rate of 86%.

4. SUMMARY

In this chapter we have discussed the challenges of estimating the prevalence rates of psychiatric disorders among Asian Americans. The major obstacles can be briefly summarized. First, there is a basic and widespread bias favoring internal validity at the expense of external validity that in some ways has discouraged the pursuit of research on ethnic minorities. Second, conducting methodologically sound epidemiological research in small populations such as Asian Americans is very costly, and as a result most studies omit studying Asian Americans or compromise the rigor of their research by using non-random sampling techniques. Third, there

216 KAREN S. KURASAKI AND ALAN K. KOIKE

are still unanswered questions regarding the validity of Western diagnostic constructs and instruments for Asian American populations.

Despite the methodological difficulties described earlier and the limitations of past research, these challenges are not insurmountable. In the second half of the chapter we described the CAPES as a model for how to overcome several of these methodological challenges. CAPES utlilized the following strategies:

1. used a modified random sampling design to deal with the challenge of studying a small population
2. selected, adapted, and translated mainstream measures
3. developed measures to assess non-Western conditions, and recruited and interviewed community participants in the three most common languages spoken among the Los Angeles County Chinese American population

Building on the experience from CAPES, great strides can be made in future epidemiological mental health research among Asian Americans.

5. REFERENCES

Abe, J. S., & Zane, N. W. S. (1990). Psychological maladjustment among Asian and White American college students: Controlling for confounds. *Journal of Counseling Psychology, 37*(4), 437-444.

American Psychiatric Association. (1980). Diagnostic and statistical manual of mental disorders (3rd ed.). Washington, DC: Author.

American Psychiatric Association. (1987). Diagnostic and statistical manual of mental disorders (3rd ed., Rev..). Washington, DC: Author.

American Psychiatric Association. (1994). Diagnostic and statistical manual of mental disorders (4th ed.). Washington, DC: Author.

Asian Week. (1991). Asians in America: 1990 Census. Classification by states. San Francisco: Author.

Chen, C.-N, Wong, J., Lee, N., Chan-Ho, M.-W., Lau, J. T.-F., & Fung, M. (1993). The Shatin community mental health survey in Hong Kong: II. Major findings. *Archives of General Psychiatry, 50*, 125-133.

Diaz, J. O. P. (1988). Assessment of Puerto Rican children in bilingual education programs in the United States: A critique of Lloyd M. Dunn's monograph. *Hispanic Journal of Behavioral Sciences, 10*, 237-252.

Hajime-Shinagawa, L. (1996). The impact of immigration on the demography of Asian Pacific Americans. In B. Ong Hing, & R. Lee, R (Eds.), *The state of Asian Pacific America: Reframing the immigration debate. A public policy report.* LEAP Asian Pacific American Public Policy Institute and UCLA Asian American Studies Center: Los Angeles.

Herrera, R. S., Delcampo, R. L., & Ames, M. H. (1993). A serial approach for translating family science instrumentation. *Family Relations, 42*, 357-360.

Hwu, H.-G., Yeh, E. K., & Chang, L. Y. (1986). Chinese Diagnostic Interview Schedule, I: Agreement with psychiatrist's diagnosis. *Acta Psychiatrica Scandinavica, 73*, 225-233.

Hwu, H.-G, Yeh, E.-K., & Chang, L. Y. (1989). Prevalence of psychiatric disorders in Taiwan defined by the Chinese Diagnostic Interview Schedule. *Acta Psychiatrica Scandinavica, 79*, 136-147.

Hwu, H.-G., Yeh, E. K., Chang, L. Y., & Yeh, Y. L. (1986). Chinese Diagnostic Interview Schedule, II: A validity study on estimation of lifetime prevalence. *Acta Psychiatrica Scandinavica, 73*, 348-357.

Kessler, R. C., McGonagle, K. A., Zhao, S., Nelson, C. B., Hughes, M., Eshleman, S., Wittchen, H-U, & Kendler, K. S. (1994). Lifetime and 12-month prevalence of DSM-III-R psychiatric disorders in the United States. *Archives of General Psychiatry, 51*, 8-19.

Kleinman, A. (1980). *Patients and healers in the context of culture: An exploration of the borderland between anthropology, medicine, and psychiatry.* Berkeley, CA: University of California Press.

ASSESSING PSYCHIATRIC PREVALENCE RATES AMONG ASIAN AMERICANS 217

Kuo, W. H. (1984). Prevalence of depression among Asian-Americans. *Journal of Nervous and Mental Disease, 172*(8), 449-457.

Marsella, A. J., Kinzie, D., & Gordon, P. (1973). Ethnic variations in the expression of depression. *Journal of Cross-Cultural Psychology, 4*(4), 435-458.

Okazaki, S. (1997). Sources of ethnic differences between Asian American and White American college students on measures of depression and social anxiety. *Journal of Abnormal Psychology, 106*(1), 32-60.

Robins, L. N., & Regier, D. A. (1991). *Psychiatric disorders in America: The Epidemiologic Catchment Area Study*. New York: The Free Press.

Snowden, L. R., & Cheung, F. K. (1990). use of inpatient mental health services by members of ethnic minority groups. *American Psychologist, 45*(3), 347-355.

Sue, S., Fujino, D. C., Hu, L. T., Takeuchi, D. T., & Zane, N. W. S. (1991). Community mental health services for ethnic minority groups: A test of the cultural responsiveness hypothesis. *Journal of Consulting & Clinical Psychology, 59*(4), 533-540.

Sue, S. (1999). Science, ethnicity, and bias: Where have we gone wrong? *American Psychologist, 54*(12), 1070-1077.

Sue, S., Kurasaki, K. S., & Srinivasan, S. (1999). Ethnicity, genders, and cross-cultural issues in clinical research. In P. C. Kendall, J. N. Butcher, & G. N. Holmbeck (Eds.), *Handbook of research methods in clinical psychology* (2nd ed., pp. 54-71). New York: J. Wiley & Sons.

Sue, S., & Sue, D. W. (1974). MMPI comparisons between Asian-American and non-Asian students utilizing a student health psychiatric clinic. *Journal of Counseling Psychology, 21*(5), 423-427.

Takeuchi, D. T., Chung, R. C-Y., Lin, K.-M.., Shen, H., Kurasaki, K., Chun, C-A., & Sue, S. (199 8). Lifetime and twelve-month prevalence rates of major depressive episodes and dysthymia among Chinese Americans in Los Angeles. *American Journal of Psychiatry, 155*,(10), 1407-1414.

Takeuchi, D. T., Kuo, H-S., Kim, K., & Leaf, P. J. (1989). Psychiatric symptom dimensions among Asian Americans and Native Hawaiians: An analysis of the symptom checklist. *Journal of Community Psychology, 17*(4), 319-329.

Takeuchi, D., & Uehara, E. (1996). Ethnic minority mental health services: Current research and future conceptual directions. In B. L. Levin, & J. Petrila (Eds.), *Mental health services: A public health perspective* (pp. 63-96). New York: Oxford University Press.

Uba, L. (1994). *Asian Americans: Personality patterns, identity, and mental health*. New York: Guilford.

Wang, C. H., Liu, W. T., Zhang, M. Y., Yu, E. S. H., Xia, Z. Y., Fernandez, M., Lung, C. T., Xu, C. L., & Qu, G. Y. (1992). Alcohol use, abuse, and dependency in Shanghai. In J. E. Helzer & G. J. Canino (Eds.), *Alcoholism in North America, Europe, and Asia* (pp. 264-286). New York: Oxford University Press.

World Health Organization (1992). *ICD-10: The ICD-10 classification of mental and behavioral disorders. Clinical descriptions and diagnostic guidelines*. Geneva, Switzerland: Author.

Yin, X.-H. (2000, May 7). Asian Americans: The two sides of America's 'model minority.' *Los Angeles Times*.

Zhang, A. Y., & Snowden, L. R. (1999). Ethnic characteristics of mental disorders in five U.S. communities. *Cultural Diversity and Ethnic Minority Psychology, 5*(2), 134-146.

Zheng, Y-P., Lin, K.-M.., Takeuchi, D., Kurasaki, K. S., Wang, Y., & Cheung, F. (1997). An epidemiological study of neurasthenia in Chinese-Americans in Los Angeles. *Comprehensive Psychiatry, 38*(5), 249-259.

Zung, W. W. K. (1965). A self-rating depression scale. *Archives of General Psychiatry, 12*, 63-70.

EDWINA S. UEHARA, NANCY FARWELL,
GREG YAMASHIRO, AND MICHAEL SMUKLER

CHAPTER 15

THE PLACE OF ETHNOGRAPHIC UNDERSTANDING IN THE ASSESSMENT OF ASIAN AMERICAN MENTAL HEALTH

1. INTRODUCTION

This chapter focuses on the role of ethnographic understanding in conducting assessments in research and clinical settings. We adhere closely to Arthur Kleinman's (1977, 1988a, 1988b) conception of the nature and purposes of mental health assessment. We begin by recounting his argument for the centrality of the ethnographic perspective to the development of valid assessments, particularly when assessor and assessed differ in cultural background. We then describe two approaches to engendering ethnographic understanding in research and clinical contexts: Byron Good's (1977; Good, Good, & Moradi, 1985) classic "semantic network analysis," and Jurg Siegfried's (1998) more recently developed "common sense reasoning" analysis. Finally, we close with some reflections on next critical steps toward enhancing ethnographic understanding in the assessment process. We call for more active, long-term collaboration among and between cross-cultural researchers and practitioners to create the capacity and knowledge bases for ethnographically informed clinical assessment.

2. ETHNOGRAPHIC UNDERSTANDING AND THE VALIDITY OF MENTAL HEALTH ASSESSMENTS

The primary point of mental health assessment, Kleinman (1988a) suggests, is not to classify disease, but rather to understand and articulate a person's experience of illness (see Sandelowski, 1996; also Siegfried, 1998). The illness experience is grounded in the client's local sociocultural context. "Symptoms" exist in a world mediated by a constellation of socially shared "values, causal connections, common sense reasons, socially relevant attributions and explanations" (Siegfried, 1998, p. 287). Illness is a culturally-shaped experience in which interpretations of symptoms—by the person, her loved ones and mental health professionals—play constitutive parts. The assessor's evaluation is not only constrained by the client's actual experiences, but is also shaped by the assessor's own cultural and professional lenses and biases, and the relationships of power (political, economic, and bureaucratic) through which mental health professionals and clients interact (Kleinman, 1988a, 1988b).

Diagnostic assessment is a fundamentally semiotic activity in which the researcher's or clinician's "analysis of one symbol system is followed by its translation into another" (Kleinman, 1988a, p. 17). Valid assessment is not simply the verification of concepts used in professionally and scientifically accepted nosologies to explain symptoms. It must also encompass the verification of the meaning of symptoms within a given social system, and avoid what cross-cultural researchers call the "categorical fallacy"—also known as the reification of one culture's diagnostic categories and their projection onto patients in another culture, where those categories lack coherence and their validity has not been established (Hughes & Okpaku, 1998; Rogler, 1993b). Thus, assessment of mental health problems should involve:

> . . . conceptual tacking back and forth between the [assessor's] diagnostic system and its rules of classification, alternative taxonomies, his [sic] clinical experience, and that of the patient, which includes the patient's interpretation. Validity is the negotiated outcome of this transforming interaction between concept and experience in a particular context (Kleinman, 1988b, p. 12).

In sum, valid mental health assessment is predicated upon an understanding of the meaning of symptoms and suffering within a local cultural field, and it is this ethnographic understanding that enables the creation of valid understanding and, ultimately, effective and humane care (Kleinman, 1977, 1988b; Kleinman & Good, 1985; Rogler, 1992, 1993a, 1993b; Twaddle & Hessler, 1985).

Despite current widespread recognition of the importance of incorporating cultural considerations in the assessment process, mental health assessments too seldom center on an ethnographic understanding of client experiences (Hughes & Okpaku, 1998). Instead, in contemporary research and treatment contexts, assessments most often comprise the assessor's recasting of the person's intimate experience of symptoms and suffering (the "illness experience") into much narrower, technical terms (the "disease"), shaped predominantly by dominant professional theories of disorder ("disease nosologies") (Kleinman, 1988a).[1] In this recasting, the intimate and psychosocial core of the person's experience of illness is

---

[1] Kleinman's definition of terms is worth repeating here: "Illness" can be viewed as the intimately human experience of symptoms and suffering—and how a sick person and members of family/network perceive, live with, and respond to symptoms and disabilities. "Illness problems" refer to the principal difficulties that symptoms and disability create in a person's life. "Disease" is what practitioners create in recasting of illness in terms of theories of disorder (1988a, pp. 3-5).

THE PLACE OF ETHNOGRAPHIC UNDERSTANDING IN THE ASSESSMENT OF 221
ASIAN AMERICAN MENTAL HEALTH

lost. It is not legitimated as a subject of clinical or scientific concern, nor does it receive an intervention (Antonovsky, 1989; Kleinman, 1988b).

Despite a substantial and expanding body of findings indicating the critical role of cultural and psychosocial factors in amplifying/damping a person's illness trajectory (see for example Park & Folkman, 1997; Pescosolido, 1991, 1992; Thoits, 1995), the mental health assessment process still tends to:

> . . . replace . . . psychosocial concerns ("soft") with the "hard," overvalued technical quest for control of symptoms. This pernicious value transformation is a serious failing of modern medicine: it disables the healer and disempowers the chronically ill (Kleinman, 1988a, pp. 9-10).

In the clinical setting, power and social status differences between practitioner and client lubricate this "pernicious transformation," as do the cost-containment imperatives underpinning most managed care schemes in which mental health care is increasingly provided. The ill effects of this transformation are often magnified in cases characterized by ethnic or cultural differences between practitioner and client (see Mechanic, 1999).[2]

Cross-cultural clinicians and researchers note that despite the best of intentions to aid the assessor in penetrating the culturally different person's phenomenologic world (Hughes & Okpaku, 1998), the published literature on cross-cultural assessment suffers from a substantial gap between the earnest plea to understand the person's lived sociocultural world and substantive guidance in how to effectively enter and understand that world (see López & Hernandez, 1986). Existing guidance to researchers and practitioners in incorporating cultural concerns into assessment tend to be pitched at "either an abstract, superficial level or fairly obvious cultural differences between social or ethnic groups—language, dress, behavior, expressed beliefs, and the like" (Hughes & Okpaku, 1998, p. 215). In the clinical setting, this state of affairs provokes many to call for more concrete and specific ethnographic methods that can be used by practitioners. In clinical settings, Hughes and Okpaku (1998) suggest:

> . . . the critical question is how can [the mental health practitioner] employ culturally relevant insights and observational skills in the interview situation itself without being an expert in specific cultural knowledge relevant to the patient. If not already ethnographically skilled, can the clinician learn anything on-the-job, so to speak, formulating from

---

[2] At the same time, as many have pointed out, it cannot be assumed that simply sharing cultural/ethnic heritage transcends problems in clinician-client understanding. As Wohl points out, "similarity is not identity: each person carries a unique version of the same culture. There is always a difference in the understanding and internalization of a culture. For this reason it can be said that all psychotherapy is transcultural or cross-cultural. There is always a gap to be traversed" (1989, pp. 343-344).

such primary encounter data new insights into the psychological and cultural construction of the patient's own world? How can the time-pressed clinician operationalize the exhortations to take cultural factors into account in the course of an intake interview? (p. 216).

Parallel sentiments and concerns are raised in research contexts, where assessors are even more pressed for time and the assessor-assessed relationship even more drastically attenuated. In our view, satisfactory responses to such issues are only partially possible within the context of "time-pressed" assessments. Skillful interviewing and careful listening to "what [people] tell us about themselves, and how they do the telling" is crucial to clinical understanding and insight (Green, 1995, p.131) and inevitably time-consuming. Moreover, ethnographic understanding requires that client narratives be understood within the framework of relevant geopolitical, historical, and sociocultural contexts.

In the case of Cambodian American survivors of the Killing Fields, for example, the researcher or clinician should be knowledgeable about such contextual factors as the history of Cambodian geopolitical conflicts and the patterns of atrocities suffered by survivors and refugees. Other factors include the medical belief systems that influence contemporary Cambodian American attributions of illness and cure (for example, Theravada Buddhism, Khmer folk religion, Chinese medicine and contemporary biomedicine), and the philosophy of syncretism or complementarity that organizes and legitimates this blend of beliefs. The researcher or clinician should understand frequently used categories of problems and attendant symptoms (for example, *kchall koo*, a life-threatening form of wind illness, in which bad wind has become "frozen" as a result of extreme exhaustion, emotional distress or spirit possession) (Frye & D'Avanzo, 1994), and the nature of causal attributions (for example, that beliefs about the causes of disease are eclectic and include imbalances in the natural or supernatural environment, offended spirits, moral transgressions, diet- or behavior-induced humoral balances and sorcery) (see Aronson, 1987).

A Cambodian client may explicitly discuss relevant contextual content in an assessment interview, but clearly cannot be expected to carry the burden of providing the historical and sociocultural framework within which his or her own illness narratives are to be understood. Rather, the burden is on the assessor to supplement skillful interviewing and careful listening with substantive knowledge of relevant contextual factors. There is no simple substitute for the acquisition of this contextual knowledge or for the skillful "negotiation" among and between diagnostic constructs and the person's experience in a particular sociocultural context.

Asian Americans are heavily comprised of immigrant and refugee groups. For members of this diverse population, personal conceptions of symptoms and illness can derive from cosmological belief systems that are quite distinct from the biomedical paradigm that dominates the mental health and larger health care systems in the U.S. A Cambodian American mental health professional in Seattle provides a classic example of how cross-cultural differences in understanding symptom expressions can easily occur. She notes that Cambodian clients in primary care

THE PLACE OF ETHNOGRAPHIC UNDERSTANDING IN THE ASSESSMENT OF ASIAN AMERICAN MENTAL HEALTH

settings often complain of experiencing symptoms of dizziness, headaches and tightness of the chest. To the physician, this presentation typically triggers thinking within a biomedical semantic network that links these symptoms to possible cardiac or respiratory system problems. However, to many Cambodian refugee clients, these same symptoms are semantically linked to *peal keutchreun* (alternatively, *koucharang*) or thinking too much, a syndrome experienced by many refugees who experienced trauma during the 1975-1979 war in Cambodia (Svy, 1996; see also Frye & D'Avanzo, 1994).

This example demonstrates the implications of local cultural context for valid mental health assessments of Asian Americans. It illustrates the importance of developing an understanding of and respect for differences in the explanatory models of professionals and lay persons (Good, 1977; Good, Good, & Moradi, 1985). It also reminds us that the person's experience of symptoms may be at least partially rooted in the historical traumas of the social body or polity. This is particularly so if the person is the survivor of war or other social catastrophes, as is the case, for example, with many Southeast Asian refugees and immigrants. In such cases, a client's suffering and manifest symptom experiences are inextricably linked to collectively experienced geopolitical atrocities. To decouple individual from social suffering—to interpret symptoms narrowly in terms of disease and individual pathology—is to risk violating the experience of sufferers and contributing to the very suffering mental health practitioners seek to remedy (see Kleinman, Das & Lock, 1997; Shay, 1995; Uehara, Farris, Morelli, & Ishisaka 1999).[3]

2.1 Enhancing Ethnographic Understanding: Two methods

The essence of developing ethnographic understanding is **empathic listening** to the person's particular and existential experience of illness and suffering, and **translating** and **interpreting** this experience in sociocultural as well as clinical context (Kleinman, 1988a; Kleinman, Das, & Lock, 1997). While there are no quick and simple substitutes for knowledge of the person's sociocultural context and history, tools that aid in enhancing ethnographic understanding are available to the researcher and clinician. These come mainly in the form of systematic approaches to the elicitation and analysis of narrative data from the client and/or ancillary sources. These tools include, for example, the ethnographic interview (an open-ended approach to clinical interviewing that places the client in the position of expert and cultural guide to his or her own illness experiences and the practitioner in the role of listener and learner) (see Green, 1995; Green & Leigh, 1989; Leigh, 1998) and various methods and strategies for eliciting and analyzing client illness narratives (for example, Cain, 1991; Cohler, 1982; Mishler, 1995; Uehara et al., 1999).

---

[3] Thus, ethnographically informed assessment of Southeast Asian survivors of trauma must involve comprehension of what Kleinman and colleagues refer to as the "sociosomatic recticulum," or the symbolic bridge between social and bodily distress (Kleinman, 1986, 1988b; Kleinman, Das, & Lock, 1997; Kleinman & Kleinman, 1994).

224 EDWINA S. UEHARA, NANCY FARWELL, GREG YAMASHIRO, AND MICHAEL SMUKLER

In this section, we illustrate how such tools can work to enhance cross-cultural understanding of illness. We do not aim to teach specific data gathering and analysis skills and strategies; instead we would point the interested reader to the growing literature on clinical ethnographic methods. We have chosen to highlight two general approaches here: the semantic network and common sense reasoning analysis. Both have great potential to enhance ethnographic understanding in clinical and research contexts but differ somewhat in focus and strategy.

2.1.1 Semantic network analysis

The impetus for the creation of Byron Good's classic ethnographic tool, the semantic network analysis, is his critique of the empiricist, biomedical paradigm that views diseases as natural entities free of cultural context and reducible to physiological terms, and diagnosis as the purely technical task of linking a person's condition to a disease category through the interpretation of disease symptoms (Good, 1977; Good, Good, & Moradi, 1985; Wartofsky, 1975). Good's aim is to support the "de-entification" of disease theory, to "explore the view that diseases are not constituted as natural entities but as social and historical realities" (Good, 1977, p. 6). Good's criticism is not that diagnosis is an unimportant mode of medical activity. Rather, he suggests, we need a new understanding of the relationship between medical language and disease—an understanding that does not reify the conception of disease or reduce medical semantics to a mere "naming" function of language. Good (1977) proposes that a disease category is powerful not because it links "symptoms" to "natural" disease entities. Rather, its meaning and power derives from its capacity to link together in a potent image a complex network of symbols, norms, values, feelings, stresses, and experiences that are deeply integrated into the structure of a community and its culture. Thus, disease categories can be understood as core symbols[4] in a semantic network—a network of words, situations, symptoms and feelings that are associated with an illness and give it meaning for the sufferer. The meaning of a disease (or illness) term is generated socially as it is used by individuals to articulate their experiences of stress, conflict and suffering, thus

---

[4] Good (1977) suggests that a culture's illness categories are what semanticists call, "core symbols"—symbols that gather their power and meaning by their capacity to link together a set or field of disparate symbols and condense them into a simple image which can 'invoke a nexus of symbolic associations". Core symbols attain their depth "not through their taxonomic generality but through their quality of 'polysemy'"—i.e., the property of a symbol to relate to a multiple range of other symbols. As core symbols, illness categories represent the very basic social experience in the society, touching upon the most basic physiological, normative, and ideological significata of the society and linking basic social and motivational elements. Illness categories thus play a crucial role in forming symbolic pathways that link "the values and aspirations of purposive action, the stresses, shames and disappointments of social contingencies, and the affective and ultimately physiological elements of the personal" (p. 38-39).

THE PLACE OF ETHNOGRAPHIC UNDERSTANDING IN THE ASSESSMENT OF ASIAN AMERICAN MENTAL HEALTH

becoming linked to typical syndromes of stress in the society (Good, 1977).[5] Core symbols and the semantic network links in which they are embedded can be evoked by eliciting from members of a local cultural system: (1) their description of illness symptoms and experiences; (2) their impressions as to causes, consequences and contingencies of those experiences; and (3) common semantic associations with causally linked terms.

To demonstrate how such a network can be constructed, Good (1977) focuses on describing the place and meaning of "heart discomfort" within the semantics of illness in Iran. He first elicits data on local concepts about the causes of heart discomfort through a health questionnaire administered to a stratified sample of 750 persons in several village locales. Respondents were asked: (1) if anyone in their family had been sick with heart distress in the past eight months; (2) if so, who/what treatments were sought and (3) what was believed to have caused the illness. Open-ended responses to these questions were content-analyzed and summarized in figure form (see Figure 1 below).

Next, Good carefully traces the common semantic associations that extend the meaning of the linked terms. For example, the contraceptive pill is identified as a cause of heart discomfort (see Figure 1). The pill, in turn is believed to make a woman appear "old"; while both being "old" and the "pill" are associated with "infertility" (see Figure 2). These semantic links are derived from a variety of sources, including respondents' statements, complaints of symptoms, and popular medicine.

Finally, he (1977) creates a comprehensive network of linked terms and associations illustrating that "infertility" is embedded in a complex of symbols and experiences. This complex, which Good labels "the problematics of female sexuality"(p. 41), comprises one of two major semantic fields within which "heart discomfort" and an array of illness symptoms, experiences and feelings are understood and given meaning. This comprehensive semantic network ultimately allows him to answer initially puzzling questions about the presentation of heart distress symptoms in Iran—for example, why seemingly diverse anxieties (contraception, pregnancy, old age, and interpersonal problems) are all associated locally with one illness (heart distress).

---

[5] An illness term is dynamic and galvanizing. As Good (1977) points out:

It is constituted as it is used in social interaction to articulate the experience of distress and to bring about action that will relieve that distress. It is in the purposive use of medical language in particular institutional and communicative contexts that semantic illness networks are generated and change.

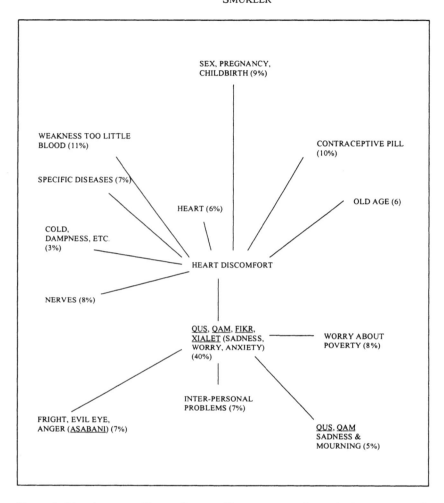

Figure 1. Listed causes of heart distress. (Percentages refer to the responses to the question: "What was the cause of the heart discomfort?"

Note: From "The heart of what's the matter: The semantics of illness in Iran," by B. Good, 1977, *Culture, Medicine & Psychiatry, 1,* p. 40.
© 1977 Kluwer Academic Publishers. Reprinted with permission.

Note that since Good's intention is to represent a local system's semantic associational network, the "goodness" of his analysis depends upon both the logic and rigor of his sampling, the accuracy of his knowledge of Iranian culture, and the logic and appropriateness of his application of knowledge to data interpretation.

Thus questions of "validity" and "reliability" enter into ethnographic as well as conventional forms of assessment.

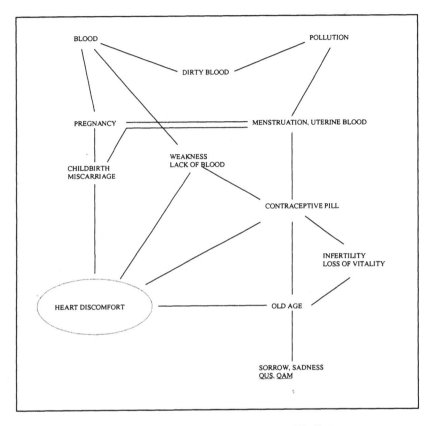

Figure 2. Female Sexuality: Potency and Pollution

Note: From "The heart of what's the matter: The semantics of illness in Iran," by B. Good, 1977, *Culture, Medicine & Psychiatry, 1,* 41.
© 1977 Kluwer Academic Publishers. Reprinted with permission.

As Svy (1996) suggests, comprehension of when and how the semantic illness networks of Asian Americans may differ from mainstream biomedical illness models is critical to valid mental health assessment. As her discussion suggests, the category, *peal keutchreun* or *koucharang*, is a core symbol in the Cambodian American illness lexicon that connects and makes coherent a set of symptoms (chest pain, palpitations, shortness of breath, and excess sleeping and so forth) and links to a series of historical and contemporary experiences. For example, in Frye and

D'Avanzo's (1994) analysis of Cambodian American conceptions of the causes and symptoms of illness, participants recognize *peul keutchreun* as a common experience among survivors of the Cambodian Killing Fields, that is associated with intrusive memories of experiences under the Khmer Rouge regime; flashbacks caused by current stress or violence in family; difficulties coping with English language and other aspects of American culture; and conflicts within the family (see Frye & D'Avanzo, 1994). Within the contemporary Cambodian semantic network, a complex structure of post-war and post-migration experiences intersect with changing gender and family roles and relations and other transformations associated with war, dislocation, and migration to lead to a typical set of stresses that many Cambodian Americans experience and articulate as "thinking too much." A mental health assessment that fails to apprehend these symptoms within the culturally and semantically appropriate network of Cambodian meanings can lead to fundamental misinterpretations of illness experience and inappropriate interventions.

2.1.2 Analysis of client common sense reasoning

Like Good's semantic network, Jurg Siegfried's (1998) approach provides analytic guidance in eliciting and analyzing local understanding of illness. Siegfried assumes the centrality of common sense reasoning to engendering ethnographic insight and cross-cultural understanding. The basis of cross-cultural assessment and therapy, he suggests, is the assessor's understanding of the assessed person's common sense language. Common sense refers to those shared, taken-for-granted, socioculturally determined patterns of making causal attributions, categorizing or topicalizing external and internal phenomena, and valuating behavior and interaction that permit people to form a successful, mutual appreciation of each others' attitudes, behaviors, and actions. It is the nature of common sense, Siegfried (1998) suggests, to assimilate and accommodate new information and to "correct itself again and again when need arises" (p. 283). Thus, communication with others may be seen "as a process of eliminating misunderstandings and doubts"—an interactive attempt "to make sense of the other's talk, behavior, or masses of sensory input by continuously eliminating false hypotheses" (p. 283). When sufficient information is given, people usually succeed in finding common ground, enabling them to share experience and understand each other.

In cross-cultural mental health research and practice, the researcher or practitioner frequently encounters unfamiliar concepts and reasoning strategies. To communicate effectively, she or he thus has "no other choice but to learn continuously the communicative practices of the local culture . . . " (Siegfried, 1998, p. 287). Viewed from this perspective, cross-cultural mental health assessment is a form of communication aimed in part at eliminating misunderstanding, understanding the client's common sense reasoning around illness, and identifying common ground on which to collaborate on a culturally acceptable treatment strategy. Understanding of a person's socioculturally formed common-sense language is the basis of cross-cultural understanding. Failure to understand such

THE PLACE OF ETHNOGRAPHIC UNDERSTANDING IN THE ASSESSMENT OF ASIAN AMERICAN MENTAL HEALTH

preconditions to treatment frequently leads to client drop out, as most cross-cultural clinicians are only too aware.

Table 1. Tibetan medical cures and behavioral counteractions to anger and jealousy (N=100)

Tibetan counteractions to anger	Mean Proportions	Tibetan counteractions to jealousy	Mean Proportions
Medical cures		*Medical cures*	
Diet	.67*	Diet	.38*
Cures for "wind" disorders	.69*	Cures for "wind" disorders	.40*
Medicine	.60	Medicine	.34*
Moxa	.43	Moxa	.27*
Medical ointment	.53	Medical ointment	.32*
Massage	.55	Massage	.18*
Religious practices		*Religious practices*	
Practice of the 10 moral principles	.93*	Practice of the 10 moral principles	.95*
Accumulation of merits	.86*	Accumulation of merits	.87*
Offering and confession	.90*	Offering and confession	.91*
Patience	.95*	Patience	.93*
Mediation on emptiness	.91*	Mediation on emptiness	.90*
Mediation on nature of mind	.89*	Mediation on nature of mind	.89*
Rituals	.96*	Rituals	.54
Guidance		*Guidance*	
Guidance	.90*	Guidance	.94*
Advice	.96*	Advice	.90*
Social activities		*Social activities*	
Cultivating of friendship	.97*	Cultivating of friendship	.84*
Lifestyle changes	.84*	Lifestyle changes	.73*
Diversion of attention	.73*	Diversion of attention	.67*
Drinking and dancing	.73*	Drinking and dancing	.44
Sexual relations	.65*	Sexual relations	.36*

*Significant deviation from random answering (p=.50)

Note: From "Common sense reasoning in the transcultural psychotherapy process", by J. Siegfried, in *Clinical Methods in Transcultural Psychiatry,* edited by S. Okpaku, 1998, Washington, DC: American Psychiatric Press.
© 1998 American Psychiatric Press. Reprinted with permission.

To comprehend a particular client's common sense reasoning in a particular problem context, the practitioner must understand broader sociocultural patterns of communication and common sense reasoning. For any particular cultural system this includes, for example, understanding how particular sets of experiences or behaviors become recognizable as "problems"; how causal attributions are made and "facts" mustered to support attributions; how attributions are challenged/supported, and what means of changing problematic behavior are culturally available.

Siegfried (1998) provides a concrete and rather elegant example of the power and importance of understanding common sense reasoning patterns. In his research on Tibetan medicine, he asks a sample of 100 Tibetan subjects what counteractions they use against the frequently topicalized problem of anger and jealousy. Siegfried summarizes responses in a simple table listing counteractions and the proportion of subjects considering a particular cure as being a normative treatment for the identified problem. This table is reproduced in Table 1.

Siegfried identifies four categories of counteractions against anger and jealousy (traditional medical cures, Buddhist religious practices, guidance, and social activities). Overall, a very wide range of counteractions are identified, from medicines and moxa to practicing of the 10 moral principles, seeking advice, cultivating friendship, and making lifestyle changes. Like Byron Good, Siegfried analyzes and makes sense out of these data by applying his intimate knowledge of Tibetan culture, society and medicine.[6] It is within this specific and detailed understanding of Tibetan culture that he is able to interpret upon these simple survey findings, and to articulate them closely with religious beliefs and every day community practices. In this example, Siegfried thus demonstrates how it is possible to gather potentially very useful data on culturally congruent problem topics (anger and jealousy) and an array of culturally available coping strategies, according to Tibetan common sense. These provide a launching point for culturally informed problem assessment and the mutual exploration of acceptable treatments. For example, these data suggest that guidance, traditional medical cures, religious practices, and some particular social activities may be culturally available tools for addressing problems in this local cultural system (Siegfried, 1998).

3. DISCUSSION

There is a growing consensus among mental health researchers and practitioners that understanding symptoms and suffering simply *qua* disease is no longer an adequate framework for mental health assessment. Following Kleinman, Rogler and others, we have argued that ethnographic understanding enhances the validity of mental health assessment, and that various ethnographic tools are available to the cross-cultural practitioner. Semantic network analysis and the analysis of common sense reasoning are just two approaches that offer assistance in developing ethnographically-informed cross-cultural assessments.

---

[6] Like Good's work, the "validity" of Siegfried's interpretations is ultimately dependent upon such factors as the adequacy of his survey and sampling methods, the depth and accuracy of his understanding of Tibetan culture, and so forth.

THE PLACE OF ETHNOGRAPHIC UNDERSTANDING IN THE ASSESSMENT OF ASIAN AMERICAN MENTAL HEALTH

We realize that the reality of time and resource limitations often make it difficult for assessors, in either research or practice contexts, to apply ethnographic tools. Moreover, the cost containment imperatives operating in most care environments support rapid and standardized assessments rather than the more time-consuming approaches we advocate here. Given the counter-pressures of contemporary practice environments, cross-cultural practitioners are especially time-pressed and challenged in incorporating ethnographic methods in assessment. Here, we suggest that the creation of long-term partnerships among cross-cultural mental health researchers and agencies that serve Asian American ethnic groups and communities could substantially contribute to progress. Such organizational partnerships might create clearing-houses to centralize and share efforts to systematically identify, translate, field-test, and disseminate compendia of tools suitable for cross-cultural assessments. Such consortia might also pool resources to identify, test, and apply the most promising tools to jointly conduct ethnographic analyses—for example, to create and continually update compendia of culture-specific medical lexicons or semantic networks, or to compile descriptions of typically topicalized mental health problems, normative solutions and patterns of common-sense reasoning among specific cultural groups. Joint efforts among mental health agencies to understand the historical and socio-cultural contexts of Asian American clients and to refine and test ethnographic assessment methods will contribute to an important aim shared by cross-cultural researchers and practitioners alike: enhancing the validity of cross-cultural mental health assessments. As many cross-cultural researchers suggest, this is a pivotal step toward the ultimate goal of assessment: the creation of treatment strategies that view the client as a whole person. Such treatments are predicated on understanding the social and cultural contexts of clients and the systemic barriers to culturally responsive relationships.

4. REFERENCES

Antonovsky, A. (1989). Islands rather than bridgeheads: The problematic status of the biopsychosocial model. *Family Systems Medicine, 7,* 243-253.

Aronson, L. (1987). Traditional Cambodian health beliefs and practices: Understanding Cambodian traditions will facilitate their care in a Western setting. *Rhode Island Medical Journal, 70,* 73-78.

Cohler, B. (1982). Personal narrative and the life course. In P.B. Baltes & O. G. Brim (Eds.), *Life-span development and behavior* (pp. 205-241). New York: Academic.

Cain, C. (1991). Personal stories: Identity acquisition and self-understanding in Alcoholics Anonymous. *Ethos, 19,* 210-253.

Frye, B., & D'Avanzo, C. D. (1994). Cultural themes in family stress and violence among Cambodian refugee women in the inner city. *Advances in Nursing Science, 16*(3), 64-77.

Good, B. (1977). The heart of what's the matter. The semantics of illness in Iran. *Culture, Medicine, and Psychiatry, 1,* 25-58.

Good, B., Good, M., & Moradi, R. (1985). The interpretation of Iranian depressive illness and dysphoric affect. In A. Kleinman & B. Good (Eds.), *Culture and Depression: Studies in the Anthropology and Cross-Cultural Psychiatry of Affect and Disorder* (pp. 369-428). Berkeley, CA: University of California Press.

Green, J. (1985). *Cultural awareness in the human services: A multi-ethnic approach.* Boston: Allyn & Bacon.

Green, J., & Leigh, J. (1989). Teaching ethnographic methods to social service workers. *Practicing Anthropology, 11,* 8-10.

Hughes, C. C. & Okpaku, S. O. (1998). Culture's role in clinical psychiatric assessment. In S. Okpaku (Ed.), *Clinical methods in transcultural psychiatry* (pp. 213-232). Washington, DC: American Psychiatric Press.

Kleinman, A. (1977). Depression, somatization, and the "new cross-cultural psychiatry. *Social Science Medicine, 11,* 3-10.

Kleinman, A. (1988a). *The illness narratives: Suffering, healing & the human condition.* New York: Basic Books.

Kleinman, A. (1988b). *Rethinking psychiatry: From cultural category to personal experience.* New York: MacMillan.

Kleinman, A. & Good, B. (Eds.). (1985). *Culture and depression: Studies in the anthropology and cross-cultural psychiatry of affect and disorder.* Berkeley, CA: University of California Press.

Kleinman, A., & Kleinman, J. (1994). How bodies remember: Social memory and bodily experience of criticism, resistance, and delegitimation following China's cultural revolution. *New Literary History, 25,* 707-723.

Kleinman, A., Das, V., & Lock, M. (Eds.). (1997). *Social suffering.* Berkeley, CA: University of California Press.

Leigh, J. (1998). *Communicating for cultural competence.* Boston: Allyn & Bacon.

López, S., & Hernandez, P. (1986). How culture is considered in evaluations of psychopathology. *Journal of Nervous and Mental Disease, 176,* 598-606.

Mechanic, D. (1999). Mental health and mental illness: Definitions and perspectives. In A. Horwitz & T.L. Scheid (Eds.), *A handbook for the study of mental health: Social contexts, theories, and systems* (pp. 12-28). Cambridge, MA: University Press.

Mishler, E. G. (1995). Models of narrative analysis: A typology. *Journal of Narrative and Life History, 5,* 87-123.

Park, C., & Folkman, S. (1997). Meaning in the context of stress and coping. *Review of General Psychiatry, 2,* 115-144.

Pescolido, B. (1991). Illness careers and network ties: A conceptual model of utilization and compliance. *Advances in Medical Sociology, 2,* 161-184.

Pescolido, B. (1992). Beyond rational choice: The social dynamics of how people seek help. *American Journal of Sociology, 97,* 1096-1138.

Rogler, L. H. (1992). Editorial. The role of culture in mental health diagnosis: The need for programmatic research. *Journal of Nervous and Mental Disease, 180,* 745-747.

Rogler, L. H. (1993a). Culturally sensitizing psychiatric diagnosis: A framework for research. *Journal of Nervous and Mental Disease, 181,* 401-408.

Rogler, L.H. (1993b). Culture in psychiatric diagnosis: An issue of scientific accuracy. *Psychiatry, 56,* 324-327.

Sandelowski, M. (1996). One is the liveliest number: The case orientation of qualitative research. *Research in Nursing & Health, 19,* 525-529.

Shay, J. (1994). *Achilles in Vietnam: Combat trauma and the undoing of character.* New York: Atheneum.

Siegfried, J. (1998). Common sense reasoning in the transcultural psychotherapy process. In S. Okpaku (Ed.), *Clinical methods in transcultural psychiatry* (pp. 279-300). Washington, DC: American Psychiatric Press

Svy, D. (1996, March). [Unpublished presentation notes on differences in semantic networks of Cambodian clients and monolingual physicians]. Seattle, WA.

Thoits, P. (1995). Stress, coping, and social support processes: Where are we? What next? *Journal of Health and Social Behavior* (extra issues), 53-79.

Twaddle, A. C., & Hessler, R. M. (1985). *A sociology of health* (2nd ed.). New York: MacMillan.

Uehara, E., Farris, M., Morelli, P. & Ishisaka, A. (1999). *'Eloquent chaos' in the oral discourses of Killing Fields survivors: An exploration of atrocity and narrativization.* Unpublished manuscript.

Wartofsky, L. (1975). Organs, organisms and disease: Human ontology and medical practice. In H. T. Englehardt, Jr. & S. F. Spicker (Eds.), *Evaluation and explanation in the biomedical sciences* (pp. 67-83). Reidel Publishing.

MAY YEH AND JOYCE WU YEH

CHAPTER 16

THE CLINICAL ASSESSMENT OF ASIAN AMERICAN CHILDREN

1. INTRODUCTION

Asian American children constitute a unique and diverse group within the Asian American population. Like adults, children have varying immigration histories, experiences, and acculturation levels. However, the potential cultural factors influencing a child's clinical presentation further include the role of children in traditional Asian cultures and additional special factors specific to youth.

Cultural factors need to be taken into consideration when interpreting information gathered with the mainstream questionnaires, projective instruments, and/or mental status examinations often used in the clinical child assessment process. This chapter reviews the limited but growing empirical literature regarding common clinical assessment tools used with Asian and Asian American children. It also discusses various cultural values and norms that may influence the child's clinical presentation in the context of the mental status examination, and highlights special considerations in the initial clinical assessment process. Case examples are also provided to illustrate specific points.[1] The focus will be upon traditional Asian values that may be relevant to clinical child assessment. Due to space limitations, we will discuss Asian cultures in a general sense and will not be able to address the great heterogeneity that exists within Asian cultures, differing acculturation levels, or issues specific to particular developmental stages. Also, the information presented reflects the greater availability of literature on some Asian cultures and Asian American groups relative to other groups. The material in this chapter is meant as an introduction to cultural factors that require consideration in the initial clinical assessment of Asian American children, with an emphasis on the role of traditional Asian values and an awareness of the need for further research. The goal is to help clinicians who conduct initial assessments and diagnostic interviews develop a preliminary cultural context from which to understand the potential range of values and clinical presentations they may encounter with Asian American children.

---

[1] Information provided from cases has been presented with client permission or has been altered to prevent client identification.

2. REVIEW OF EMPIRICAL LITERATURE

Little research has been conducted to test the validity of standardized clinical assessment instruments with Asian or Asian American children. However, some empirical literature describe the use of various instruments with specific Asian or Asian American groups and comparisons to mainstream American culture.

2.1 Checklists

The Child Behavior Checklist (CBCL) (Achenbach, 1991) is available in several Asian languages (Vignoe, Berube, & Achenbach, 1999) (e.g., Cambodian, Chinese, Japanese, Korean, Tagalog, and/or Vietnamese, depending on the CBCL version). Several empirical studies, which we review here, provide information about its cross-cultural use with Asian and Asian American children.

Li, Su, Townes, and Varley (1989) reported cross-cultural differences between Chinese samples on the CBCL parent and teacher versions when compared to U.S. norms. Chinese mean behavior problem scale T-scores were generally lower than those of the U.S. norms, and in addition, use of the CBCL clinical cut-off score reflected a high false negative rate with the Chinese sample in the study. However, Li et al. (1989) found that scores of Chinese children with attention deficit disorder with hyperactivity were significantly different from Chinese controls, indicating some utility in differentiation for that disorder. Su and her colleagues (Su, Li, Wan, Yang, & Luo, 1996; Su, Li, Luo, Wan, Yang, 1998) have developed norms and revisions of the CBCL specifically for Chinese children, with reports available in the Chinese language literature.

Weisz et al. (1993) compared Thai and American adolescent behavior and emotional problems using the CBCL and the Thai Youth Checklist, which is a Thai-language instrument that includes comparable CBCL items. They found that while total problems scores did not differ notably, 45 of the 118 individual problems showed significant cultural effects, with Thai adolescents displaying more overcontrolled behavior problems. Thai adolescents scored significantly higher than American adolescents on total overcontrolled behavior scores, but did not differ significantly on total undercontrolled behavior scores. In terms of undercontrolled problems, Thai adolescents reported more indirect, subtle behaviors, while American youth had more interpersonally aggressive behaviors, suggesting a possible cultural influence on the expression of aggression.

Chang, Morrissey, and Koplewicz (1995) reported that Chinese-American children from a weekend Chinese school in New York City scored significantly lower on the CBCL Total problem, Internalizing problem, Externalizing problem, Total Competence, Activities, and Social scales when compared to the CBCL's reported norms by age and gender. Chang et al. (1995) postulated that these lower scores may have been due to factors such as respondent underreport of problems, actual differences in symptom scores, characteristics specific to the selected sample, cultural intolerance of acting-out behavior, or other cultural influences. Total number of years in the United States was not significantly correlated with the results. In addition, Chang et al. (1995) compared the sample's scores to norms obtained from a Chinese sample of boys (Li et al., 1989, described above) and found that the Chinese-American boys in the New York City sample scored significantly higher than the Chinese boys on the Withdrawn, Anxious/Depressed, Social Problems, Thought Problems, and Aggressive Behavior scales. They also scored significantly lower on Total Competence, Activities, and Social Competence Scores. Chang et al. (1995) suggested these findings might have resulted from stressors related to acculturation and minority status in the United States. Taken as a whole, the studies summarized above suggest that the CBCL and its versions are useful with Asian American populations, but that profile interpretation with existing norms may require special consideration of cultural influences.

Chen and Yang (1986) compared Chinese American youth scores on the Offer Self-Image Questionnaire to scores obtained from standard Chinese and United States samples. They report that the Chinese American youth scores were generally similar to Offer's normed sample, but with a significant difference in Sexual Attitudes, in which Chinese Americans (CA) tended to be more conservative. When compared to the general U.S. sample (GS), low levels of significance were found for the Body-and Self-Image Scale (CA lower than GS), Morals Scale (CA higher than GS), and the Psychopathology scale (CA higher than GS). In general, Chinese American self-image scores were more similar to those of the general American sample than to the Chinese sample. Overall, the Chinese American scores were significantly different from the Chinese scores, with Chinese American scores falling between those of the general Americans and Chinese. However, there were no significant differences between the Chinese American and Chinese samples on the Morals, Family Relationships, and Superior Adjustment Scales.

When comparing child samples in Singapore and in those in England on the junior Eysenck Personality Questionnaire, Eysenck and Long (1986) found that while personality dimensions were similar in the two samples, differences between the samples were found on the personality factors. Notably, the Singapore sample showed elevated Social Desirability.

2.2 Projective Tests

When comparing 20 Japanese child Rorschach location profiles to Exner's (1982, as cited in Takeuchi & Scott, 1986) norms from Americans, Takeuchi and Scott found twice as many responses given by Japanese subjects as compared to the original normed sample, a larger range of content covered by the Japanese children, and three location trends that suggest a high mental maturity in the Japanese sample. Lower Japanese scores on form quality may have reflected cultural differences, as the scoring system was based on American conventionality (Takeuchi & Scott, 1986).

Nuttall, Chieh, and Nuttall (1988) compared kinetic family drawings of Chinese and U.S. elementary school children and found that the Chinese youth included parents and grandparents more often than did the U.S. youth. In addition, U.S. youths' pictures reflected individualism more so than did the drawings of their

Chinese counterparts. In a comparison of Japanese and Filipino children with the Kinetic Family Drawing Test (KFD) (Burns, 1980, as cited in Cabacungan, 1985), cultural differences were apparent in several areas, including the actions of the major figures, communication and nurturance levels, depicted actions, and actual family size drawn (Cabacungan, 1985).

When scoring tests that involve drawing components, it is important to consider the cultural role of spontaneous, creative drawing. Gardner (1989) has observed that, in the United States where exploratory, creative drawing may be highly valued at an early age, Chinese cultures place a greater early emphasis upon acquiring basic skills through being taught and through practice. Such cultural influences may then affect the nature of the figures and illustrations produced in drawing tests.

The available literature supports the viability of the Roberts Apperception Test for Children (RATC) (McArthur & Roberts, 1982) for use with Asian American youth (Roberts, 1994). Cadavid-Hannon (1988) compared 120 well-adjusted pre-adolescent children from four ethnic groups (Anglo, Armenian, Mexican-Hispanic, and Korean) and found that all of the groups scored within the originally normed average range for children without clinical difficulties. However, significant differences were found among the four groups on some scales or sub-scales, even within the average range. Specifically relevant to this chapter, the Korean group scored lower on Reliance on Others (asking for help from others) than the Mexican-Hispanic children and the Armenian children; lower on Aggression than the Mexican-Hispanic children; higher on Limit Setting from parents as perceived by children than all of the other groups; lower on the Anxiety 1 subscale (apprehension and fear) than the Anglo children; and higher on the Rejection 2 subscale (scored on responses dealing with physical separation themes) than the Anglo as well as the Mexican-Hispanic children. In a separate small study of 40 youth, Lee-Oh (1994) found that Korean-American early adolescents scored significantly higher than the RATC norms on the Anxiety and Depression scales. In the same study, American-Korean early adolescents' scores on the Anxiety and the Depression scales of the RATC were correlated with different parenting behaviors as indicated by the Cornell Parent Behavior Inventory.

Chu (1968a, 1968b) describes a Thematic Apperception Test remodified for Chinese children of primary school age and indicates that this "remodified" version provides relevant information for differentiating "problem" children from "normal" children. Chu's (1968a) version of the TAT contains a set of drawings developed to reflect themes and relationships important to Chinese children.

3. CULTURAL VALUES AND THE MENTAL STATUS EXAMINATION

In this section, we will highlight areas of the mental status examination in which the clinical presentation of youth may require special consideration of the child's cultural context. General topic areas of the mental status examination as suggested by Sattler (1992) will be used as the overall framework for this discussion; that is, we discuss the areas of appearance and behavior, speech and communications, content of thought, cognitive functioning, emotional functioning, and insight and

THE CLINICAL ASSESSMENT OF ASIAN AMERICAN CHILDREN 237

judgment.[2] For each selected topic, cultural values that may underlie clinical presentation will be described, with possible resulting presentation styles presented. Case examples from the authors' clinical experiences are included to illustrate specific points. Because presentation styles may vary greatly depending on the cultural background and acculturation level of the youth, the following are offered primarily as general considerations for developing hypotheses to be evaluated by the clinician, rather than as steadfast rules.

3.1 Appearance and Behavior

Values upon hierarchical relationships, social desirability, and situationally-appropriate responses may influence the child's appearance and behavior during a clinical interview. Traditional Asian cultures place great importance upon hierarchies and deferential behavior by children to authority figures (Yee, Huang, & Lew, 1998). Because adults by nature assume an authority role to children in traditional Asian cultures, a clinical intake interview in which an adult stranger is evaluating the child may elicit responses appropriate to an authority figure. Culturally congruent deferential behavior may include limited eye contact with the clinician, a restraint of emotions, and limited initiation of interaction. Thus, when such behaviors are displayed, the clinician must determine whether they indicate respect towards the clinician rather than avoidance, resistance, or some other clinical symptom.

In traditional Asian cultures, a high value is placed upon socially desirable behavior (Doi, 1973, as cited in Nakakuki, 1994). Therefore, in clinical interviews, Asian American children may respond in such a way as to appear well-behaved and obedient. Such a social norm, coupled with a desire to save the family's face may also promote limited disclosure of the youth's or the family's problems (Chan, 1998). There is a saying in Chinese culture that, "We shouldn't spread out the family ugliness" (translation from Chinese). Therefore, presentation in the interview may reflect culturally-influenced, socially-desirable behavior and a lack of orientation towards informing the clinician about problems or distress.

Although the clinical interview setting may create apprehension in most children, this experience in Asian American children may be compounded by a culturally-influenced desire to be situationally appropriate and an unfamiliarity with the concept of counseling in general. Past research has shown that Asian Americans may possess certain skills that may not be manifested in certain situations (Ayabe, 1971; D. Sue, Ino, & D. W. Sue, 1983). For example, it is possible that a child may possess the skills to be initiating or verbal, but she may not exhibit these to the examiner in the belief that such behavior is not appropriate in the interview setting. A value upon "saving face" may further encourage a greater vigilance to situational appropriateness. Therefore, it is important to investigate the child's appearance and behavior across multiple settings and/or situations.

---

[2] We have decided to omit the topic of Sensory and Motor Functioning in this discussion.

CASE EXAMPLE. During the initial interview, a teen-aged Japanese American youth was initially unresponsive and nonverbal. His facial expression and motoric inactivity suggested depressive symptoms. In order to increase understanding of whether the youth's appearance and behavior reflected a consistent presentation or were responses to the perceived situational cues of the clinical interview, the examiner initiated the playing of board games with the youth. The youth responded with great interest, participation, and animation. Such a change in interview format not only provided valuable information to the examiner, but also gave the youth new situational cues with which to reframe his interactions with the examiner.

3.2 Speech and Communications

Parenting styles, traditional Asian values, a value upon nonverbal communication, and bilingual capabilities all require consideration in evaluating the speech and communication of Asian American children. In traditional Asian cultures, parents encourage their children to be obedient instead of being assertive (Uba, 1994). For example, O'Reilly, Tokuno, and Ebata (1986) found that Japanese American parents valued a child who "behaves well" as the most important attribute in social competence while White Americans endorsed being "self-directed" as the most important. Such cultural values may influence the degree to which children take initiative with interviewers.

In order to preserve interpersonal harmony, overt confrontations are avoided in traditional Asian cultures while indirect, nonverbal, and subtle communication styles are valued (Chan, 1998; Shon & Ja, 1982; D. W. Sue, 1990). In addition, parenting practices in traditional Asian cultures emphasize physical contact in parenting instead of vocalization, with infants often being carried by caregivers (Chan, 1998). Thus, children may be less direct and verbose in their responses to interviews and may rely more upon nonverbal, indirect communication.

There is anecdotal information suggesting that for Asian American children, selective mutism symptoms may occur with greater frequency, and in many cases, resolve without clinical intervention. In such largely self-resolving cases, Asian American parents, typically of immigrant background, report that their children exhibited selective mutism symptoms lasting approximately 6 months to 1 year upon entering either pre-school, kindergarten, or first grade. These children reportedly behaved normally in the home and performed well on their paperwork at school. However, in addition to displaying noticeable shyness at school, they were mute in classes, especially to teachers. In these anecdotal cases, the functioning level of these children was generally acceptable. Time, understanding support, and limited teacher and parent intervention were sufficient to bring the children to their expected levels of interaction in the school setting, with no formal clinical involvement necessary. It is possible that such behaviors are culturally unique to Asian American children because of their cultural background or high sensitivity to shame, shyness,

THE CLINICAL ASSESSMENT OF ASIAN AMERICAN CHILDREN   239

or embarrassment. In the absence of studies regarding selective mutism in the Asian American population, it is suggested that suspected cases involve a thorough evaluation of functioning levels in other areas outside of the mute presentation to determine the appropriateness of clinical interventions.

For bilingual children, fluency in the language of the interview must be taken into account in evaluating such factors as communicativeness and expressiveness. In addition, the choice of language by bilingual children may at times provide clinically meaningful information.

> CASE EXAMPLE. A fluently bilingual (Chinese, English) teen-aged female was interviewed along with her mother, who spoke Chinese exclusively. Although the examiner was also bilingual, the client chose to use English during the examination. During the course of the interview, it became apparent that the youth's decision to use English was an act of distancing her mother and expressing anger towards her mother by excluding her from the conversation. The examiner's sensitivity to this situation promoted rapport building with the youth and facilitated an accurate assessment of the issues to be addressed in treatment.

3.3   Content of Thought

Traditional Asian families place an extremely high value upon the avoidance of familial shame. In addition, there is a clear boundary between what is kept private within a family and what is told to others outside of the family. Therefore, Asian American children may not be forthcoming about familial information in an effort to protect the family. This may be further complicated by the reliance of some immigrant parents upon their children to communicate with mainstream American society if their children are more versed in English. In such situations, youths may feel an even greater responsibility to be protectors of the family's privacy and reputation. Thus, when evaluating Asian American children, it is important to discern whether a limited production of information reflects culturally-motivated restraint and hesitation rather than difficulties in processing thoughts.

A high sensitivity to the perceptions of others and a great concern about what others may think about them may produce a culturally-influenced belief that others are also talking about them. Although such a phenomenon may appear to be an idea of reference, it is recommended that a shame-oriented cultural basis for such a belief be evaluated concurrently. (The cultural basis of such an orientation towards other persons is described in detail below in the Emotional Functioning section.)

3.4   Cognitive Functioning

When briefly examining a child's cognitive functioning, it is important to consider the traditional Asian value of saving face. The desire to avoid loss of face may influence children to avoid guessing upon answers, elaborating upon responses, or providing a confidently delivered statement. In addition, it is not appropriate for

240 MAY YEH AND JOYCE WU YEH

children to boast about their abilities in traditional Asian cultures (Okano, 1994). Thus, children may avoid answering questions in a way that may be perceived as self-displaying or flaunting such as telling elaborate stories or giving multiple responses for definitions. These response styles may have implications for the evaluation of cognitive functioning. In Asian cultures, a reply of "I don't know" is not taken as a certainty that someone truly does not know how to do something. It may reflect modesty or an uncertainty about the response.

3.5 Emotional Functioning

Restraint of emotions is a culturally-mandated sign of maturity in traditional Asian societies. Several Chinese sayings help to illustrate this point. "If you are too happy, that will lead to sadness." "If you get too much of what you want, you forget your shape." The second saying implies that if a person becomes too excited, a person will lose control of him/herself and get in trouble. Thus, a limited range of emotion during clinical interviews may reflect such values.

There is a consensus in the literature that Asian cultures contain a greater sensitivity to the feeling of shame than is apparent in Western cultures (Cheung, 1986; Ha, 1995; Okano, 1994). Hong Kong Chinese and Asian Americans in Hawai'i tend to score higher on an Embarrassability scale than do Caucasians Americans (Singelis, Bond, Sharkey, & Lai, 1999), and shame or shyness related behaviors such as blushing are more apparent in Japanese cultures (Okano, 1994). In addition, some have observed that the Japanese and Taiwanese experience a higher frequency of shyness than do those in some Western populations (Pilkonis & Zimbardo, 1979). Although a biologically-determined tendency for shyness has been proposed (Kagan, Reznick, & Snidman, 1988), this hypothesis has not yet been thoroughly examined for Asian Americans. However, in terms of other influences, it is clear that Asian cultures view shame or embarrassability (Singelis et al., 1999) differently from Western cultures (Ha, 1995; Okano, 1994). According to Okano (1994), "It even seems as if something in the Japanese culture is actively promoting, facilitating, or at least allowing people to show manifestations of the experiences of shame and related feelings such as shyness, secretiveness, embarrassment, and a sense of inferiority" (p. 326-327). In Chinese culture, it is a severe insult to say of a person that, "He/she does not have shame" (translation from Chinese). In teaching their children right from wrong, parents with traditional Asian values (e.g., parents in China) often use shame as a negative consequence, and affective manipulation may be used as a primary socialization tool (Wilson, 1981). For example, parents may use shame to prevent children from performing an undesirable action (e.g., parents tell children that they will be shamed if the child behaves a certain way). This socialization process sensitizes the child to the feelings of others such as family members (e.g., you are going to make mom feel very sad and lose face) and other observers (e.g., you'll be ridiculed by other people). Thus, answering questions regarding one's own feelings may be difficult due to this focus upon the feelings of others and also the interdependence of one's own feelings upon those of others. A clear understanding of how Asian culture views the affect of shame is very

THE CLINICAL ASSESSMENT OF ASIAN AMERICAN CHILDREN 241

important in the assessment of Asian American children, not only in discerning culturally-normal shyness, non-assertiveness, and self-effacing behaviors, but also in differential diagnosis, as can be seen in the following case example.

CASE EXAMPLE. A 7-year-old Korean American female was exhibiting unusual behaviors such as squinting, wrinkling her face, and covering her face with either one or both hands. At times, her hands became stiff, her body twisted as if in a spasm, and she would pull the collar of her shirt or jacket up and shrink her head into her clothes. Because of her odd behavior, poor communication, lack of verbal expression, social awkwardness, and inattentiveness, school staff suspected an Autistic Disorder.

In conducting this evaluation, it was important to be sensitive to the potential for culturally influenced, situation-specific behaviors. Through information gathering at the school, it became apparent that the behaviors occurred whenever attention was called upon the child either by introducing her to a new person or asking her to answer a question. Her physical behaviors suggested extreme discomfort and an appearance of wanting to disappear. In contrast to school reports, the child's mother reported her to be very affectionate with immediate family members and other relatives as well as very verbally expressive, suggesting situationally-constrained social discomfort. Furthermore, her responses to the Roberts Apperception Test for Children (McArthur & Roberts, 1982) indicated tight and logical thought process with age appropriate and realistic thought content. An Autistic Disorder diagnosis was not supported. In addition, although the child was anxious or uncomfortable at school or at public or social settings, there was a lack of avoidant behaviors typical of Social Phobia. She in fact reported liking school and was not mute across all situations in the school setting. The examiner concluded that the child was displaying selective, culturally-influenced, shame-based, attention-phobic psychopathology. The child responded well to a behavioral program and supportive environment.

When evaluating an older Asian American youth's affect, it is important to note that cultural factors may underlie an apparent incongruence between affect and speech. For example, a teen-aged female may smile or laugh when talking about abuse or pain. Such a behavior may occur because the youth feels that she is burdening the interviewer and feels apologetic for doing so. In addition, because the self is not important in traditional Asian cultures, the youth may not want the interviewer to feel burdened on her behalf. Thus, such ostensible inappropriate affect may require further consideration.

3.6 Insight and Judgment

In traditional Asian cultures, there is a strong belief that life events are controlled by external forces (Cheung, 1986). In summarizing literature on internal/external loci of control, Yang (1986) indicates that Chinese subjects had higher external locus of control scores than did Anglo-American subjects. Thus, if something negative occurs, the thought is that someone or something else is in control of it. The development of learned helplessness or depression in traditional Asian cultures is normally counteracted by a second, complementary philosophy regarding internal coping styles. According to Confucius, "If you miss the target, don't blame the target, examine yourself" (translation from Chinese), which means, when bad circumstances exist, change yourself. Brickman et al. (1982) indicated that there is a distinction between responsibility for the cause of the problem and responsibility for its solution. Thus, when a child expresses a lack of control over the ability to control events, it may be necessary to inquire further about the child's perception of competence to cope with the events when evaluating for depressive symptomatology.

The cultural norms of the parent-child relationship may also become important influences in the child's responses regarding problems and their causes. A statement by Confucius indicates the importance of filial piety: "In case someone sees his parent's wrong doing, he should suggest to him very slightly. If the parent does not listen to him, he should respect the parent without any disobedience, and labor for the parent without any complaints" (translation from Chinese). In addition, Mencius says, "For a son to criticize his father, it is like a thief to steal from a merciful giver" (translation from Chinese). In traditional Asian cultures, parents, especially mothers, sacrifice themselves for their children (Nakakuki, 1994). They live for the next generation and consider children to be the "root of their life" who will, as they have, pay their parents back for their efforts. A common Chinese saying is that "To raise children is like storing up grain; you don't have to worry about getting old or getting hungry" (translation from Chinese). Just as parents sacrifice themselves for their children, they also expect children to do the same for them. These cultural inclinations may mean that Asian American children from highly traditional families may not feel comfortable criticizing their parents or commenting negatively about them, particularly to a person outside of their family. Combined with the sense of internal responsibility mentioned above, children may then blame themselves for their problems, saying that it is because they themselves are bad or need to be changed. Thus, it is important to include additional assessment tools and collateral information beyond the clinical interview if the clinician believes that the child may be avoiding negative reports about the family due to cultural factors. This may be particularly important if the child may not be reporting serious problems that are putting the child at risk (e.g., abuse, substance abuse, etc.).

In traditional Asian culture, the self is defined by relationships and not by self-attributes. Singelis et al. (1999) propose that two kinds of esteem exist in both Eastern and Western cultures: independent self-esteem and interdependent self-esteem. Traditional Asian cultures would reflect a greater emphasis upon interdependent self-esteem. Thus, a question such as, "What are you good at?" may

THE CLINICAL ASSESSMENT OF ASIAN AMERICAN CHILDREN   243

be difficult to answer. Children may say, "Nothing. I can't think of anything." In addition, cultural emphasis is not put upon the self, but on virtue, with children esteemed not for their attributes but for their virtues (Jung, 1998). Comparing oneself to be better than others would not be considered a virtue (Wang, Meredith, & Tsai, 1996). In addition, children may express self-demeaning statements that are culturally appropriate. Thus, children may be uncomfortable with self-regard statements, such as judging how they feel, and voicing special competence in an area (e.g., sports) may be culturally incongruent.

Due to a strong value upon maintaining interpersonal harmony, traditional Asian cultures may promote behaviors that would limit the possibility for jealousy or competitiveness from others (Okano, 1994). These behaviors may include an unwillingness to contradict a person publicly, restraint from assertion of one's own desires, and modesty. In a study of college students in Hong Kong, those students giving self-effacing attributions were more liked than those providing self-enhancing attributions (Bong, Leung, & Wan, 1982, as cited in Singelis et al., 1999). Such behavior in the clinical setting should be evaluated within the cultural context.

Furthermore, it has been observed that children in Western cultures make comparisons based on the average person, whereas mainland Chinese children compare themselves to the best person (Wang et al., 1996). An unwillingness to voice competence at a task does not necessary reflect low self-esteem or depression but rather may be reflections of culturally-based humility, differential standards of comparison, and/or interdependent self-esteem.

4. SPECIAL FACTORS TO BE CONSIDERED IN THE CLINICAL ASSESSMENT OF CHILDREN

4.1 Acculturation

When determining the acculturation level of children, parental influences must be taken into consideration. Parents may differ in the degree to which they encourage acculturation to the "American way of life," with some parents desiring their children to retain a strong Asian cultural identity and others wanting their children to become as "Americanized" as possible as a perceived means to societal success. In addition, parents may endorse certain American values while promoting an overall adherence to traditional Asian values (Nguyen & Williams, 1989). Furthermore, because countries of origin may be themselves changing (Nakakuki, 1994; Yang, 1986) and increasingly influenced by Western culture, a child who immigrates to the United States from a particular Asian country may be more acculturated to Western values in some ways than would perhaps a US-born child whose parents immigrated with more traditional Asian values and instilled these in the child. The child's acculturation information must be interpreted within the context of the acculturation level of other family members, such as parents. Thus, the clinical assessment of Asian American children must contain a thorough understanding of the child's history, values, and cultural background. Preliminary information suggests that the Asian American Family Conflicts Scale (Lee, Choe,

244 MAY YEH AND JOYCE WU YEH

Kim, & Ngo, 2000) may aid assessment of Asian American generational parent-child conflicts and bears further research.

4.2 Voluntary Broken Family Phenomenon

This section will highlight a frequent occurrence in Asian/Asian American families that we will call "voluntary broken family phenomenon." This phenomenon has significant clinical implications. Voluntary separation of family members has long-standing, cultural roots for Asian families. Traditionally, these separations have been made for career, financial, or academic reasons. For example, historically, Chinese fathers ventured away from home in the countryside to the cities in order to take examinations for official positions or for work and may not have returned home for many years. Chinese laborers who came to the United States for financial gains in the mid-19th century through early 20th century left their wives and children behind and stayed in the U.S. for years before returning to China or sending for their families. This practice of separating fathers from their families continues today for similar reasons.

A recent, additional form of voluntary family separation exists whereby minors come to the United States without their parents. There are thousands of Asian children who are sent to the United States while their parents, or, in many cases, their fathers, maintain employment and residence in their native countries (Lin, 1998b). Parental reasons for sending youth to the United States are many and include wanting children to have a better chance for higher education and better socioeconomic status, a desire for sons to avoid mandatory military service, concerns regarding the political stability of the country of origin, to demonstrate high socioeconomic status, and to separate the child from unwanted societal influences in the country of origin (Hong, 1998; Jen, 1998; Kim, 1998; Leung, 1998; Lin, 1998b; Masuda, 1998). Usually, these minors range from 6 to 18 years of age and are attended by their mothers, siblings, relatives, friends, guardians, or sponsor families. Parents typically travel back and forth between the United States and their native country in order to maintain "remote control" over the children. This group of people are referred to informally as "astronaut parents" and "parachute kids" (Fu, 1994, as cited in Lin, 1998b). In an exploratory study, Huang (1998) observed some negative consequences of father absence in four pairs of Chinese siblings from Taiwan whose fathers were absent for 7 to 16 years during their elementary to high school years. Cheng (1998) found significantly higher levels of depression in children who were unaccompanied when compared to those who immigrated with at least one parent. Both accompanied and unaccompanied groups had higher levels of depression than that of the average American teenager. (For further information regarding these unaccompanied children from China, Taiwan, Hong Kong, Japan, and Korea, see Lin, 1998a.)

Another form of the voluntary broken family phenomenon involves highly educated or motivated Asian couples who come to the United States while leaving their young children, often infants, behind in their native country, often sending for them after they are more established in the United States. In other cases, Asian

THE CLINICAL ASSESSMENT OF ASIAN AMERICAN CHILDREN   245

American couples who are married in the United States send their infant children to their native countries to be raised by grandparents or other relatives. The children are brought back to the United States upon reaching school age. The motivations behind these trends may be positive and involve a combination of values upon education, a desire to become financially secure in order to provide for the family, and the hope of the child to retain values from the country of origin. Parents may believe that if they think it would be beneficial for the children, the children will not be adversely affected and will even be grateful for the separation. In addition, parents may assume that children either do not feel the hurt or that their feelings at this time do not matter. Finally, they may believe that if a child is too young to remember the event in later years, then the event has no influence on his/her life.

The disruption in attachment to primary caregivers caused by such voluntary separations may render the child more vulnerable to emotional and behavioral problems as suggested by attachment theories (Bowlby, 1973; Cassidy & Shaver, 1999). In extreme cases, such disruption may be manifested in the disturbed or inappropriate social relatedness of Reactive Attachment Disorder of infancy or early childhood (American Psychiatric Association, 1994). While such severe cases may not be common, the factors placing these kinds of children at risk for psychological disorders may include the following: 1) Immediate placement of the child in a full-time day care center after unification with the parents. In such a case, the child may not have had the opportunity to mourn for his/her loss of the original guardians (e.g., grandparents) or to re-establish bonding with the parents. 2) Having a sibling or siblings who have never been separated from the parents and who are then more naturally attached to the parents. 3) Marital or family conflicts. The quality of care and parental understanding of the child's feelings and resolution of those feelings after the unification are critical factors in the child's adjustment process.

In her clinical practice of close to 20 years with Asian American children, one of the authors has found close to 70% of her public caseload and 30% of private clinical cases to have experienced some sort of early voluntary familial separation. The following example is typical of those cases.

> CASE EXAMPLE. Singaporean American immigrant parents desired for their child to partake of educational opportunities in the United States. In order to establish themselves financially in the U.S. to make this education possible, it was necessary for both parents to be employed, creating a need for childcare. When the child was one year of age, the parents decided to send him to Singapore to be raised by his grandparents. The parents believed that as the first grandchild in the family, the child would be a particular joy to the grandparents and would have a better chance of retaining strong Singaporean roots and values. Upon arrival to Singapore, the child regressed developmentally, including a loss of his previously acquired ability to walk. He cried frequently upon waking, asked for his parents often, had difficulty eating and drinking, displayed a dysphoric mood, and suffered weight loss for a period of 6 months to a year before the symptoms dissipated. When the child reached the age of five, he returned to the United States to begin his education. During the

intervening years, the parents had given birth to a second child (a boy), and given their improving financial situation, had kept this second child with them in the United States to be cared for at a daycare. The parents assumed that the elder child's familial bonds with them would be natural and strong despite the separation. They also did not allow the child time to mourn the loss of relationship with his grandparents who had assumed his primary care for the past four years. In addition, the younger son was very unhappy with the arrival of the older brother and the sharing of parental attention, creating conflict within the home. The older child's early attachment disruption, confusion regarding removal from the grandparents at age five, jealousy of the younger child's relationship with his parents, and a lack of feeling understood and accepted by the parents, placed the child at high risk for psychopathology. The older child eventually became physically abusive to the younger child and maintained a hostile attitude towards his parents. However, at school, no atypical behavior was noted, and the child was an excellent student. Initially, the family hid the violent situation from others, and concurrently, were unable to correct the child's behavior. As the child grew into his teen years, his physical violence extended to his parents, at which point mental health services were sought.

4.3 Cultural Norms in Parenting as They Relate to Child Abuse

When evaluating Asian American children for child abuse, it is important to understand the types of behaviors that are normative in the child's culture. Corporal punishment is not only allowed but also endorsed in traditional Asian cultures, especially in China (Ho, 1986), Korea, Vietnam, and Cambodia. There is a Chinese saying that, "Without being spanked, a child will not become anything useful" (translation from Chinese). In addition, Okamura, Heras, and Wong-Kerberg (1995) describe shaming behaviors such as name calling, severe criticisms, or asking the child to kneel, as expressions of the parent's love in Asian cultures through the correction of misbehaviors. Because some normative Asian parenting practices may be seen as emotional abuse by legal and social institutions within Western cultures, the task of evaluating child abuse in Asian American families is particularly challenging. Certainly, parenting practices that are uncontrolled, irrational, frequent, out of proportion, and physically injurious would be considered to be out of both Asian and Western cultural norms. Consultation with cultural experts is recommended and may assist the clinician in determining abuse.

It is also important to assess the meaning of parenting practices for youth who have been raised in the United States. For example, the shaming behaviors described above may be intended by parents as expressions of parental love and discipline in traditional Asian cultures, but they may not be interpreted as such by youth who are highly acculturated to American values regarding self-esteem. In such cases, it may be clinically appropriate for clinicians to assess and educate the parent regarding the

THE CLINICAL ASSESSMENT OF ASIAN AMERICAN CHILDREN 247

meaning of the practice to their child, as well as its legal and psychological ramifications.

Certain traditional Asian health-related practices may also be misconstrued as abuse. For example, according to Chan (1998), dermabrasion is a common health-related treatment among Southeast Asian groups. Chan (1998) further describes "coining" or *cao gio* (scratch wind) as a common practice that:

> involves first covering the affected area with a medicated ointment such as Tiger Balm, then gently rubbing the area with the edge of a coin (or spoon) downward and away from the head, until dark marks that look like bruises can be seen. This procedures allows the 'toxic wind' to be brought to the body surface and released...These practices [including pinching and cupping] all typically produce welts and superficial bruises that may last a few days and can be easily mistaken as signs of physical abuse (p. 309).

Consultation with cultural experts may be necessary to determine the context of a behavior under evaluation for abuse.

5. CONCLUSION

The competent clinical assessment of Asian American children requires a clear understanding of each child's individual, familial, and cultural context. The utility of standardized, Western clinical tools may vary with Asian American child populations, and further research in this area is certainly necessary. Cultural variables may affect the child's clinical presentation, with both the presence and absence of apparent symptomatology requiring thorough information gathering and hypothesis testing. We have only begun to understand the complex cultural variables that may affect the mental health of Asian American children, and it is hoped that the needs of this population will be addressed as a whole, as well as one child at a time.

6. REFERENCES

Achenbach, T. M. (1991). *Manual for the Child Behavior Checklist and 1991 profile.* Burlington, VT: University of Vermont Department of Psychiatry.

Ayabe, H. (1971). Deference and ethnic difference in voice levels. *Journal of Social Psychology, 85,* 181-185.

American Psychiatric Association. (1994). *Diagnostic and statistical manual of mental disorders* (4th ed.). Washington, DC: Author.

Bowlby, J. (1973). *Attachment and loss, II: Separation.* New York: Basic Books.

Brickman, P., Rabinowitz, V. C., Karuza, J., Jr., Coates, D., Cohn, E., & Kidder, L. (1982). Models of helping and coping. *American Psychologist, 37,* 368-384.

Cabacungan, L. F. (1985). The child's representation of his family in Kinetic Family Drawings: A cross-cultural comparison. *Psychologia, 28,* 228-236.

Cadavid-Hannon, E. B. (1988). *A study of children's adaptive adjustment across multi-cultural groups using the Roberts Apperception Test for Children.* Unpublished Doctoral Dissertation, California School of Professional Psychology, Los Angeles, CA.

Cassidy, J., & Shaver, P. R. (Eds.) (1999). *Handbook of attachment: Theory, research, and clinical applications.* New York: Guilford Press.

Chan, S. (1998). Families with Asian roots. In E. W. Lynch & M. J. Hanson (Eds.), *Developing cross-cultural competence: A guide for working with children and their families* (pp.251-344). Baltimore: Paul H. Brookes Publishing Co.

Chang, L. Y., Morrissey, R. F., & Koplewicz, H. S. (1995). Prevalence of psychiatric symptoms and their relation to adjustment among Chinese-American youth. *Journal of the American Academy of Child and Adolescent Psychiatry, 34,* 91-99.

Chen, C. L., & Yang, D. C. (1986). The self-image of Chinese-American adolescents: A cross-cultural comparison. *International Journal of Social Psychiatry, 32,* 19-26.

Cheng, C.-H. (1998). Assessment of depression among young students from Taiwan and Hong Kong: A comparative study of accompanied and unaccompanied minors. In J. C. H. Lin (Ed.), *In pursuit of education: Young Asian students in the United States* (pp. 95-112). El Monte, CA: Pacific Asia Press.

Cheung, F. M. C. (1986). Psychopathology among Chinese people. In M. H. Bond (Ed.), *The psychology of the Chinese people* (pp. 171-212). Hong Kong: Oxford University Press.

Chu, C.-P. (1968a). The remodification of TAT adapted to Chinese primary school children: I. Remodification of pictures and setting up the objective scoring methods. *Acta Psychologica Taiwanica, 10,* 59-73.

Chu, C.-P. (1968b). The remodification of TAT adapted to Chinese primary school children: II. The application and evaluation of pictures. *Acta Psychologica Taiwanica, Mar. 10,* 74-89.

Eysenck, S. B. G., & Long, F. Y. (1986). A cross-cultural comparison of personality in adults and children: Singapore and England. *Journal of Personality and Social Psychology, 50,* 124-130.

Gardner, H. (1989). Learning, Chinese-style. *Psychology Today, 23,* 54-56.

Ha, F. (1995). Shame in Asian and Western cultures. *American Behavioral Scientist, 38,* 1114-1131.

Ho, D. Y. F. (1986). Chinese patterns of socialization: A critical review. In M. H. Bond (Ed.), *The psychology of the Chinese people.* Hong Kong: Oxford University Press.

Hong, K.-H. (1998). Overseas study by unaccompanied Korean minors: Current issues and future strategies. In J. C. H. Lin (Ed.), *In pursuit of education: Young Asian students in the United States* (pp. 27-43). El Monte, CA: Pacific Asia Press.

Huang, T. L. (1998). Effects of father absence in Chinese American families. In J. C. H. Lin (Ed.), *In pursuit of education: Young Asian students in the United States* (pp. 76-94). El Monte, CA: Pacific Asia Press.

Jen, T. (1998). After the parachute lands: Young students from China. In J. C. H. Lin (Ed.), *In pursuit of education: Young Asian students in the United States* (pp. 62-74). El Monte, CA: Pacific Asia Press.

Jung, M. (1998). *Chinese American family therapy: A new model for clinicians.* San Francisco: Jossey-Bass Publishers.

Kagan, J., Reznick, J. S. & Snidman, N. (1988). Biological basis of childhood shyness. *Science, 240,* 167-171.

Kim, S. C. (1998). Young Korean students in the United States. In J. C. H. Lin (Ed.), *In pursuit of education: Young Asian students in the United States* (pp. 44-54). El Monte, CA: Pacific Asia Press.

Lee, R. M., Choe, J., Kim., G., & Ngo, V. (2000). Construction of the Asian American family conflicts scale. *Journal of Counseling Psychology, 47,* 211-222.

Lee-Oh, J. (1994). *A study of the effect of the parenting style by Korean-American parents on their adolescent children's psychological adjustment.* Unpublished Doctoral Dissertation, California School of Professional Psychology, Los Angeles, CA.

Leung, A. C. N. (1998). "Home alone": The Chinese version - Unaccompanied minors from Hong Kong. In J. C. H. Lin (Ed.), *In pursuit of education: Young Asian students in the United States* (pp. 18-26). El Monte, CA: Pacific Asia Press.

Li, X.-R., Su, L.-Y., Townes, B. D., & Varley, C. K. (1989). Diagnosis of attention deficit disorder with hyperactivity in Chinese boys. *Journal of the American Academy of Child and Adolescent Psychiatry, 4,* 497-500.

Lin, J. C. H. (Ed.) (1998a). *In pursuit of education: Young Asian students in the United States.* El Monte, CA: Pacific Asia Press.

Lin, J. C. H. (1998b). Young Taiwanese students in the United States. In J. C. H. Lin (Ed.), *In pursuit of education: Young Asian students in the United States* (pp. 4-17). El Monte, CA: Pacific Asia Press.

Masuda, G. I. (1998). International students from Japan. In J. C. H. Lin (Ed.), *In pursuit of education: Young Asian students in the United States* (pp. 55-61). El Monte, CA: Pacific Asia Press.

McArthur, D. S. & Roberts, G. E. (1982). *Roberts Apperception Test for Children: A manual.* Los Angeles: Western Psychological Services.

Nakakuki, M. (1994). Normal and developmental aspects of masochism: Transcultural and clinical implications. *Psychiatry, 57,* 244-257.

Nguyen, N. A., & Williams, H. L. (1989). Transition from East to West: Vietnamese adolescents and their parents. *Journal of the American Academy of Child and Adolescent Psychiatry, 28,* 505-515.

Nuttall, E. V., Chieh, L., & Nuttall, R. L. (1988). Views of the family by Chinese and U.S. children: A comparative study of kinetic family drawings. *Journal of School Psychology, 26,* 191-194. (From *PsycINFO,* Abstract)

Okamura, A., Heras, P., & Wong-Kerberg, L. (1995). Asian, Pacific Island, and Filipino Americans and sexual child abuse. In L. A. Fontes (Ed.), *Sexual abuse in nine North American cultures: Treatment and prevention* (pp.67-96). Thousand Oaks, CA: SAGE Publications, Inc.

Okano, K.-I. (1994). Shame and social phobia: A transcultural viewpoint. *Bulletin of the Menninger Clinic, 58*(3), 323-338.

O'Reilly, J. P., Tokuno, K. A., & Ebata, A. T. (1986). Cultural differences between Americans of Japanese and European ancestry in parental valuing of social competence. *Journal of Comparative Family Studies, 17,* 87-97.

Pilkonis, P. A., & Zimbardo, P. G. (1979). The personal and social dynamics of shyness. In C. E. Izard (Ed.), *Emotions in personality and psychopathology* (pp. 133-160). New York: Plenum.

Roberts, G. E. (1994). *Interpretive handbook for the Roberts Apperception Test for Children.* Los Angeles: Western Psychological Services.

Sattler, J. M. (1992). *Assessment of children: Revised and updated* (3rd ed.). San Diego, CA: Jerome M. Sattler, Publisher, Inc.

Shon, S., & Ja, D. (1982). Asian families. In M. McGoldrick, J. Pearce, & J. Giordano (Eds.), *Ethnicity and family therapy* (pp. 208-229). New York: Guilford Press.

Singelis, T. M., Bond, M. H., Sharkey, W. F., & Lai, C. S. Y. (1999). Unpackaging culture's influence on self-esteem and embarrassability: The role of self-construals. *Journal of Cross-Cultural Psychology, 30,* 315-340.

Su, L., Li, X.-R., Wan, G., Yang, Z., & Luo, X. (1996). The Hunan norms of Achenbach's Child Behavior Checklist. *Chinese Journal of Clinical Psychology, 4,* 24-28. (From *PsycINFO,* Abstract)

Su, L., Li, X.-R., Luo, X., Wan, G., & Yang, Z. (1998). Standardization of newly revised Child Behavior Checklist (CBCL) and validity test. *Chinese Mental Health Journal, 12,* 67-69. (From *PsycINFO,* Abstract)

Sue, D. W. (1990). Culture-specific strategies in counseling: A conceptual framework. *Professional Psychology: Research and Practice, 21,* 424-433.

Sue, D., Ino, S., & Sue, D. W. (1983). Nonassertiveness of Asian Americans: An inaccurate assumption? *Journal of Counseling Psychology, 30,* 581-588.

Takeuchi, M., & Scott, R. (1986). Educational productivity and Rorschach location responses of preschool Japanese and American children. *Psychology in the Schools, 23,* 368-373.

Uba, L. (1994). *Asian Americans: Personality patterns, identity, and mental health.* New York: The Guilford Press.

Vignoe, D., Berube, R. L., & Achenbach, T. M. (1999). *Bibliography of published studies using the Child Behavior Checklist and related materials: 1999 edition.* Burlington, VT : University of Vermont Department of Psychiatry.

Wang, A., Meredith, W. H., & Tsai, R. (1996). Comparison in three Chinese cultures of scores on the self-perception profile for children. *Perceptual and Motor Skills, 82,* 1087-1095.

Weisz, J. R., Suwanlert, S., Chaiyasit, W., Weiss, B., Achenbach, T. M., & Eastman, K. L. (1993). Behavioral and emotional problems among Thai and American adolescents: Parent reports for ages 12-16. *Journal of Abnormal Psychology, 102,* 395-403.

Wilson, R. W. (1981). Conformity and defiance regarding moral rules in Chinese society: A socialization perspective. In A. Kleinman & T.Y. Lin (Eds.), *Normal and abnormal behavior in Chinese people* (pp. 117-136). Dordrecht, The Netherlands: D. Reidel Publishers.

Yang, K.-S. (1986). Chinese personality and its change. In M. H. Bond (Ed.), *The psychology of the Chinese people.* Hong Kong: Oxford University Press.

Yee, B. W. K., Huang, L. N., & Lew, A. (1998). Families: Life-span socialization in a cultural context. In L. C. Lee & N. W. S. Zane (Eds.), *Handbook of Asian American psychology* (pp. 83-135). Thousand Oaks, CA: Sage.

JONATHAN SANDOVAL

CHAPTER 17

EXAMINING THE ROLE OF CULTURE IN EDUCATIONAL ASSESSMENT

1. INTRODUCTION

Educators and psychologists working in the schools continually struggle with the issue of how culture should be taken into account in the psychoeducational assessment of children and youth. When psychoeducational assessments are culturally informed, children are more likely to receive needed services and well-timed, effective educational interventions. When they are not, these assessments may fail to identify the problem correctly and lead to inappropriate interventions, resulting in children not being educated to their full potential. To maximize our ability to conduct culturally informed assessment, it is appropriate to return to and examine our basic assumptions. In this chapter I will focus on two fundamental questions: 1) why do we use tests in the first place? and 2) how can we accomplish the purposes of assessment and still be responsive to the cultural background of the test-taker?

Demographic changes over the last two decades reflect an increase in the diversity of American society. Over the next 30 years, the US population is expected to increase by 72 million to reach 335 million in 2025 (U.S. Bureau of the Census, 1996). Sixty-one percent of the population growth will come from Hispanic and Asian groups, who together will increase from 14% to 24% of the national population (U.S. Bureau of the Census, 1996). More than ever before, psychologists who perform psychoeducational evaluations will make decisions based on tests that were not developed for use with many of the individuals taking them. The use of tests with norms and constructs derived primarily from individuals of European ancestry will be increasingly inappropriate as a foundation for decision-making, such as for diagnosis, for assignment to special educational programs, for employment selection and so on. So why will we likely continue to use tests?

2. WHY WE USE TESTS

The flip answer to this question is that we use tests because we are required to for legal or regulatory reasons, or to be reimbursed from insurance or managed care. We use tests because the results may lead to eligibility for additional or more

251

252 JONATHAN SANDOVAL

appropriate services for our clients. Sometimes we deliver those services, and the test leads us to select a particular treatment intervention. However, let us dig deeper.

Why use tests, not some other form of data gathering such as an informal interview? A more complex answer is that we use tests because they are efficient, standardized, and give us a basis of comparison through the use of norms. The idea of tests being standardized emerged at the beginning of the century as a result of the development of experimental psychology. Early psychologists such as Binet and Whitmer believed that standardization was important so that the results of individual test performance could be comparable across test-takers and norms could be developed (Sandoval, 1993). We use tests because we have norms against which we can evaluate our client's performance. But what if the assessments have been administered to individuals who diverge in significant ways from the norm group? Can we assume this is a meaningful comparison? Often times we cannot.

A test is thought to be good or valid when it measures a particular construct for each score it yields. If the test is found to be valid, it can be relied upon to provide accurate information about an individual difference that is important for intervention or treatment. But if a test is developed on one group of individuals will it be valid for a sub-group who comes from a different cultural background? In many cases, this is not an easy question to answer.

3. CULTURAL CONSIDERATIONS

The key issue for the psychologist to consider when using a test with an individual who is not from the culture within which the test was developed is construct irrelevant variance. Construct irrelevant variance is the degree to which a test measures something extraneous to the construct the test was designed to measure. Some percentage of the variance in test scores may be attributed to the intended construct, some is traditionally assigned to error, but with some tests there may be other irrelevant factors being assessed. A classic example is a reading comprehension test. In addition to measuring reading comprehension, it may also be measuring such irrelevant constructs as familiarity with the subject matter, an emotional reaction to the content, or decoding speed and skill. If a reading comprehension test has a great deal of construct irrelevant variance, a low score will be especially difficult to interpret, because it will not be clear whether the score earned is the result of poor reading comprehension or construct irrelevant variance. For example, a child who cannot decode English orthography will be found to have poor reading comprehension, even when his reading comprehension in Chinese may be excellent. Furthermore, on educational tests, reading skill is often assumed, and thus may contribute to construct irrelevant variance. For example on a history test, individual reading skill that is lower than the level required to understand a history test will contribute to construct irrelevant variance.

Another important contributor to construct irrelevant variance is opportunity to learn the construct. Many tests are intended to assess what an examinee knows as a result of formal instruction or informal learning. Achievement tests are of this type, but even tests such as the Wechsler scales have items assessing general information

EXAMINING THE ROLE OF CULTURE IN EDUCATIONAL ASSESSMENT 253

and cultural comprehension. If children have not grown up in the United States or in the dominant western culture, or if children have been educated in substandard schools with un-credentialed teachers (as is the case in many urban school districts), they will not have had the same opportunity to learn. In these cases, lack of background knowledge will contribute to construct irrelevant variance.

Much of the concern in Asian American mental health assessment is on whether tests developed in the United States have too much irrelevant construct variance or whether they are even measuring the same construct when they are administered to Asian Americans. One area where both of these concerns are especially apparent is in the assessment of individuals for whom English is a second language.

One of the more complex challenges for psychologists is the reliable and valid assessment of skills of persons from non-English backgrounds who might be limited in their English proficiency, who communicate effectively in a language other than English, and are the product of a non-mainstream US culture. What inferences can be drawn when the tests have been administered so that the instructions or the substance and content of the task may not have been completely understood by the examinee? All tests normed on native speakers of English are, to some degree, measures of English competency and proficiency. Thus when used with English speakers, English proficiency is not likely to account for significant variance in the total score. (An exception would be a test of English grammar or vocabulary). In contrast, when used with non-native speakers, a test in English must be interpreted as measuring English proficiency in addition to the constructs it was designed to measure.

In any testing situation, but particularly in high stakes assessments, examinees must have an opportunity to demonstrate the competencies, knowledge or attributes being measured. The inability to understand directions and the content of items is clearly a barrier to demonstrating competence. As a result, an assessment of an individual in a language he or she cannot comprehend will almost always be a poor measure of the construct. The same problem may also apply to individuals from a different culture for whom English *is* a first language. In this instance, test content may have a culturally derived meaning that was not present in the group with which the test was developed.

Perhaps a brief story of unknown authorship will illustrate this point:

Sherlock Holmes and Watson were on a camping trip. They had gone to bed and were lying there looking up at the sky.

Holmes said, "Watson, look up. What do you see?

Watson answered, "Well, I see thousands of stars."

Holmes: "And what does that mean to you?"

Watson: "Well, I suppose it means that of all the planets and suns and moons in the universe, that we are truly the one most blessed with the reason to deduce theorems to make our way in this world of criminal enterprises and blind greed. It means that we are truly small in the eyes of God but struggle each day to be worthy of the senses and spirit we have been blessed with. And, I suppose, at the very least, in the meteorological .sense, it means that it is most likely that we will have another nice day tomorrow. What does it mean to you, Holmes?"

Holmes: "To me, it means someone has stolen our tent."

Holmes and Watson come from two different cultures, perhaps, or at least from two different frames of reference. The story is intended to illustrate how one item can be answered correctly from two different cultural perspectives.

It is tempting, when faced with a client who does not fit the population for whom the test was developed and normed, for the psychologist to forsake testing altogether for alternative strategies such as interviewing. In many instances this action will be the correct course to take. We often do not leap to this solution automatically, however, because we know that human judgment is subject to powerful biases. Choosing not to test often means using alternative measures or methods that are even less satisfactory than standardized tests. In addition the decision not to use a test may also lead to the denial of services or opportunity to those who are deserving, or, alternatively, the provision of services or opportunities to those who cannot use them.

4. COGNITIVE BIASES

It is well accepted that strategies and heuristics that are prone to error influence human decision-making. Cognitive psychology has identified a number of heuristics judges use in making decisions which lead to biased outcomes (Sandoval, 1998). Human judges have difficulty evaluating the representativeness of information, especially the failure to consider accurately base-rate and sample size information. Another phenomenon is the disposition to confirm existing cognitive schemas. Decision-makers make errors by detecting a correlation when none exists while failing to detect a correlation when one does exist (Chapman & Chapman, 1967; Friedlander & Phillips, 1984; Kurtz & Garfield, 1987). They make data fit existing ideas and ignore data that conflicts with their existing preconceptions. A third general phenomenon is the tendency to be influenced by recently activated schemas, a phenomenon called the availability bias or the anchoring bias (Tversky & Kahneman, 1974). In encountering new information or new clients, professionals are over-influenced by what they have encountered in the recent past or by particularly vivid information.

An especially troubling bias in human cognition is related to the tendency to confirm expectations, because psychologists are often presented with a great deal of information they must sort through in making a judgment. Expectancies based on status are at the heart of prejudice, and may not be in awareness. Psychologists must acknowledge that stereotyping is a difficult problem to overcome. It seems innately human to categorize the world, and to form concepts about groups of individuals who have something in common. On the basis of these classifications individuals develop schemas or complex concepts and constructs concerning the members of categories, schemas which include feelings, beliefs and expectations for behavior for the members of the categories. A problem, called the fallacy of stereotyping (Scriven, 1976), occurs when we act on an element of the schema as if it applied to all members of the classification.

Stereotypes based on ethnicity are among the most pervasive in our society. Individuals at an early age quickly learn the stereotypes applicable to their own ethnicity as well as to others. Individuals both high and low in prejudice have detailed knowledge of attributions of ability, talent, values, taste, etc. of different ethnic groups. Some of the questions discussed in this volume have to do with the stereotypes of Asian Americans as the model minority—performing well in mathematics while performing less well in verbal pursuits, valuing family above self, striving to save face, and somaticizing anxiety. How influenced are we by these stereotypes when we meet a new client?

Seldom do individuals perfectly match all of the features of a prototype, although they may match several and exemplify one or two. Schemas for different diverse groups may be simple or complex, depending on our experiences. Interpreting tests when a schema for the examinee has been activated requires psychologists to be particularly careful. The schema test that users have developed around particular minority groups of clients may be complex or simple, depending on their exposure to the culture. Schemas permit individual to act efficiently and correctly much of the time, but if they are automatically applied in every situation, individuals will make bad judgments.

Tests were developed to be more objective than individual, subjective judgment. Binet originally developed his test because teachers could not be relied upon to evaluate children accurately who needed help, because of biases related to social class (French & Hale, 1990). John Gardner writes of educational tests first introduced in this country: "The tests couldn't see whether the youngster was in rags or in tweeds, and they couldn't hear the accents of the slums" (Gardner, 1961, p 48). Tests have served this purpose to some extent, but they have not "levelled the playing field."

For many purposes, as Paul Meehl has demonstrated, the actuarial approach to diagnosis based on test results is superior to a clinical approach using non-test information (Dawes, Faust, & Meehl, 1989; Meehl, 1954). Decisions based on a well developed and validated test may be superior to decisions based on professional intuition. According to Faust, "It is possible that, other things being equal, the more a test reduces freedom to vary on the basis of clinical impression, the better it performs" (Faust, 1986, p. 424). To the extent that tests are useful tools to help us avoid the biases in subjective judgment we should use them.

256 JONATHAN SANDOVAL

5. ACCOMPLISHING THE PURPOSES OF ASSESSMENT WHILE BEING RESPONSIVE TO THE CULTURAL BACKGROUND OF THE TEST-TAKER

A number of recommendations evolve out of a consideration of bias and the need for critical thinking. Cognitive limitations and biases are certainly going to affect practitioners in working with Asian American or any minority clients. There are several steps to accomplishing the goal of culturally sensitive assessment and avoiding cognitive bias.

5.1 Identify preconceptions

First it is important to try to identify some of the conceptions and points of view practitioners have about Asian Americans or others, both positive and negative and recognize that they exist. Self-awareness is the first step in gaining the capacity to understand other's point of view (Sue et al., 1998).

5.2 Develop complex schemas or conceptions of client groups

Second, it is important for practitioners to gain a more complex schema about Asian Americans they may encounter in practice. The point of cultural sensitivity training is not to create stereotypes, but rather to build new and more complete and accurate schemas that will help test users understand individuals functioning within a particular context. Practitioners must recognize that changing their conceptions about diverse groups will not be an easy or automatic task.

5.3 Triangulation

Third, psychologists must always look for corroborating evidence from different sources. Assessors ideally have multiple measures and multiple sources of information about key constructs so that there is convergence and cross validation. Psychologists might ask: "Have I tested in both L1 (first language) and L2 (second language)?" Have I genuinely tested alternative or competing hypotheses that might bear on the interpretation of test results and help render a more valid professional judgment? Have I used multiple measures and found consistency? Am I incorrectly dismissing inconsistencies in performance?

5.4 Actively Search for Disconfirmatory Evidence as Well as Confirmatory Evidence.

Fourth, because of the confirmatory bias, it is imperative in making judgments based on tests or on other information that practitioners learn to search constantly for disconfirming evidence and for alternative explanations for initial hunches about the client. Clinicians must constantly attend to negative information, information incompatible with the working hypothesis, and not simply try to explain away

EXAMINING THE ROLE OF CULTURE IN EDUCATIONAL ASSESSMENT 257

anomalous findings (Gambrill, 1990). They must not always see difficulties as attributable to internal states of the client; instead they must look to environmental causes as well. They can learn to shift the frames of reference they use (Gambrill, 1990) by asking: "What is missing from this case information?" Or they can ask questions that completely reverse their perspective (Gambrill, 1990), such as: What if B caused A rather than the reverse?

5.5 Resist a Rush to Judgment

Fifth, practitioners must learn to resist impulsivity and reserve judgment. They must wait for all the facts to present themselves and not give undue weight to vivid data, personally relevant data, or recent data. They must beware of the regression to the mean effect and not over interpret shifts from extremely high or extremely low scores.

5.6 Seek Supervision

Sixth, practitioners must get feedback on decision making with Asian American clients. In working with new kinds of clients, they must feel comfortable consulting with a colleague with experience with the population. Of course it is also important for practitioners to recognize when they are not competent to make a judgment about an individual or a situation, so that they make appropriate referrals.

5.7 Distrust Memory

Seventh, it is useful for practitioners to find ways to minimize the role of memory. Memory is a process involving construction (Bartlett, 1932) and highly subject to the confirmatory bias. Psychologists should make recordings, take notes, and document impressions through counts, checklists or other objective means.

5.8 Be Conservative in Interpreting Tests

When dealing with test data on Asian Americans, practitioners must consider that the test has provided some information about performance. If the comparison to the norm group doesn't make sense, practitioners should be comfortable not using it. Scores should be labeled "estimates" (Sattler, 1988). On the other hand, test data does represent some minimal performance, and does represent the interplay of many forces in the client's life.

5.9 Consider Construct Irrelevant Variance

Consistent with the issues of language fluency and acculturation raised by Comas-Diaz and Grenier (1998), psychologists must constantly ask: "In evaluating the performance of this person on the test, have I made sure that this test is a measure of the construct in question as opposed to a test of some other irrelevant construct such as English language fluency?" Have I taken the acculturation of the test taker into account? Are their acculturation measures available to use with this population? Psychologists should be aware that culture and language are related but not perfectly correlated. It is important to ask: "Are the testing process and the material familiar to the test taker?" Has the examinee had an opportunity to learn the knowledge or skills called for by the test? Have I done sufficient training (as permitted) and coaching to reduce the influences of other irrelevant constructs, which may result from low acculturation, contributing to performance? In addition, they must ask: "Have I taken other cultural and language-related variables into account?" Speed of response, for example, may be influenced by cultural norms and by the cognitive effort involved in dual language processing. Has there been sufficient time for the examinee to demonstrate competency? Is there evidence of fatigue? Have we established rapport?

6. OPTIONS IN TESTING

If a test is invalid and has only construct irrelevant variance for a particular group, it should be abandoned; that much is plain. However, in the educational arena test users often encounter situations where tests have an unknown amount of construct irrelevant variance. Instead of abandoning tests they have often looked for ways to cope with this uncertainty in doing educational assessment. The test may have some validity, but the test user cannot be sure how much. It is then useful to consider some options to explore in the educational assessment of Asian Americans, particularly those who do not speak English fluently (Sandoval & Duran, 1998).

6.1 Using Mainstream Tests in English Developed for Mainstream English Language Speakers

At what point on the continuum of bilingualism or proficiency in English as a second language (L2) does one use with confidence a test with content or instructions in English? Unfortunately there is little empirical evidence to guide the psychological professional, particularly in working with young children where language proficiency is developing.

Even if the individual is proficient in English, if they have a different first language (L1), there still may be a need to consider if the outcome of the test has been depressed by factors related to language, particularly for younger children with smaller vocabularies.

There is some consensus that the extra time needed by bilingual individuals to process two languages also needs to be taken into account. The time and effort needed to process information from one language to another suggests that a reasonable accommodation in testing would be to extend time limits or give non-speeded tests and to allow more frequent breaks in testing to recover from the mental

EXAMINING THE ROLE OF CULTURE IN EDUCATIONAL ASSESSMENT

effort. Of course, if the construct being measured involves speed, such an accommodation might not be appropriate.

Particular care must be taken if the responses to a test are given orally. Even if an individual is competent in English, the individual's speech may be highly accented. Accents are usually more pronounced in adults than in children. Comprehending accented English, even from an examinee who was reared in an English speaking location such as Glasgow, Scotland, is no easy chore for most American psychologists. In the case of a test that yields a spoken response, the examiner's listening comprehension of the accent will be very important for both rapport and understanding. If the psychologist were unable to understand an accent, it would be better to make a referral to a colleague who does.

An important factor, as mentioned earlier, is whether English proficiency is related to the reason for assessment. For example, if the assessment is to determine entrance into college where English is the language of instruction, test scores in English usually correlate better with success in college humanities and social science coursework than do test scores in another language.

One modification that is possible with the directions to a test is to give them bilingually. If the examiner is bilingual and a translation is available, the directions to the test might be given in both English **and** the examinee's first language. The effects of such a modification should be investigated empirically, however.

6.2 Alternatives to English Language Testing

6.2.1 Translation of tests or other assessment devices into L1

Perhaps the first option that comes to mind to psychologists as well as others (such as the courts) when faced with a non- or limited English proficient speaker is to have the test of interest translated into the language of the test taker, and the examinee's responses translated into English. It is best to take time and effort and translate the test prior to using it, but in many situations a translator, often a layperson competent in the non-English language, is drafted to translate questions or responses in situ. Both translating tests and the use of the translator in testing are fraught with hazards and issues.

6.2.2 Test translation or adaptation

Translating a test from one language to another at the same time preserving the content, difficulty level, reliability and validity is a daunting undertaking. It is rarely done successfully at the local level. An adaptation may be oriented to making the test suitable for use in a different culture or in a different language or both. Geisinger (1994) points out that the term test adaptation has replaced test translation to emphasize the need to adapt to the culture of the examinee, to make changes in content and in wording as well as to translate the language itself.

6.2.3 Working with interpreters

Clearly it would be best for an assessment of non-English speakers to be done by a psychologist with demonstrated second language proficiency. The availability of trained speakers in some languages, such as Cantonese or Spanish, may someday be sufficient, but given the large number of languages spoken in the U.S., making it a requirement that individuals be assessed by native speakers of their language is impractical. Instead, psychologists need to be prepared to work with interpreters. This training can come from workshops or from consultation with an experienced psychologist in which a set of competencies have been worked out.

6.2.4 Using Asian tests

Tests may be available in the first language of the individual to be tested. Tests in languages other than English have been produced by publishers in the United States for the U.S. market but few in Asian languages.

If used with a US population who have grown up in this country, there may be problems in language and cultural context of the tests developed elsewhere. Hong Kong born Chinese do not necessarily share common referents with Taiwan immigrants. This diversity will have to be taken into account in the interpretation.

6.2.5 Nonverbal tests

In some domains, such as intellectual functioning, it may be possible to use nonverbal tests. Tests vary in the amount of language used in the directions and in the items. Items may be presented pictorially, symbolically or numerically yet measure the same constructs as items presented verbally. A good nonverbal test begins with items so simple that test takers immediately realize what is being asked of them without being told. Among nonverbal tests, some are more culturally loaded than others. Picture tests such as the Peabody Picture Vocabulary Test are culturally loaded because they tap information associated with mainstream American culture, however symbolic tests such as the Raven's Progressive Matrices, Digit Span, and Maze tests are less culturally loaded because they tap information more neutrally associated with a particular culture. An examiner will wish to find a test with the following characteristics: A nonverbal performance test with pantomime instructions which offers opportunities for practice; items which are abstract figural in nature but which require an oral response or gestural response; and a power test which reflects non-scholastic skills involving solving novel problems. Some such tests exist.

There is a long history of using nonverbal tests in the U.S. In the cognitive domain, in addition to the Army Alpha test, the Army Beta test was developed during the First World War with the aim of assessing limited English speakers and illiterate English speakers. Both group tests and individual tests are available. For example in individual tests, the Wechsler Scales have long had performance tests that are language reduced, and most modern scales measuring intellectual functioning have nonverbal tests (the Differential Ability Scales, the Kaufman tests, the Stanford Binet). Better measures are appearing all the time, some requiring only gestural directions and permitting extensive practice and coaching prior to testing.

EXAMINING THE ROLE OF CULTURE IN EDUCATIONAL ASSESSMENT

In personality assessment, many projective devices use nonverbal pictorial materials. Projective devices such as the Rorschach may reveal useful information, but these measures still have high cultural loadings and little research has been done on normative responses by limited English speakers.

It must be pointed out that there are a number of disadvantages in using nonverbal tests. It is almost always the case that verbal tests will predict verbal abilities and verbal performance better than nonverbal assessment. Ability to use language is an important feature of academic performance, job performance and social competency in the mainstream culture. Nonverbal tests may not have the same degree of validity for many purposes as verbal measures.

Another problem is the abstract and symbolic nature of many nonverbal tests. The stimulus materials and tasks may be quite unfamiliar to examinees and represent an artificial testing context. Performance in authentic and context rich environments may yield more valid results for some test takers.

6.2.6 Performance Testing

A final option for assessing Asian Americans is to examine performance in more naturalistic settings with assessments that authentically capture desired competencies. Genesee & Upshur (1996) have discussed achievement testing in classrooms. They describe the use of observation, informal objectives-referenced testing, conferencing and portfolios to derive important information about achievement and other constructs.

Jitendra and Rohena-Diaz (1996) suggest the use of curriculum-based dynamic assessment. Dynamic assessment involves determining improvement over time on tasks that are carefully taught to the examinee. Changes in performance when mediated in a one-to-one environment can be used to estimate ability.

Valid use of performance assessments with Asian Americans requires attention to the same concerns as for valid use of standardized tests (American Educational Research Association, American Psychological Association, National Council on Measurement in Education, 1999). Establishing the accuracy and reliability of scores and classifications on performance assessments is essential. Further, it is important to assure that the construct irrelevant factors on performance assessments do not lead to inappropriate inferences regarding examinees' competency in the construct areas under assessment. This can be a challenge. For example, in education, many of the new forms of performance assessment in subject matter areas, such as mathematics or science, include performance criteria requiring that examinees demonstrate their ability to communicate how they go about solving problems in writing. Fair and valid assessments in such circumstances may require accommodations such as allowing students more time to respond, writing responses in a non-English language, or oral responses in English or the non-English language. It is important to note that assessment users have the responsibility for determining whether such accommodations alter the intended constructs under measurement.

262   JONATHAN SANDOVAL

7. CONCLUSION

Clinicians, with the help of competent peers, must constantly examine their work, evaluate it for effectiveness, and judge whether they are living up to the standards of best practice. It is through this review process that critical thinking can occur. It is important to guard against stereotyped and simplistic thinking when assessing Asian American and other individuals from minority groups. So many factors may be involved in an interpretation such as culture, poverty and acculturation, not to mention the more usual irrelevant factors of emotion and developmental status, that makes drawing inferences about culturally and linguistically different clients especially difficult. Nevertheless psychologists are usually charged with making judgments that impact lives and they cannot shirk their responsibility.

8. REFERENCES

American Educational Research Association, American Psychological Association, & National Council on Measurement in Education. (1999). *Standards for educational and psychological testing.* Washington, DC: American Educational Research Association.

Bartlett, F. C. (1932). *Remembering.* Cambridge, UK: Cambridge University Press.

Chapman, L. J., & Chapman, J. P. (1967). Genesis of popular but erroneous psychodiagnostic observations. *Journal of Abnormal Psychology, 74,* 271-280.

Comas-Diaz, L. & Grenier, J. R. (1998). Migration and acculturation. In J. Sandoval, C. L. Frisby, K. F. Geisinger, J. D. Scheueneman, and J. R. Grenier (Eds.), *Test interpretation and diversity: Achieving equity in psychological assessment* (pp. 213-240). Washington: APA.

Dawes, R. M., Faust, D., & Meehl, P. E. (1989). Clinical verses actuarial judgment. *Science, 243,* 1668-1674.

Faust, D. (1986). Research on human judgment and its application to clinical practice. *Professional Psychology: Research and Practice, 17,* 420-430.

French, J. L. & Hale, R. L. (1990). A history of the development of psychological and educational testing. In C. R. Reynolds and R. W. Kamphaus (Eds.), *Handbook of psychological and educational assessment of children: Intelligence and achievement* (pp. 3-28). New York: Guilford.

Friedlander, M. L., & Phillips, S. D. (1984). Preventing errors in clinical judgment. *Journal of Consulting and Clinical Psychology, 52,* 366-371.

Gambrill, E. (1990). *Critical thinking in clinical practice: Improving the accuracy of judgments and decisions about clients.* San Francisco: Jossey-Bass.

Gardner, J. W. (1961). *Excellence.* New York: Harper & Row

Geisinger, K. F. (1994). Cross-cultural normative assessment: Translation and adaptation issues influencing the normative interpretation of assessment instruments. *Psychological Assessment, 6(4),* 304-312.

Genesee, F., & Upshur, J. A. (1996). *Classroom-based evaluation in second language education.* New York: Cambridge University Press.

Jitendra, A. K., & Rohena-Diaz, E. (1996). Language assessment of students who are linguistically diverse: Why a discrete approach is not the answer. *School Psychology Review, 25(1),* 40-56.

Kurtz, R. M., & Garfield, S. L. (1978). Illusory correlation: A further exploration of Chapman's paradigm. *Journal of Consulting and Clinical Psychology, 46,* 1009-1015.

Meehl, P. E. (1954). *Clinical versus statistical prediction; a theoretical analysis and a review of the evidence.* Minneapolis: University of Minnesota Press.

Sandoval, J. (1993). The history of interventions in school psychology. *Journal of School Psychology, 31,* 195-217.

Sandoval, J. (1998). Critical thinking in test interpretation. In J. Sandoval, C. L. Frisby, K. F. Geisinger, J. D. Scheueneman, and J. R. Grenier, J. R. (Eds.), *Test interpretation and diversity: Achieving equity in psychological assessment* (pp. 31-49). Washington, DC: APA.

EXAMINING THE ROLE OF CULTURE IN EDUCATIONAL ASSESSMENT 263

Sandoval, J., & Duran, R. P. (1998). Language. In J. Sandoval, C. L. Frisby, K. F. Geisinger, J. D. Scheueneman, and J. R. Grenier, J. R. (Eds.), *Test interpretation and diversity: Achieving equity in psychological assessment* (pp. 181-212). Washington, DC: APA.

Sattler, J. (1988). *Assessment of children* (3rd ed.). San Diego, CA: Author.

Scriven, M. (1976). *Reasoning*. New York: McGraw-Hill.

Sue, D. W., Carter, R.T., Casas, J. M., Fouad, N. A., Ivey, A. E., Jensen, M., LaFromboise, T. Manese, J. E., Ponterotto, J. G., & Vazquez-Nutall, E. (1998*). Multicultural counseling competencies*. Thousand Oaks, CA: Sage Publications.

Tversky, A., & Kahneman, D. (1974). Judgment under uncertainty: Heuristics and biases. *Science, 185*, 1124-1131.

U.S. Bureau of the Census (1996). *Warmer, older, more diverse: State-by-state population changes to 2025* (PPL-47). Washington, DC: U.S. Department of Commerce.

FREDERICK T. L. LEONG AND MEI TANG

CHAPTER 18

A CULTURAL ACCOMMODATION APPROACH TO CAREER ASSESSMENT WITH ASIAN AMERICANS

1. INTRODUCTION

This chapter will present a cultural accommodation approach to address the emerging need for better theoretical models to guide career assessment with culturally diverse populations. Based on a recent integrative model of cross-cultural counseling and psychotherapy proposed by Leong (1996), this cultural accommodation approach is flexible and can be applied to enrich existing career theories which are primarily Eurocentric. The chapter will have three sections: 1) introduction of the cultural accommodation approach; 2) brief literature review on the career development and assessment of Asian Americans; and 3) illustration of how this cultural accommodation model can be applied to guide career assessment research and practice with Asian Americans. We should point out that we will be using the term "cross-cultural" in the broadest sense throughout this chapter and the related terms of cross-racial, cross-ethnic, and cross-national are subsumed under cross-cultural in our usage.

2. CULTURAL ACCOMMODATION APPROACH

With the increasing diversity of the American population, and as more minority members enter the world of work, it becomes inevitable that counselors and researchers will encounter various problems that are atypical of mainstream culture and therefore neglected by career development theories (Leong, 1995). As Leong and Brown (1995) pointed out, four major and interrelated criticisms have plagued current career choice theories: 1) they are based upon a restricted range of persons; 2) they are based upon assumptions of limited scope; 3) they confuse or inappropriately define terms such as race, ethnicity, and minority; and 4) they tend to ignore or limitedly address the socio-political, socio-economic, social psychological, and socio-cultural realities of minority individuals. These problems have led some scholars either to dismiss current theories as models for understanding the career behavior of diverse groups or to call for re-articulations that would render the theories more cross-culturally relevant (cf., Brooks, 1991). Leong and Brown (1995) also observed that most theories of career choice make five assumptions, the validity of which appear particularly suspect when considered from

265

a cross cultural perspective: 1) career development is continuous, uninterrupted, and progressive; 2) decision-makers possess the psychological, social, and economic means of effecting their choices; 3) there is dignity in all work; 4) there exists a free and open labor market; and 5) most career choices flow essentially from internal (viz., personality) factors.

Although cross-cultural studies of psychology and vocational behavior have made commendable progress in recent decades, comprehensive and integrative theoretical models for cross-cultural counseling are still underdeveloped. The limits of the unidimensional nature of the career development theories confine the benefits of the counseling services for minority members, including Asian Americans. The following discussion focuses on using a cultural accommodation approach in expanding current theories to make them more culturally relevant for racial and ethnic minorities in general, and Asian Americans in particular.

Leong's (1996) recent multidimensional and integrative model of cross-cultural counseling and psychotherapy used Kluckhohn and Murray's (1950) tripartite framework. Leong (1996) proposed that cross-cultural counselors and therapists need to attend to all three major dimensions of human personality and identity, namely the Universal, the Group, and the Individual dimensions. The Universal dimension is based on the knowledge-base generated by mainstream psychology and the "universal laws" of human behavior that have been identified (e.g., the universal "fight or flight" response in humans to physical threat). The Group dimension has been the domain of both cross-cultural psychology as well as ethnic minority psychology and the study of gender differences. The third and final dimension concerns unique Individual differences and characteristics. The Individual dimension is more often covered by behavioral and existential theories where individual learning histories and personal phenomenology are proposed as critical elements in the understanding of human behavior. Leong's (1996) integrative model proposes that all three dimensions are equally important in understanding human experiences and should be attended to by the counselor in an integrative fashion.

Leong (1996) used a famous quote from Kluckhohn and Murray's (1950) influential article on "The Determinants of Personality Formation" published in their book *Personality in Nature, Society, and Culture*, as the beginning point for his integrative model. The quote was: "Every man is in certain respects: a) like all other men, b) like some other men, and c) like no other man" (p. 35). In this quote, Kluckhohn and Murray are pointing out that some of the determinants of personality are common features found in the genetic makeup of all people. This addresses the biological aspect of the biopsychosocial model generally used in today's medical sciences. For certain other features of personality, however, Kluckhohn and Murray (1950) state that most men are like some other men, showing the importance of social grouping, whether that grouping is based on culture, race, ethnicity, gender, or social class. Lastly, they said that "Each individual's modes of perceiving, feeling, needing, and behaving have characteristic patterns which are not precisely duplicated by those of any other individual" (p. 37). Each person's individuality, often the focus of social learning theories and models, is thus expressed in the last part of the quote. It accentuates the fact that all persons have distinct social learning experiences that can influence their values, beliefs, and cognitive schemas.

According to Leong (1996), the Universal. component of personality is reflected in Kluckhohn and Murray's (1950) observation that "all persons are like all other persons" in some respects. This statement accentuates the idea that all human beings share some characteristics, whether they are physical or psychological. There is much evidence to support this notion, as all humans develop physically in similar fashions, learn to talk in similar fashions, and learn to think in similar fashions (e.g. Piaget's conservation experiments). This notion has been thoroughly accepted by the medical community, whereas Group and Individual differences are often not seen as important in medical treatment. This Universal component of human personality has also been accepted by many in the psychological community, as exemplified by the common factors model (Frank, 1961) which points out that the effective aspects of counseling and psychotherapy are shared by many cultures.

In their search for universal laws of human behavior, psychologists are looking for these universal elements of human personality. The concept of cultural validity as articulated by Leong and Brown (1995) is concerned with these universal principles. Each psychological construct or model needs to be examined in regard to its cultural validity. Until its cultural validity is evaluated, cross-cultural extensions and applications of a construct or model beyond the cultural population upon which it has been developed need to proceed cautiously. As pointed out by Leong and Brown (1995), much of the work of cross-cultural psychology is concerned with the assessment of the cultural validity of psychological constructs and models that have been developed primarily within the Western cultural context.

On the other hand, simply focusing on the Universal dimension completely ignores the Group and Individual components that are absolutely necessary for a complete understanding of human behavior. While the Universal dimension in counseling is very important to the integrative model, it is necessary but not sufficient (Leong, 1996). According to Leong (1996), the Group component of human personality is equally important as the Universal component. These groupings may be based on culture, race, ethnicity, social class, occupation, or gender. All persons in one group share some type of bond with other members of the group, and this bond will distinguish the group members from members of other groups. It is further believed that belonging to a group will be a major determinant of a person's personality.

Membership in a group can affect an individual in many ways, and these ways can become the focus of counseling and psychotherapy. For example, persons who have suffered from oppression because of their religion or race will need to address these feelings. They will no longer be speaking from a Universal perspective, as their experiences have not been shared by all persons. A therapist who tries to relate to these clients on a Universal level will be doing them a disservice, and this will most likely lead to premature termination of the therapeutic relationship.

The Group .component of personality is especially important when discussing cross-cultural counseling and psychotherapy. There have been many models of racial identity that focus on the Group component. Other important constructs related to the Group dimension include racial/ethnic identity, acculturation, and value preferences. A competent counselor must be able to look at all these variables from the standpoint of his or her client, especially if the client is a member of a different group. Not doing so would make it impossible to accurately conceptualize the client's psychological state, which in turn would make effective therapy impossible.

There has been much research looking at the experiences of different groups. There are many dynamics that must be taken into consideration in counseling situations involving a client and therapist of different cultural backgrounds. Each person must have some awareness of the experiences of the other in order to be able to form a relationship. This is especially true for the therapist. A therapist operating only at the Universal level may alienate his/her client. Although the two may not have shared experiences in their backgrounds, the counselor must be able to address issues that involve groups other than his/her own. Leong (1996) pointed out that using only the Universal dimension to understand people is severely limited due to the importance of group differences such as cultural differences. Indeed, Leong and Brown (1995) have proposed that when problems occur in establishing the cultural validity of a construct or model, culturally specific variables (often referred to as "indigenous" variables in cross-cultural psychology circles) can add greatly to our understanding of human behavior. It is important to note here that human behavior always occurs within a specific cultural context. In other words, the integrative combination of the Universal and Group dimensions of human personality provides a richer model with which to understand human beings. This in turn requires us to examine issues of both cultural validity and cultural specificity in the advancement of career developmental theories.

Finally, there is the Individual component of human personality within Leong's (1996) integrative model. While it is true that we all share some commonalities, as reflected by the Universal component, no two persons are identical in every way. Kluckhohn and Murray (1950) said "Each individual's modes of perceiving, feeling, needing, and behaving have characteristic patterns which are not precisely duplicated by those of any other individual" (p. 37). Kluckhohn and Murray seem to be referring to an idea akin to the concept of the "psychological environment" (Lewin, 1951), which referred to the idea that although two people may share the same physical space, they may not share the same psychological space. To neglect the Individual component would be to run the danger of stereotyping persons from various cultural groups due to over-generalizations from the Group dimension. The Individual component of human personality is equally as important as the Universal or Group components, but it will not be dealt with directly in the current chapter since we are concerned primarily with the issues of cultural validity and cultural specificity.

The integrative model of cross-cultural counseling proposed by Leong (1996) has as one of its fundamental bases the notion that the individual client must exist at three levels, the Universal, the Group, and the Individual. The problem with much of the past research in the field of cross-cultural counseling is that the focus has been on only one of the three levels, ignoring the influence of the other levels in the counseling situation. Leong's (1996) integrative model includes all three dimensions of personality as well as their dynamic interactions, and thus will have better incremental validity than any model that only focuses on only one of the three

A CULTURAL ACCOMMODATION APPROACH TO CAREER ASSESSMENT WITH ASIAN AMERICANS

levels. The integrative model for cross-cultural counseling and psychotherapy was conceived to provide a more complex and dynamic conception of human beings.

The cultural accommodation approach, based on this.integrative model, is proposed to be superior to both the universalist and the culture assimilation approaches to psychological theories. In ignoring the cultural dimension, the universalist approach is only culturally valid for the original group on which the theory was developed (i.e., White European Americans) but of limited cultural validity for racial and ethnic minority groups. In minimizing the role of cultural factors, models based on a culture assimilation approach will also be of limited value cross-culturally and when applied to racial and ethnic minority groups. Both the universalist and culture assimilation approaches suffer from many cultural gaps and blind spots.

The proposed cultural accommodation approach involves three steps: (a) identifying the cultural gaps or cultural blindspots in an existing theory that restricts the cultural validity of the theory; (b) selecting current culturally specific concepts and models from cross-cultural and ethnic minority psychology to fill in the cultural gaps and accommodate the theory to racial and ethnic minorities; and (c) testing the culturally accommodated theory to determine if it has incremental validity above and beyond the culturally unaccommodated theory. In the next section, we will identify some of the cultural gaps in our career assessment with Asian Americans and also discuss the various culturally specific constructs and elements that should go into a model of career assessment that is culturally accommodated to Asian Americans.

3. CAREER ASSESSMENT OF ASIAN AMERICANS

In order to identify existing gaps in our knowledge-base and useful culture-specific variables, this section reviews essential constructs in career assessment literature and their relevance to Asian Americans. The occupational constructs both at individual and group levels are reviewed below.

3.1 The Assessment of Individual Differences Variables

3.1.1 Interests
Earlier studies of Asian Americans' occupational interests found that they evidence higher interest in physical sciences and lower interest in social sciences (D. W. Sue & Kirk, 1972, 1973; D. W. Sue & Frank, 1973). However, when Leong (1982) examined Asian American students' expressed interests (based on self-reported results) as opposed to their measured interests (based on profiles of an interest inventory), he found that although more than 50% of the Asian American students expressed interests in Investigative areas, only 30% had measured interests in the same area. The Investigative area is one of six types of work personalities

postulated by Holland (1985). The same pattern of discrepancy existed between expressed and measured interest in social occupations. Leong (1986), in his literature review, has summarized that Asian Americans express more interest in physical science, technical trades, and business occupations, and less interest in social, sales, business contacts, and verbal-linguistic occupations. In the recent normative samples of the Strong Interest Inventory (Harmon, Hansen, Borgen, & Hammer, 1994), Asian Americans in various occupations are found to have similar interests to the General Reference Sample. However, Asian American samples have a larger proportion of representation in the engineering and physical fields than their ethnic representation in the U.S. population (Fouad, Harmon, & Hansen, 1994). Haverkamp, Collins and Hansen's (1994) analysis of the structure of interest of Asian American college students has shown that it is similar to that of White Americans. However, the typical RIASEC (Realistic-Investigative-Artistic-Social-Enterprising-Conventional) order on hexagon of Holland's (1985) model is not supported for Asian Americans males. For Asian American females, the Conventional and Enterprising types are in the reverse order (RIASCE).

3.1.2 Occupational Values and Needs

Traditional Asian values emphasize collectivism and interdependence. Authority has been reserved for older people and a hierarchical relationship of family members and society is assumed (Fong, 1973; Moy, 1992). These cultural values are also reflected in career development areas. For instance, Leong's (1991) study on the occupational attributes of Asian American and White American students has found that Asian Americans have more extrinsic and pragmatic values than do White Americans. Asian Americans also valued financial security more than did White Americans. Similarly, the 1992 NCDA (National Career Development Association) Gallup survey (Brown & Minor, 1992) found that for Asian and Pacific Island Americans, higher pay and more recognition were major incentives to accomplishing more on their jobs.

Cultural influences were found to be associated with Chinese-American students' work value orientation two decades ago (Tou, 1974). More recently, in the Leong and Tata (1990) study, the Ohio Work Values Inventory (OWVI) and the Suinn-Lew Asian Self-Identity Acculturation Scale (SL-ASIA) were administered to 177 Chinese-American children. The results showed that the participants viewed money and task satisfaction as the most important values and object orientation and solitude as the least important values of work. When these children were divided into low, medium, and high acculturation groups, significant acculturation differences were found only for self-realization. High-acculturation Chinese American children valued self-realization more than did low-acculturation Chinese American children.

3.1.3 Personality Variables

A major theme of career development theories is about the relationship between the personality of an individual and the characteristics (or personality) of the work

A Cultural Accommodation Approach to Career Assessment with Asian Americans 271

environment. There are very few studies about the relationships between Asian Americans' personality and their vocational behaviors. In Leong's (1985) review of the career development literature, three personality variables recurred across many studies. The three variables were locus of control, social anxiety, and intolerance of ambiguity. Asian Americans were found to be less autonomous, more dependent, and more obedient to authority (D. W. Sue & Kirk, 1972, 1973). Asian Americans were found to experience greater social anxiety and be emotionally withdrawn, socially isolated, and verbally inhibited (S. Sue & D. W. Sue, 1974). D. W. Sue and Kirk (1973) also found that Asian Americans had lower tolerance of ambiguity and uncertainty in novel-experimental situations. They were socially introverted and less socially concerned.

3.1.4 Career Maturity and Development

Asian Americans show higher levels of dependent decision-making styles than White Americans (Leong, 1991, 1995). In the same study, Leong found that Asian Americans had lower levels of career maturity (i.e. individuals successfully accomplish developmentally appropriate tasks in career domains) but did not differ in terms of vocational identity (an awareness of specifying one's characteristics in relation to career choice). He attributed the above differences to the cultural characteristics of Asian Americans. Due to the collectivistic value orientation, it is not uncommon for Asian Americans to consider the needs and expectations of family members when important life decisions are made. Unfortunately, Leong's (1991) study only used the total score of the Career Maturity Inventory (CMI; Crites, 1978) instead of the five subscale scores. Using the subscale scores would provide more accurate findings about the career maturity patterns of Asian Americans.

3.1.5 Career Adjustment

Asian Americans have experienced similar work adjustment problems as other minority groups, but they also have a set of unique concerns (Leong, 1998). Due to the relatively lower scores on verbal parts of standardized tests, as compared to the higher achievement in mathematics, Asian Americans are often perceived to be less competent in positions requiring verbal skills. This could mean that they would be passed up for promotion or that they would receive less favorable performance reviews. Traditional Asian culture does not encourage a person to advocate for oneself; instead, one should be modest about one's accomplishments. In contrast, Western culture views such modesty as indicative of less competence.

Asian Americans also experience variety of stress related to job or job settings. A national study conducted by Gallop Poll revealed that Asian Americans did perceive themselves to be underemployed at work (Brown, Minor, & Jepsen, 1991). Brown et al. (1991) reported that Asian Americans, more than any other minority group, experienced stress on the job. Other kinds of career-related stresses experienced by Asian Americans include income levels, particularly if they cannot provide for

272 FREDERICK T. L. LEONG AND MEI TANG

extended family members (Yu & Wu, 1985; Kincaid & Yum, 1987), fear of "losing face" in organizations (Redding & Ng, 1982), and restricted occupational mobility (Kincaid & Yum, 1987; Tang & O'Brien, 1990). For immigrants and refugees from Southeast Asia, the adjustment problems are identified as inconsistent occupational status between homeland and U.S. (Tang & O'Brien, 1990), lack of English proficiency, lack of information about the labor market, being restricted to pursue license due to lack of American educational credentials, and lack of an established ethnic support community (Anh & Healy, 1985).

3.1.6 Career Outcome Expectation

Outcome expectation is defined as a judgment about the likely consequences of certain behaviors (Betz, 1992). For instance, an Asian American student may want to be a physician because it is expected that most physicians have a higher income than average. In other words, one's expectations about the consequences of a particular job choice are referred to as career outcome expectations. Little work has been done on the assessment of outcome expectations (Betz, 1992). The limited findings related to the outcome expectations of Asian Americans show that Asian Americans are likely to choose careers that are more financially secure and more prestigious in social status (Tang, Fouad, & Smith, 1999). In a study investigating the variables affecting the career aspirations, Leung, Ivey, and Suzuki (in press) found that Asian Americans considered occupations of higher prestige than the White American students did. It is argued that Asian Americans are more inclined to choose prestigious occupations because they think such occupations would bring them financial reward and security.

3.1.7 Career Self-Efficacy

Unlike outcome expectations, career self-efficacy is a judgment about one's ability or competence to accomplish a career-related task, such as making career choices, work performance, and job persistence (Betz & Hackett, 1986). Bandura (1986) suggests that there are four sources of information that influence one's perceived self-efficacy: performance attainments, vicarious learning, verbal persuasion and physiological states. There are also three levels of outcome based on perceived self-efficacy: choice (making efforts versus avoidance), performance (doing well versus doing poorly) and persistence (persistence of choice versus withdrawing).

Bandura's (1986) work has been the guideline for developing instruments to measure self-efficacy. The assessment of self-efficacy has been conducted in specific career-related domains such as career decision-making self-efficacy (Taylor & Betz, 1983), occupational task self-efficacy (Rooney & Osipow, 1992), career self-efficacy for women (Betz & Hackett, 1981) and academic domains (Lent, Brown & Larkin, 1984). Tang et al. (1999) investigated the role of career self-efficacy in career choice behaviors among Asian Americans. The study found that the highest levels of self-efficacy for Asian Americans were in Social, Conventional,

A Cultural Accommodation Approach to Career Assessment with Asian Americans

273

and Investigative types of occupations; and that self-efficacy have a mediating impact of acculturation on Asian Americans' career choices.

3.2 Analysis of Group Level Variables

3.2.1 Family Influence

When Asian Americans make plans about their future career choices, they tend to consider the needs and expectations of their parents. Leong and Leung (1994) have argued that because some Asian Americans feel obligated to support the family, they have a strong desire to go into occupations that provide financial stability. Asian American parents also tend to have high expectations about the educational and occupational achievements of their youngsters (Leong & Gim, 1995; S. Sue & Okazaki, 1990). The response of Asian Americans to the expectations of their family is a function of their level of acculturation and ethnic identity (S. Sue & Morishima, 1982).

Although family influence is recognized by researchers in Asian-American psychology as having important implications for career choice process and career assessment of Asian Americans, there are few empirical studies studying the relationship between family influence and career development behaviors of Asian Americans. One recent study (Tang et al., 1999) studied the impact of family socioeconomic status and family involvement on career choices of Asian American college students. The family involvement in Asian American students' career choice was related to career choice while the family SES had a mixed relationship with career choice.

3.2.2 Occupational Stereotyping and Segregation

Stereotypes of occupational distribution among Asian Americans have been widespread. Leong and Hayes (1990) presented various vignettes to college students and asked them to indicate who had more ability and opportunity to succeed in various careers. The profile of personal characteristics was exactly the same except for ethnic background; some were White Americans and some were Asian Americans. The results showed that Asian Americans were seen by White American students to be more likely to succeed as engineers, computer scientists, or mathematicians and to be less successful in sales. Leong and Hayes (1990) have argued that such stereotyping may initially serve as an external barrier to vocational exploration for Asian Americans but it later could become an internal barrier as Asian Americans internalize the stereotyped message. Asian Americans who do well in math and science are unable to take credit for their achievements because stereotyping suggests that Asian Americans have a natural ability to excel in these areas (Fukuyama & Cox, 1992). Leong and Chou (1994) suggest that Asian Americans may react to such stereotypes differently, depending on their acculturation levels.

274 FREDERICK T. L. LEONG AND MEI TANG

Occupational segregation has been evident in the unbalanced occupational distribution of Asian Americans in the workforce (U. S. Bureau of the Census, 1993). Asian Americans have been over-represented in some jobs, such as physician, medical scientist, physicist, engineer, and biological life scientist, and underrepresented in other jobs, such as lawyers, judges, and chief executive officers. Tang et al. (1999) used Hsia's (1988) Representation Index (RI) to calculate the occupational representativeness of the Asian American college students' career choices in their study. They found that the three most frequent choices among these participants were engineer (RI =244), physician (RI = 426), and computer scientist (RI = 275), with an RI of 100 reflecting proportionate distribution; and RI above 100 reflecting overrepresentation. This finding demonstrates occupational stereotyping and segregation among Asian Americans.

Leong (1998) noted that this pattern of occupational segregation among Asian Americans into science and engineering fields may have significant effects on promotion and advancement. It is most commonly through rising into the administrative ranks that individuals are able to advance their careers in terms of both salary and prestige. However, occupational stereotyping and segregation may affect promotion for Asian Americans since they are viewed as lacking social and managerial skills.

4. APPLICATION OF CULTURAL ACCOMMODATION TO CAREER ASSESSMENT OF ASIAN AMERICANS

The application of the proposed cultural accommodation approach includes three steps: 1) identifying the cultural gaps or cultural blind spots in an existing theory that restricts the cultural validity of the theory; 2) selecting culturally-specific concepts and models from cross-cultural and ethnic minority psychology to fill in the cultural gaps and accommodate the original theory to racial and ethnic minorities; and 3) testing the culturally accommodated theory to determine if it has incremental validity above and beyond the original (culturally unaccommodated) theory (Leong & Serafica, in press). A culturally accommodated theory would be helpful for assessing the occupational constructs discussed in the previous section and also provide more appropriate approaches to study the issues such as discrepancies between inventoried interests and expressed interests, occupational stereotypes and segregation, and the relationship between interests, self-efficacy, values, and career choices.

Instead of developing a whole new approach to career assessment just for Asian Americans, there are a few variables that can be incorporated into existing career assessment tools to make the assessment process and outcome more culturally valid. In other words, the cultural accommodation approach is not trying to abolish the current practice of conducting career assessment with Asian Americans. However, the deficiencies of the current career assessment process need to be identified, and at the same time, the variables that address specific cultural groups need to be added to the existing models of career assessment. This is the essence of the cultural accommodation model that we propose will be more relevant, valid and predictive of

A CULTURAL ACCOMMODATION APPROACH TO CAREER ASSESSMENT WITH ASIAN AMERICANS

the career development and vocational behavior of Asian Americans than an unaccommodated model. In the following section, we will review several culturally relevant constructs and discuss how these constructs can be applied in career development of Asian Americans.

4.1 Cultural Identity

A major perspective on cultural identity for Asian Americans involves the concept of acculturation. In applying Leong's (1996) integrative model to provide career services to Asian Americans, counselors need to recognize how acculturation links the Group and Individual dimensions as it moderates cultural and individual differences. At the Group or cultural level, for example, Asian Americans (e.g., Chinese-, Japanese-, and Korean-Americans) may share certain cultural values, norms, and beliefs. Concurrently, as individuals, Asian Americans differ from each other. Understanding acculturation level helps the counselor to understand how each Asian American (or other minority group member) differs from another.

Step one of the cultural accommodation model, then, should incorporate assessment of the client's acculturation level. This, in turn, would guide the counselor in determining whether and how to modify subsequent steps (e.g., in terms of selecting, sequencing, and interpreting assessment instruments). Major issues related to ethnic minority vocational behavior and career development, relative to acculturation level include occupational segregation, stereotyping, discrimination, prestige, mobility, attitudes, aspirations and expectations, stress, satisfaction, choice and interest (Leong, 1985; Leong & Serafica, 1995).

To the extent that acculturation level is an important component of cultural identity, Leong and Chou (1994) have already delineated some possible relationships between career variables and acculturation for Asian Americans. In providing an overview of the research and theoretical literature in Asian American ethnic identity and acculturation, Leong and Chou (1994) proposed an integration of these two areas. They argued that even though Berry's (1980) model is considered an acculturation model, it actually deals more directly with cultural identity. According to Berry's model, individuals who hold positive views of both their own culture and the host culture are Integrationists who attempt to have the best that both cultures have to offer. Assimilationists, the second possible acculturation outcome, hold a positive view of the host culture, but a negative view of their own culture (Berry, 1980). Individuals who view their host culture negatively and their own culture positively are Separationists (Berry, 1980). Finally, Berry's model includes a group that is not recognized by the other models, namely Marginal persons who hold a negative view of both host and own culture.

Using this integrated model of cultural identity, Leong and Chou (1994) went on to propose significant relationships between Asian Americans' cultural identity and various career variables such as occupational segregation, stereotyping, discrimination, prestige, mobility, attitudes, aspirations and expectations, stress, satisfaction, choice and interest (see Leong, 1985; Leong & Serafica, 1995). For example, they proposed that Asian Americans with a Separationist Identity are more susceptible to occupational segregation, while those with an Assimilationist Identity are less susceptible to occupational segregation. This pattern could be the result of the cultural background (Fong, 1973) of less acculturated Asians or stereotyped tracking of Asians by the majority-dominated working world.

Leong and Chou (1994) also proposed that occupational stereotyping would follow the pattern of occupational segregation for Asian Americans. Leong and Serafica (1995) have explained that Asian Americans are stereotyped as more qualified in the physical, biological, and medical sciences and less qualified or likely to be successful in verbal, persuasive, or social careers. They have proposed that Asian Americans who hold Separationist Identity may believe occupational stereotypes to be more valid. At the same time, Separationist Asian Americans may be more subject to occupational stereotyping. Assimilationists and Integrationists, on the other hand, may be more resistant to such stereotypes and therefore more likely to enter non-traditional career fields (e.g., law, sales, and social work).

Leong and Chou (1994) also proposed that Assimilationist Asian Americans will perceive and experience the least amount of occupational discrimination (e.g., existence of glass ceilings) because they will tend to attribute lack of success of Asian Americans to individual lack of ability and not to discrimination. In addition, Leong and Chou proposed that Asian Americans who are Assimilationists and Integrationists will view their job in much the same way European Americans do (e.g., as more of a virtue in and of itself), and thus choose occupations based on what they enjoy (Leong & Tata, 1990), whereas Separationist Asian Americans will view careers more as a means to an end (e.g., financial security). However, Assimilationists may tend to choose occupations traditionally closed to Asian Americans (e.g., politics, media) to "prove" to European Americans they are not stereotypically Asian.

Finally, Leong and Chou (1994) proposed that Asian Americans who hold Separationist Identity may exhibit less self-efficacy in career choice, interest, or expectations because of the strong reverence and respect of parental authority in Asian cultures. These individuals may choose their careers based more on family desires or needs than on their own desires or interest. Therefore, these individuals may experience more stress (A. M. Padilla, Wagatsuma, & Lindholm, 1985) and less job satisfaction. Recent research is beginning to find support for Leong and Chou's (1994) proposition that acculturation or cultural identity is a significant factor in understanding the career behavior of Asian Americans. For example, Tang, Fouad, and Smith (1999) applied a path model to 187 Asian American college students' career choices and found that acculturation plays a significant role in influencing career self-efficacy and career choice.

4.2 Cultural Values

There are many instruments assessing individuals' values in the current career assessment literature. The widely used ones include the Value Scale (Nevill & Super, 1989), and the Minnesota Importance Questionnaire (Gay, Weiss, Hendel,

A CULTURAL ACCOMMODATION APPROACH TO CAREER ASSESSMENT WITH ASIAN AMERICANS

Dawis & Lofquist, 1971). These inventories tend to measure the occupational values of people from a White, middle class, male perspective. The profiles are also based on norm groups mainly derived from such populations. While these inventories provide very useful information about individuals' preference for what is important in their work settings, there is a deficit for minority members who may not necessarily share the same kind of work values. For instance, both of the inventories mentioned above focus more on individualistic values that relate to the ways that people view themselves in the work environment (e.g., whether they can get promoted, whether they can use their abilities, whether they can get their needs met, and so on) rather than on collectivistic values that relate to people's views about the impact of work on their families or associated group (e.g. how people view what work can bring to their family or others who are important in their lives).

Using the cultural accommodation model, the career assessment of occupational values should incorporate culturally relevant values. For Asian Americans, what is important in work is not just what brings personal benefits. If a person cares only about her/his gains and losses from work, this person is perceived in traditional Asian culture as being selfish, because she/he does not consider others' benefits first. The "others" can be family members, or other members in the group or community. Since the traditional culture values center more on interdependence, deference to authority and senior people, family unity and conformity with social norms (Moy, 1992), Asian Americans value different sets of job qualities than White Americans, on whom many vocational instruments are based.

Of the various values that have been examined, Individualism-Collectivism has received the most research attention during the last two decades. Individualism-collectivism represents a value orientation that plays a potentially significant role in career development and vocational behavior (Hartung, Speight, & Lewis, 1996; Leong, 1993). An individualistic orientation in work values leads people to be more inclined to self-expression and self-actualization. The ultimate goal of individualism is independence. This contrasts with collectivist-oriented cultures that emphasize the collaborative benefits for everybody in the group. Because of this difference, career choices for Asian Americans may not be solely an individual choice based on personal interests and preference; instead, they are choices that fulfill the responsibility of individuals caring for the family (Leong & Chou, 1994).

Sometimes Asian Americans have to compromise their career choices with their familial responsibilities and expectations in order to benefit both themselves and their families. The three dimensions of human personality proposed by Leong (1996) would help to scrutinize the functions of individualism/collectivism values in Asian American career assessment. Consideration of the Universal level of humans' pursuit of careers (e.g. the assessment of interests, occupational values, abilities, etc.) would be the necessary variables to be examined for career planning. These traits are as important for Asian Americans as they are for other ethnic groups. However, the assessment results of those variables may have different meanings for Asian Americans because of their cultural heritage and the stronger collectivist orientation in their value systems. For instance, a profile for an Asian American high school student indicates he has interest and talent in occupations that are related to people interactions such as social worker, counselor, and school teacher. His parents, however, want him to go to engineering school instead. If the career counselor neglects the cultural factors which are the Group level of Leong's (1996) integrated model of cross-cultural counseling, two outcomes are possible. One is that the student is advised to follow his own preference and then gets into trouble with his parents. The other is that the student is advised to listen to his parents' idea and then feels frustrated because he doesn't like engineering. The first outcome suggests that the counselor fails to acknowledge the interdependence of family members, or, in other words, fails to attend to the Group dimension. The second outcome indicates that the counselor focuses only on the Group level, thinking that all Asian Americans are the same and that they all value more collective benefits, in this case, the familial expectations. The student's individuality is totally ignored. It is no surprise that the student would feel frustrated.

When evaluating the results of career assessment, cultural factors such as collectivism need to be considered from three dimensions—Universal, Group, and Individual. In this case, the counselor needs to closely study the profiles to see if there is some areas in which the student has some interests and abilities and which can lead to an occupation that satisfies both his own and his parents' aspirations.

4.3 Construals of the Self

Asian Americans with more collectivistic values may conceive of the self as interdependent, whereas persons from individualistic cultures may view the self as independent (Markus & Kitayama, 1991). Such a self-conception may make career decision making a much more interpersonal process for collectivists than for individualists. For the latter, career decision making may be an individual matter based mainly on personal interests, values, and aspirations (Hartung et al., 1996). As discussed earlier, such value differences can easily lead counselors to culturally inappropriate counseling process and culturally inappropriate goals. Therefore, assessing the client's self-construal is another important aspect in the cultural accommodation approach of career assessment.

According to Markus and Kitayama (1991), the independent self has the core need to strategically express or assert the internal attributes of the self; the interdependent construal formulates self in relation to others. Being unique is very critical for the independent self and fitting-in is very important for the interdependent self. The basis of self-esteem for the independent self is the ability to express the self and to validate internal attributes. For the interdependent self, the basis of self-esteem is the ability to adjust, restrain self, and maintain harmony with social context (Markus & Kitayama, 1991).

These concepts are very helpful in understanding the vocational behaviors of Asian Americans in work settings. Asian Americans are often passed-up for promotion or tenure (Leong & Serafica, 1995) because of a perceived lack of managerial skills, which needs further investigation. One possibility may be because the self-construal of Asian Americans leads them to behave differently from what is expected in the typical method of evaluating job performance (i.e. one has to

A Cultural Accommodation Approach to Career Assessment with Asian Americans

279

present/express onself to let others know that one has done an excellent work). Asian Americans' quietness and modesty are often mistakenly viewed as lack of confidence or ability.

The culturally appropriate way of assessing Asian Americans' work performance should incorporate the self-construal into the evaluation process. Again, one should not assume that every Asian American acts the same way, or narrowly focus on the Group level only. Counselors using the cultural accommodation approach would equally consider a variety of elements that play a role in Asian Americans' career development.

5. SUMMARY

According to the cultural accommodation model, the gaps in the existing career assessment of Asian Americans can often be reduced by incorporating culture-specific variables into career assessment to make it more relevant and useful for racial and cultural minorities. By using Leong's (1996) integrative model of examining Universal, Group, and Individual dimensions of human personality, one can increase the cultural validity of the cultural accommodation approach discussed in this chapter. Furthermore, the cultural accommodation approach needs to recognize the importance of using the person-environment interaction model rather than just focusing on the person and ignoring the cultural context variables in the lives of racial and ethnic minorities.

The value of the proposed cultural accommodation approach is in providing a guideline for conducting career assessment of Asian Americans. More studies are needed to investigate whether the culture specific variables (e.g., cultural identity) can account for significant amounts of variance in vocational behavior of racial and ethnic minority individuals in this cultural accommodation process. Also, future research is needed to demonstrate incremental validity where culture specific variables account for additional variance above and beyond those accounted for by the variables in the current career assessment models which are not accommodated to the culture-specific attitudes, values, beliefs and needs of Asian American clients.

6. REFERENCES

Anh, N. T., & Healy, C. C. (1985). Factors affecting employment and job satisfaction of Vietnamese refugees. *Journal of Employment Counseling, 22*, 78-85.

Bandura, A. (1986). *Social foundations of thought and action: A social cognitive theory.* Englewood Cliffs, NJ: Prentice Hall.

Berry, J. W. (1980). Acculturation as varieties of adaptation. In A. M. Padilla (Ed.), *Acculturation: Theories, models and some new findings* (pp. 9-25). Boulder, CO: Westview Press.

Betz, N. E. (1992). Career Assessment: A review of critical issues. In S. D. Brown & R. W. Lent (Eds.), *Handbook of counseling psychology* (2nd ed.). New York: John Wiley & Sons.

Betz, N. E., & Hackett, G. (1981). The relationship of career-related self-efficacy expectations to perceived career options in college women and men. *The Journal of Counseling Psychology, 28*, 399-410.

280   FREDERICK T. L. LEONG AND MEI TANG

Betz, N. E., & Hackett, G. (1986). Applications of self-efficacy theory to understanding career choice behavior. *Journal of Social and Clinical Psychology, 4,* 279-289.

Brooks, L. (1991). Recent developments in theory building. In D. Brown, L. Brooks et al. (Eds.), *Career choice and development* (2nd ed., pp. 364-394). San Francisco: Jossey-Bass.

Brown, D., Minor, C. W., & Jepsen, D. A. (1991). The opinions of minorities about preparing for work: Report of the second NCDA national survey. *The Career Development Quarterly, 40,* 5-19.

Brown, D., & Minor, C. W. (Eds.). (1992). *Career needs in a diverse workforce: Implications of NCDA Gallup Survey.* Alexandria, VA: The National Career Development Association.

Crites, J. O. (1978). *Theory and research handbook: Career Maturity Inventory.* Monterey, CA: McGraw-Hill.

Fong, S. L. M. (1973). Assimilation and changing social roles of Chinese Americans. *Journal of Social Issues, 29,* 115-127.

Fouad, N. A., Harmon, L. W., & Hansen, J. C. (1994). Cross-cultural use of the Strong. In L. W. Harmon, J. C. Hansen, F. H. Borgen, & A. L. Hammer (Eds.), *Strong Interest Inventory: Application and technical guide.* Palo Alto, CA: Consulting Psychologists Press.

Frank, J. D. (1961). *Persuasion and healing.* Baltimore: John Hopkins University Press.

Fukuyama, M. A., & Cox, C. I. (1992). Asian-Pacific Islanders and career development. In D. Brown & C. W. Minor (Eds.), *Career needs in a diverse workforce: Implications of the NCDA Gallup Survey* (pp. 27-50). Alexandria, VA: The National Career Development Association.

Gay, E. G., Weiss, D. J., Hendel, D. D., Dawis, R. V., & Lofquist, L. H. (1971). Manual for Minnesota Importance Questionnaire. *Minnesota Studies in Vocational Rehabilitation, 28* (6, Serial No. 83).

Harmon, L. W., Hansen, J. C., Borgen, F. H., & Hammer, A. C. (1994). *Strong Interest Inventory.* Palo Alto, CA: Consulting Psychologist Press.

Hartung, P. J., Speight, J. D., & Lewis, D. M. (1996). Individualism-collectivism and the vocational behavior of majority culture college students. *Career Development Quarterly, 45,* 87-96.

Haverkamp, B. E., Collins, R. C., & Hansen, J. C. (1994). Structure of interests of Asian-American college students. *Journal of Counseling Psychology, 41,* 256-264.

Holland, J. L. (1985). *Making vocational choices: A theory of vocational personalities and work environments.* Englewood Cliffs, NJ: Prentice-Hall.

Hsia, J. (1988). *Asian Americans in higher education and at work.* Hillsdale, NJ: Erlbaum.

Kincaid, D. L., & Yum, J. O. (1987). A comparative study of Korean, Filipino and Samoan immigrants to Hawai'i: Socioeconomic consequences. *Human Organization, 46,* 70-77.

Kluckhohn, C., & Murray, H. A. (1950). Personality formation: The determinants. In C. Kluckhohn & H.A. Murray (Eds.), *Personality in nature, society, and culture* (pp. 35- 48) New York: Alfred A. Knopf.

Lent, R. W., Brown, S. D., & Larkin, K. C. (1984). Relation of self-efficacy expectations to academic achievement and persistence. *Journal of Counseling Psychology, 31,* 356-362.

Leong, F. T. L. (1982). *Differential career development attributes of Asian American and White college students.* Unpublished master's thesis, University of Maryland.

Leong, F. T. L. (1985). Career development of Asian-Americans. *Journal of College Student Personnel, 26,* 539-546.

Leong, F. T. L. (1991). Career development attributes of occupational values of Asian American and White American college students. *Career Development Quarterly, 39,* 221-230.

Leong, F. T. L. (1995). *Career development and vocational behavior of racial and ethnic minorities.* Hillsdale, NJ: Lawrence Erlbaum Associates.

Leong, F. T. L. (1996). Toward an integrative model for cross-cultural counseling and psychotherapy. *Applied and Preventive Psychology, 5,* 189-209.

Leong, F. T. L. (1998). Career development and vocational behaviors. In L. C. Lee & N. W. S. Zane (Eds.), *Handbook of Asian American psychology* (pp.359-398). Thousand Oaks, CA: Sage.

Leong, F. T. L., & Brown, M. (1995). Theoretical issues in cross-cultural career development: Cultural validity and cultural specificity. In W. B. Walsh & S. H. Osipow (Eds.), *Handbook of vocational psychology* (pp. 143-180) (2nd ed.). Hillsdale, NJ: Lawrence Erlbaum.

Leong, F. T. L., & Chou, E. L. (1994). The role of ethnic identity and acculturation in the vocational behavior of Asian Americans: An integrative review. *Journal of Vocational Behavior, 44,* 155-172.

Leong, F. T. L., & Gim, R. H. C. (1995). Career assessment and intervention with Asian Americans. In F. T. L. Leong (Ed.), *Career development and vocational behavior of racial and ethnic minorities* (pp. 193-226). Hillsdale, NJ: Lawrence Erlbaum Associates.

A CULTURAL ACCOMMODATION APPROACH TO CAREER ASSESSMENT WITH ASIAN AMERICANS

Leong, F. T. L., & Leung, S. A. (1994). Career assessment with Asian Americans. *Journal of Career Assessment, 2,* 240-257.

Leong, F. T. L., & Hayes, T. J. (1990). Occupational stereotyping of Asian Americans. *The Career Development Quarterly, 39,* 143-154.

Leong, F. T. L., & Serafica, F. (1995). Career development of Asian Americans: A research area in need of a good theory. In F. T. L. Leong (Ed.), *Career development and vocational behavior of racial and ethnic minorities* (pp. 67-102). Hillsdale, NJ: Lawrence Erlbaum.

Leong, F. T. L., & Serafica, F. (in press). Cross-cultural perspective on Super's career developmental theory: Career maturity and cultural accommodation. In F. T. L. Leong & A. Barak (Eds.), *Contemporary models in vocational psychology: A volume in honor of Samuel H. Osipow.* Mahwah, NJ: Lawrence Erlbaum Associates.

Leong, F. T. L., & Tata, S. P. (1990). Sex and acculturation differences in occupational values among Chinese-American children. *Journal of Counseling Psychology, 37,* 208-212.

Leung, S. A., Ivey, D., & Suzuki, L. (in press). Factors affecting the career aspirations of Asian Americans. *Journal of Counseling and Development.*

Lewin, K. (1951). *Field theory in social science: Selected theoretical papers.* New York: Harper & Row.

Markus, H. R., & Kitayama, S. (1991). Culture and the self: Implications for cognition, emotion, and motivation. *Psychological Review, 98,* 224-253

Moy, S. (1992). A culturally sensitive, psychoeducational model for understanding and treating Asian-American clients. *Journal of Psychology and Christianity, 11,* 358-369.

Nevill, D. D., & Super, D. E. (1989). *The Value Scale: Theory, application and research.* Palo Alto, CA: Consulting Psychologists Press.

Padilla, A. M., Wagatsuma, Y., & Lindholm, K. J. (1985). Acculturation and personality as predictors of stress in Japanese and Japanese-Americans. *The Journal of Social Psychology, 125,* 295-305.

Redding, S. G., & Ng, M. (1982). The role of "face" in the organizational perceptions of Chinese managers. *Organization Studies, 3,* 201-219.

Rooney, R. A., & Osipow, S. H. (1992). Task-specific Occupational Self-efficacy Scale: The development and validation of a prototype. *Journal of Vocational Behavior, 40,* 14-32.

Sue, D. W., & Frank, A. C. (1973). A typological approach to the psychological study of Chinese and Japanese American college males. *Journal of Social Issues, 29,* 129-148.

Sue, D. W., & Kirk, B. A. (1973). Differential characteristics of Japanese-American and Chinese-American college students. *Journal of Counseling Psychology, 20,* 142-148.

Sue, D. W., & Kirk, B. A. (1972). Psychological characteristics of Chinese-American students. *Journal of Counseling Psychology, 19,* 471-478.

Sue, S., & Morishima, J. K. (1982). *The mental health of Asian Americans.* San Francisco: Jossey-Bass.

Sue, S., & Okazaki, S. (1990). Asian-American education achievements: A phenomenon in sea:ch of an explanation. *American Psychologist, 45,* 913-920.

Sue, S., & Sue, D. W. (1974). MMPI comparisons between Asian American and non-Asian students utilizing a student health psychiatric clinic. *Journal of Counseling Psychology, 21,* 423-427.

Tang, M., Fouad, N. A., & Smith, P. L. (1999). Asian Americans' career choices: A path model to examine factors influencing their career choices. *Journal of Vocational Behavior, 54,* 142-147.

Tang, J., & O'Brien, T. P. (1990). Correlates of vocational success in refugee work adaptation. *Journal of Applied Social Psychology, 20,* 1444-1452.

Taylor, K. M., & Betz, N. E. (1983). Applications of self-efficacy theory to the understanding and treatment of career indecision. *Journal of Vocational Behavior, 22,* 63-81.

Tou, L. A. (1974). A study of work orientations of Chinese American and White American students of the 7th and 8th grades in Catholic elementary schools. (Doctoral Dissertation, Catholic University of America, 1974). *Dissertation Abstracts International, 35,* 831A.

U. S. Bureau of the Census (1993). *1990 Census of Population: Asian and Pacific Islanders in the United States.* Washington, DC: U.S. Department of Commerce.

Yu, L. C., & Wu, S. (1985). Unemployment and family dynamics in meeting the needs of Chinese elderly in the United States. *The Gerontologist, 25,* 472-476.

RICHARD M. LEE AND ADAM J. DARNELL

CHAPTER 19

THEORY AND METHOD OF MULTICULTURAL COUNSELING COMPETENCY ASSESSMENT

1. INTRODUCTION

In 1973, the American Psychological Association's (APA) Vail Conference stated that "the provision of professional services to persons of culturally diverse backgrounds by persons not competent in understanding and providing professional services to such groups shall be considered unethical" (Korman, 1973, p. 105). Almost a decade later, a framework for standards of multicultural counseling competency (MCC) was proposed by leading scholars in the field (D.W. Sue, et al., 1982). These MCC standards have since gone through several revisions and each time a call to the profession has been made to officially recognize them (Arrendondo et al., 1996; D. W. Sue, Arrendondo, & McDavis, 1992). APA eventually established a set of service provider guidelines for working with ethnic, linguistic, and culturally diverse populations (APA, 1993), but failed to incorporate these guidelines into their official ethical standards and principles (APA, 1987). Graduate training programs in psychology, initially slow to respond to the call for multiculturalism, have made a concerted effort in recent years to better train future clinicians for the provision of culturally competent services. Surveys of counseling, clinical, community, and school psychology programs have found an increase in the number of multicultural coursework offerings, a greater recruitment and retention of minority students and faculty, and an increase in multicultural and cross-cultural research (Constantine, Ladany, Inman, & Ponterotto, 1996; Hills & Strozier, 1992; S. M. Quintana & Bernal, 1995; Suarez-Balcazar, Durlak, & Smith, 1994). It is less known, however, if these policy and programmatic changes ensure the development of culturally competent practitioners (Ponterotto & Casas, 1991). There also is little consensus on how to best assess the MCC of mental health professionals and trainees working with diverse cultural populations (Ponterotto, Rieger, Barrett, & Sparks, 1994).

This chapter will examine current conceptualizations of and assessment procedures for MCC with special consideration for treating the Asian American population. We focus on MCC as it relates to Asian Americans because this racial group, to a great extent, has been an invisible minority in society. Asian Americans have been perceived as the model minority situated or wedged between the White majority and other racial minorities (Takaki, 1989). The public view of Asian

284 RICHARD M. LEE AND ADAM J. DARNELL

Americans as the well-adjusted minority who remains a foreign presence within America reflects an "orientalist" notion of Asian Americans by the dominant White culture as an object of both desire and aversion (Lee, 1999; Said, 1979). This racially oppressive image of Asian Americans is gradually changing in society, but there remains a tremendous lack of knowledge about this ethnically diverse population. The inadequacy of mental health care for Asian Americans is another disconcerting result of the model minority myth (Uba, 1994). This lack of mental health services for Asian Americans persists despite repeated studies that demonstrate Asian Americans do experience high amounts of psychological distress, present with serious mental health problems, and continue to under-utilize counseling services (Snowden & Cheung, 1990; S. Sue, Fujino, Hu, Takeuchi, & Zane, 1991). With this specific cultural population in mind, we begin with an operational definition and framework of MCC to understand the complexities of this construct. We proceed to examine empirical support for MCC in counseling and psychotherapy. The main body of the chapter reviews the different approaches to assessing MCC, followed by a discussion of their limitations and areas of future research. We conclude with a recommendation for the use of portfolios as a complementary approach to assess competency via demonstration.

2. DEFINING MULTICULTURAL COUNSELING COMPETENCY

Multicultural competency, as it pertains to counseling and psychotherapy, was operationally defined by D.W. Sue and colleagues in 1982 and subsequently revised in 1992. According to these leading scholars, MCC has several key characteristics or domains: cultural self-awareness, understanding the worldview of the client, and culturally relevant interventions, strategies and techniques. These three MCC characteristics can further be described as having three dimensions - beliefs and attitudes, knowledge, and skills - for a total of nine competency areas (3 characteristics x 3 dimensions). Sodowsky, Taffe, Gutkin, and Wise (1994) added a fourth dimension, "the counselor's interactional process with the minority client, such as the counselor's trustworthiness, comfort levels, stereotypes of the minority client, and worldview" (p. 142). This relationship-oriented dimension increases the total competency areas to twelve (3 characteristics x 4 dimensions).

The MCC operational definition and framework were revisited recently at The National Multicultural Leadership Summit, held in Newport Beach, CA on January 1999. The Summit participants represented the leading scholars in the field of multicultural counseling and together they ratified the following MCC standards in practice. APA's Divisions 17, 35, and 45 have subsequently accepted these standards. The practicing psychologist shall: (1) make a lifelong commitment to maintaining cultural expertise; (2) develop awareness of issues of discrimination and oppression and how these issues relate to presenting psychological concerns; in addition, find ways to address and dismantle oppression; (3) pay special attention to the unique worldviews and cultural backgrounds of clients; (4) recognize the client-in-context; (5) be aware that contextual therapy may require non-traditional interventions; (6) examine traditional practice interventions for their cultural appropriateness; (7) receive on-going feedback and assessment of personal cultural competence; (8) affirm the importance of empirical research to culturally competent practice.

3. EMPIRICAL SUPPORT FOR MULTICULTURAL COUNSELING COMPETENCY

There is growing empirical evidence that multiculturally-sensitive counseling approaches are perceived to be more effective than mainstream, humanistic approaches, particularly when working with racial and ethnic minority populations (Atkinson & Lowe, 1995). One early study involving Asian Americans by Atkinson, Maruyama, and Matsui (1978), for example, examined Asian American and Caucasian American college students' perceptions of a rational, directive counseling approach compared to an affective, non-directive approach. Asian Americans consistently rated audiotapes of counselors who used the directive approach to be more credible and approachable. Expanding on this earlier study, Atkinson and Matsushita (1991) developed audiotapes of simulated counseling with Japanese American and Caucasian American counselors using directive and non-directive approaches. Japanese American young adults and college students were most willing to see a Japanese American counselor using a directive style, although some individual within-group differences were found. Using a videotape analog study design, Sodowsky (1991) found that Asian Indian international students rated culturally consistent counselors higher on counselor expertness and trustworthiness than mainstream counselors who were not culturally consistent. Coleman (1998) similarly found that psychology graduate and ethnic minority undergraduate students rated videotapes of multiculturally sensitive counselors treating Fijian and Chinese American clients higher on both general and multicultural counseling competencies, compared to counselors who used mainstream, humanistic counseling skills. Asian American students also consistently preferred vignettes of counselors who exhibited an ability to facilitate the use of indigenous support systems and willingness to serve as a consultant (Atkinson, Kim, & Caldwell, 1998). These preferred counselor characteristics are consistent with culture-specific helper roles for Asian Americans.

4. ASSESSMENT OF MULTICULTURAL COUNSELING COMPETENCY

The assessment of MCC can be divided into two distinct approaches or categories (Coleman, 1996). The first approach to assessing MCC relies upon idiographic (e.g., mentorship, supervision) and pedagogical (e.g., required coursework) methods. The second approach to assessing MCC is through the use of quantitative surveys administered to trainees, counselors, and supervisors. We discuss the relative advantages and disadvantages of each approach and recommend some ways to improve them.

4.1 Assessment of MCC in Graduate Training Programs

Many multicultural or cross-cultural training models have been proposed over the years (e.g., D'Andrea & Daniels, 1991; Pedersen, 1977; Sue, 1991; Torres, Ottens, & Johnson, 1997; Vázquez, 1997). These programs expose students to a culturally diverse faculty, students, research, coursework, and client populations. This hands-on exposure is designed to encourage graduate students to explore their own cultural history, critically examine the role of the dominant culture in psychology, question the legitimacy of oppression and colonization, seek to understand the experiences of the culturally different, and develop culture-specific counseling skills through supervised practica (LaFromboise & Foster, 1992). Surveys of graduate programs in counseling, clinical, school, community psychology, and internship sites suggest that progress has been made in incorporating such training into the curriculum (Bernal & Castro, 1994; Bernal & Padilla, 1982; Lee et al., 1999; Murphy, Wright, & Bellamy, 1995; S. M. Quintana & Bernal, 1995; Rogers, Ponterotto, Conoley, & Wiese, 1992; Speight, Thomas, Kennel, & Anderson, 1995; Suarez-Balcazar et al., 1994). The findings across specialty programs are remarkably consistent in that 50 to 60 percent of most programs now require at least one multicultural counseling course and many offer additional multicultural courses. Counseling psychology programs appear to be most likely to require such coursework.

And yet this is not enough. Multicultural training remains at many graduate programs an ancillary training goal, making a systematic and formal assessment of MCC difficult to achieve. But there is very little assessment of the effectiveness of the multicultural training in promoting MCC. There seems to be an implicit understanding that students will naturally develop MCC by taking the required courses and working with diverse populations, yet not all students enroll in multicultural counseling courses, few faculty truly integrate or infuse cultural materials into their general courses, and many students do not have enough client contact hours with culturally different populations (Allison, Crawford, Echemendia, Robinson, & Knepp, 1994; Bernal & Castro, 1994). When an assessment of a student's MCC does occur, it is generally done informally through clinical supervision (Lee et al., 1999; Speight et al., 1995). This reliance on supervisors to be responsible for the assessment of a student's MCC concerns us because it shifts the responsibility away from the core faculty, who should hold the primary responsibility over a student's readiness as a professional. Furthermore, there is evidence to suggest that supervisors are not necessarily prepared or competent to assess MCC in graduate students.

In one of the larger studies on MCC in graduate training programs, Allison and colleagues (1994) asked 259 counseling and clinical psychologists about their graduate training and competency with specific racial and cultural groups. Allison and his colleagues found that 46 percent of respondents never or infrequently asked about cultural issues in supervision. Only 31 percent felt that supervision of work with diverse clients was "excellent" or "good." By contrast, 34 percent reported that such supervision was "poor" or "inadequate." This finding is consistent with Constantine's (1997) smaller survey of 30 matched pairs of supervisors and

THEORY AND METHOD OF MULTICULTURAL COUNSELING COMPETENCY ASSESSMENT

supervisees. Forty percent of supervisees felt their supervisors were reluctant to bring up multicultural issues. Another 13 percent of supervisees felt that supervisors did not process cultural differences between supervisor and supervisee. By contrast, none of the supervisors reported the need to bring up multicultural issues more often in supervision. Thirteen percent of the supervisors did recognize the need to address cultural differences between supervisor and supervisee, but 30% of supervisors placed the onus on the supervisee to get more minority clients or raise the issue in supervision.

Allison et al. (1994) also found that only 16% of the respondents reported feeling "extremely or very competent" working specifically with Asian American clients, despite 46% of the respondents having worked with Asian American training cases in the past. Twenty percent of the respondents reported that they are currently seeing Asian American clients. The competency ratings working with European American (97%), African American (38%), and Hispanic (26%) were higher, and only competency working with Native Americans (8%) was lower. In short, Allison et al.'s findings suggest that MCC training still has a long way to go. It particularly challenges the legitimacy of training programs relying upon individual supervisors to assess the MCC in their graduate students. The study also demonstrates the continued lack of awareness and understanding of Asian Americans as a visible racial minority group. It is clear that pedagogical reform is necessary to ensure that graduate training programs are successful in the development and assessment of MCC, particularly as it applies to Asian Americans.

Ponterotto and colleagues (1995; 1997) have developed two self-report instruments to assist training directors and faculty in the development and assessment of MCC within training programs. The instruments are designed to evaluate the multicultural training components and the training effectiveness at promoting MCC. They also serve as a starting point for a more formal assessment of MCC in graduate training programs.

4.1.1 The Multicultural Competency Checklist

Ponterotto, Alexander, and Grieger (1995) developed the Checklist as a quick and easy way for counseling training directors to self-assess their efforts to establish MCC. The brief 22-item checklist uses a forced choice rating system ("met" or "not met") to assess competency in minority representation among students and faculty, curriculum issues, counseling practice and supervision, research considerations, student and faculty competency evaluations, and physical environment. The checklist has been administered to both graduate students (Constantine, Ladany, Inman, & Ponterotto, 1996) and faculty or program directors (Ponterotto, 1997) to assess relative strengths and weaknesses of existing training. The checklist does not however contain information on training with specific racial and cultural groups. It will be important for programs to modify the checklist to ask about training with specific racial and cultural groups, such as Asian Americans. Programs then can carefully address their training deficiencies for working with each racial and cultural group.

288 RICHARD M. LEE AND ADAM J. DARNELL

4.1.2 The Multicultural School Psychology Counseling Competency Scale (MSPCC)

Rogers and Ponterotto (1997) developed the MSPCC for school psychology training directors and faculty to self-assess the effectiveness of the multicultural training in their programs. In constructing the scale nine experts in the field rated each item candidate using a 5-point Likert-type scale to establish content validity. The final scale consists of 11-items that refer to the extent to which graduate students in a given program possess MCC at the time of graduation (e.g., "Aware of her/his own cultural heritage and values"). The statements are rated on a 4-point Likert-type scale, ranging from "not at all" to "very much." Internal reliability for the MSPCC was strong (α = .88) and inter-item correlations were moderate in size (r's = .37 - .74). Items were retained if they had an average rating of 4 or higher. A principal components analysis revealed one unidimensional construct, assessing multicultural awareness/sensitivity, thus establishing preliminary construct validity. No other research has been conducted with the MSPCC to validate its utility, but it appears to complement the Multicultural Competency Checklist. In particular, the MSPCC provides training directors with a means to estimate the effectiveness of the overall training program at promoting MCC in recent graduates.

4.2 Assessment of MCC in Individuals

The Multicultural Counseling Checklist and the MSPCCS provide an assessment of MCC at the programmatic level, but they are not precise enough to assess MCC at the individual level. It therefore has been argued that standardized individual assessment measures of MCC are necessary to hold psychologists and trainees accountable. Advocates of standardized instruments also argue that these instruments facilitate the development of MCC and provide an objective method to determine if MCC has been achieved (Ponterotto, Rieger, Barrett, & Sparks, 1994). For a detailed comparison of many of these instruments, readers are referred to comprehensive reviews by Ponterotto et al. (1994), Ponterotto and Alexander (1996), and Pope-Davis and Dings (1995).

4.2.1 The Cross-Cultural Counseling Inventory-Revised (CCCI-R)

The CCCI-R, developed by LaFromboise, Coleman, and Hernandez (1991), is considered the first measure of MCC. The CCCI-R consists of 20 items that are rated by an evaluator or supervisor along a 6-point Likert-type scale, ranging from "strongly disagree" to "strongly agree." The CCCI-R has demonstrated excellent internal reliability (α = .95). For additional reliability, three experts in the field viewed 12 videotapes of analog counseling sessions, rated the videotaped counselors using the CCCI-R, and obtained an inter-rater reliability coefficients of .84. A single factor emerged from a principal components analysis, suggesting the CCCI-R reflects a general measure of MCC. It has sometimes been used in conjunction with measures of general counseling effectiveness (Coleman, 1998), such as the Counselor Rating Form (Barak & LaCrosse, 1975) or Counselor Effectiveness

Rating Scale (Atkinson & Wampold, 1982). The CCCI-R remains the most widely used measure of MCC (Ponterotto, Rieger, Barrett, & Sparks, 1992), particularly in analog research studies (e.g., Atkinson, Casas, & Abreu, 1992; Ramos-Sánchez, Atkinson, & Fraga, 1999). Gim, Atkinson, and Kim (1991) found that Asian American college students rated hypothetical counselors higher on the CCCI-R when they were introduced as Asian American and when they were portrayed as more culturally sensitive.

4.2.2 Cross-Cultural Critical Incident Quality Index (CCIQI)

Byington, Fischer, Walker, and Freedman (1997) developed the CCIQI for assessing the case conceptualization skills of rehabilitation counselors. The CCIQI consists of nine items that address different MCC criteria. Cultural experts or supervisors using a Likert-type scale, ranging from "not present" to "excellent", rate the counselor on each criterion. The internal reliability estimate using Spearman-Brown formula was .86. In their particular study, graduate students participated in a 2-day workshop on multicultural ethics and assessment. Students were presented with a vignette of an Asian American client with an amputated arm seeking rehabilitation counseling at the start and end of the workshop. Pre-post changes in the CCIQI were not significantly different, although post-workshop scores were slightly higher. It is difficult to fully assess the reliability and validity of the CCIQI because limited information on its scale construction is available. Its focus on the assessment of case conceptualization skills, however, provides another form of assessment that is not adequately measured by the CCCI-R, thus potentially serving as a complementary tool for supervisors.

4.2.3 The Multicultural Awareness-Knowledge-and-Skills Survey (MAKSS)

The MAKSS developed by D'Andrea, Daniels, and Heck (1991) is a 60-item self-report measure that assesses three categories of competencies: awareness of personal attitudes toward minority clients, knowledge about minority clients, and cross-cultural communication skills. Items are rated using Likert-type scales, ranging from "strongly disagree" to "strongly agree" or "very limited" to " very aware". The internal reliability for the three subscales are adequate to strong (Awareness α = .75; Knowledge α = .90; Skill α = .96). Separate factor analyses were performed for each subscale to establish construct validity. This is an unusual psychometric procedure, because scale items are traditionally analyzed together to determine the construct validity of the original subscales. Nevertheless, D'Andrea and others reported that MAKSS Awareness subscale appears to have three distinct factors, whereas the MAKSS Knowledge and Skills subscale have unidimensional single factors. Changes in pre-post scores on the MAKSS after students completed a multicultural training course provided preliminary evidence of criterion-related validity. A later study by Neville et al. (1996) compared the impact of multicultural training on White racial identity attitudes and MCC. They also found that multicultural training positively affected scores on the MAKSS Knowledge and

290   RICHARD M. LEE AND ADAM J. DARNELL

Skills subscales, up to a year later. White racial identity status was also significantly correlated with MAKSS subscales.

4.2.4 Multicultural Case Conceptualization Ability (MCCA)

Ladany, Inman, Constantine, and Hofheinz (1997) developed the MCCA to assess multicultural case conceptualization ability. Multicultural experts use a five-point scoring system across two domains: etiology of client's problem and effective treatment strategy. A score of 0 signifies no indication of race in the conceptualization of client's problem; 3 signifies two or more indications of potential racial issues in the conceptualization; and 5 signifies three or more mentions of potential racial issues in the conceptualization. Inter-rater reliability was .86 for the etiology rating and .87 for the treatment rating. In their study, Ladany et al. had participants conceptualize a vignette about an African American college student. A small correlation was found between MCCA-etiology and participant's racial identity status. The MCCA was not, however, correlated with the CCCI-R, suggesting the need for continued validation of this rating system.

4.2.5 The Multicultural Counseling Awareness Scale-B (MCAS-B)

The MCAS-B developed by Ponterotto, Sanchez, and Magids (1991) is a 45-item self-report measure that consists of two subscales: Knowledge/Skills and Awareness. Items are rated along a 7-point Likert-type scale, ranging from "not at all true" to "totally true". The internal reliability for the two subscales is adequate to strong (Knowledge/Skills α = .78 - .93; Awareness α = .67 - .78). Content validity was established using quantitative and qualitative methods. Construct validity was demonstrated by both exploratory and confirmatory factor analyses. Criterion-related validity was also established by comparing MCAS scores between multicultural counseling experts and trainees, as well as between individuals with varying levels of multicultural training experience (Ponterotto et al., 1996).

4.2.6 The Multicultural Counseling Inventory (MCI)

The MCI developed by Sodowsky, Taffe, Gutkin, and Wise (1994) is the most psychometrically sound self-report MCC measure available, according to Pope-Davis and Dings (1995). The MCI is a 40-item self-report measure that assesses four categories of competencies: multicultural counseling skill, multicultural awareness, multicultural counseling knowledge, and the multicultural counseling relationship. The items reflect the MCC operational definition by Sue et al. (1992) and Sodowsky et al (1994), and the four corresponding subscales were derived from factor analysis. Items are rated along a 4-point Likert-type scale, ranging from "very inaccurate" to "very accurate." The internal reliability for the subscales are adequate to good (Skills α = .81 - .83; Awareness α = .81 - .83; Knowledge α = .78 - .79; and Relationship α = .71 - .72). Content validity for the MCI was established through expert evaluations of item clarity and classification of items into subscale categories. Construct validity was established through exploratory and confirmatory factor

THEORY AND METHOD OF MULTICULTURAL COUNSELING COMPETENCY ASSESSMENT

analyses. Surprisingly, inter-correlations between the subscales were low to moderate ($r = .16 - .41$). Higher scores on MCI by students with more multicultural training and professionals with multicultural counseling experience demonstrated criterion-related validity. One survey of 344 graduate students in counseling and clinical psychology found that counseling psychology graduate students identified themselves as more culturally competent in domains of skills, awareness, and knowledge than clinical psychology graduate students (Pope-Davis, Reynolds, Dings, & Nielson, 1995). Sodowsky et al. (1994) cited evidence for concurrent validity between the MCI and MAKSS, but did not present validity coefficients. Pope-Davis and Dings (1994) administered the MCI and MCAS-B to 92 predoctoral interns at university counseling centers. They found that the MCAS-B Knowledge/Awareness subscale was moderately correlated with the MCI Knowledge ($r = .58$) and MCI Awareness ($r = .55$) but only slightly correlated with MCI Skills ($r = .27$). The MCI has also been examined in comparison to White racial identity. According to racial identity scholars, psychologists and trainees with more internalized White racial identities should have greater MCC. Somewhat consistent with this hypothesis, Ottavi, Pope-Davis, and Dings (1994) found that only the Pseudo-Independence racial identity status uniquely contributed to all four MCI subscales, above and beyond demographic and educational and clinical experiences.

4.2.7 The Multicultural Counseling Ethics and Assessment Competency Scale (MCEACS)

The MCEACS, developed by Byington et al. (1997), is the most recently developed self-report measure of MCC. The MCEACS is a 17-item measure that is designed to assess three areas: sociopolitical, ethics, and assessment. The scale items are rated on one of two 5-point Likert type scales. Eight counseling professionals rated the original 36 items as "essential," "useful but not essential," or "not essential" to establish content validity. Further refinement led to the final 17-item measure, which had an internal reliability estimate of .92 (α). Preliminary criterion validity was established by examining pre-post scores on the MCEACS after graduate students participated in a 2-day workshop on multicultural ethics and assessment. Concurrent validity was established by correlating the MCEACS with the MAKSS ($r = .69$).

4.3 Psychometric Evaluation of MCC Instruments

The standardized MCC instruments for program directors, supervisors, and student trainees provide a relatively quick and easy means to assess a program's or an individual's MCC. Despite the ease of administration, Constantine et al. (1996) and Ponterotto et al. (1997) found that only 20 to 23 percent of counseling psychology graduate training programs reported using self-report instruments to assess MCC. Even more striking, Lee, et al. (1999) found that only 2 of 48 counseling center pre-doctoral internship sites highly emphasized the use of self-report instruments to assess MCC. While some training programs may consciously choose to not use the instruments as an assessment tool for MCC, it may be that the low utilization rate is due to a simple lack of knowledge of their existence and utility. As is often the case with multicultural issues in graduate education, only professionals deeply committed to MCC are likely to employ such instruments as a training device.

We readily acknowledge the difficulty of creating an instrument to quantify MCC. At the same time, we were struck by the lack of psychometric rigor in the development of some of these instruments. The instruments purportedly measure multicultural knowledge, awareness, and skills across the three domains of self, other, and strategies. Factor analyses on the various scales, however, have failed to support the multidimensional model of MCC. We suspect that it may not be possible, nor reasonable to expect, to measure fully all the dimensions and characteristics of MCC, but the available data suggests that perhaps the original operational definition is insufficient and needs to be revisited. It also may be that the self-report measures focus too heavily on the more superficial aspects of multicultural knowledge, awareness, and skills. There is likely to be more apparent overlap between constructs at this surface level. It therefore may be too difficult to assess the depth of one's competency - where differentiation between constructs is likely to occur - using paper and pencil inventories.

Another psychometric concern is the possibility of social desirability in participant responses. That is, people may respond positively to multicultural-related items because it is expected. They also may over-estimate their perceived competencies. That is, it is easier for individuals to self-evaluate their multicultural knowledge and awareness than to assess one's actual performance or skills working with specific ethnic or racial groups. Only the MCAS-B attempted to account for social desirability to any extent. The possibility of social desirability is a valid reason for why the self-report instruments should be completed in conjunction with the supervisor-rated instruments, such as the CCCI-R. Although these two types of measures are not identical in content, they provide supervisor and supervisee a chance to discuss discrepancies, including issues of social desirability, during the assessment.

The stability or test-retest reliability of the instruments over time also has not been adequately studied. Little is known about which MCC dimensions or characteristics are more amenable or resistant to change. While studies have examined pre-post differences on the measures after a multicultural course or training (e.g., D'Andrea, Daniels, & Heck, 1991), control groups need to be more frequently employed to determine if training has an actual effect. In a related vein, there is no research on which aspects of multicultural training contribute to MCC. Systematic studies need to be conducted to understand exactly how multicultural awareness, knowledge, and skills are developed.

Concurrent validity between the different MCC instruments is necessary. Pope-Davis and Dings (1994) conducted one of the few studies that examined the relationship between two of the measures - MCI and MCAS-B, and found that they seem to be measuring different constructs. Concurrent validity should be established using multi-trait/multi-methods. For example, MCC scores on the MCI can be compared and contrasted with qualitative interviews with trainees and supervisors. Divergent validity is also necessary to ensure that the self-report instruments are not simply measuring related constructs, such as general counseling competency, racial attitudes, cognitive flexibility, and ego-strength.

We also agree with Ponterotto and Casas (1991) as well as Betz and Fitzgerald's (1993) earlier critiques of many MCC studies that they rely too heavily on analog experimental designs. These studies use an 'analog' of actual counseling, such as a videotaped session or a vignette, followed by the administration of a counseling competency instrument. Analog research designs allow a researcher to control for confounds and other extraneous factors, but the design can be too artificial to generalize beyond the laboratory setting (Heppner, Kivlighan, & Wampold, 2000). As S. Sue (2000) notes, psychology researchers are often too concerned with internal validity at the expense of external validity. One study has stood out as going beyond analog designs. Merta, Ponterotto, and Brown (1992) studied Asian foreign students who participated in a university orientation program. They found that highly acculturated Asian foreign students rated authoritative peer counselors higher on overall counselor effectiveness, whereas, low acculturated Asian students rated collaborative peer counselors higher.

If these MCC instruments are to be useful beyond training, outcome research is necessary to determine if counselors who score high on MCC instruments are in effect better multicultural counselors. For example, analog and more importantly service delivery studies need to examine the relationship between counselor's MCC and objective client outcome measures, such as increased level of functioning. Another direction of outcome research would be to compare self-report measures of MCC with ethnic/racial matching between counselor and client. It may be, however, that MCC is the more salient, underlying construct than ethnic/racial matching. S. Sue and Zane (1989), for instance, posited the importance of counselor credibility when working with Asian American clients. Atkinson, Wampold, Lowe, Matthews, and Ahn (1998) also found that Asian American college students consistently preferred a counselor with similar values and attitudes, as well as similar personality and age, over an ethnically similar counselor.

Additionally, the self-report instruments fail to differentiate ethnic and racial minority groups. Respondents simply rate their competency working with "a minority group," "a culturally different group," or "a recent immigrant." While these terms provide a way to quickly assess general multicultural competency, high general competency scores do not ensure one's competency working with specific cultural groups. The CCCI-R appears to be more adaptable for use with specific cultural groups, because the supervisor can rate a supervisee on his or her effectiveness working with individual clients from different cultural backgrounds.

Finally, norms for the MCC instruments need to be established in order to assess one's current MCC status. López et al. (1989), for instance, proposed a developmental model for culturally sensitive psychotherapists. The culturally unaware therapist does not understand the importance of culture and does not entertain cultural hypotheses. The therapist eventually develops a heightened awareness of culture but is unprepared to work with culturally different clients. As the therapist begins to address cultural issues in treatment, he or she may also begin to feel burdened by this responsibility. In the final stage, the culturally sensitive therapist is able to entertain cultural hypotheses, carefully test them, and develop appropriate and effective strategies. It would be helpful if this developmental sequence could be measured using the MCC instruments. The norms would allow supervisors to assess specific areas of deficiency, set realistic training goals, and track the overall progress of their trainees and themselves.

Despite these limitations, we encourage the continued use of such instruments, particularly for research purposes. We also acknowledge that even with future item refinement and scale validation, these instruments only provide a superficial assessment of MCC. We particularly doubt their practical use to assess one's multicultural counseling skills and performance.

4.4 Portfolio Assessment: A Complimentary Approach

Coleman (1996) proposed a portfolio approach to MCC assessment that addresses many of the shortcomings found in our review of relying on graduate training programs and standardized instruments. The portfolio concept has been used primarily in the field of education in order to assess the competency of students and teachers in given domains. It requires that the teacher or student actually demonstrate his or her competency rather than assess his or her ability to simply identify examples of competency, as is the case with standardized instruments. Coleman (1996) summarizes, "portfolios are an effective way of helping students and teachers determine the important information and skills that are necessary to acquire within a particular context and then demonstrate the degree to which an individual has acquired that information and skills" (p. 219). The portfolio generally consists of a collection of student materials that tell a story of his or her efforts and achievements in a given competency domain. In the case of MCC, the materials might include case reports, clinical presentations, videotapes of therapy, workshop proposals, papers and publications, research projects, even a score report from one of the objective measures described above. Graduate faculty and supervisors subsequently evaluate these materials and provide students with constructive feedback.

The portfolio approach has a number of advantages to traditional assessment methods. To begin, it is context-dependent. This emphasis on context allows for the assessment of competency with specific ethnic and racial groups, such as Asian Americans. Supervisor and supervisee also can work together in determining goals and outcome as they relate to this given population. This collaboration allows supervisor and supervisee to have in-depth discussions of cultural issues, moving beyond the superficial assessment found in standardized instruments. In the case of Asian Americans, the projection of prevailing stereotypes (e.g., model minority myth) by a culturally insensitive therapist can be discussed with a supervisor in a constructive manner. The use of case reports and clinical presentations in the portfolio also ensures that MCC will be assessed on a more regular basis. Lee, et al.'s (1999) survey of training directors from predoctoral counseling center internship sites, for example, found case reports and clinical presentations to be the second and third most used approach toward assessing MCC, following direct supervision. By contrast, standardized MCC instruments were the least frequently used to assess competency.

Coleman (1996) does caution, however, that the portfolio approach has some limitations. In particular, the reliability in scoring or evaluating portfolios still needs to be addressed. A number of steps can be taken to safeguard against inconsistent or incompetent evaluations. The most important step is the use of multiple experts to evaluate the portfolios. As with clinical supervision, MCC can only be assured when experts in the field are evaluating the quality of the work. Multiple people also should evaluate the material in order to increase inter-rater reliability. Likewise, portfolios should be regularly compared with other students in order to maintain a consistent standard. The complementary use of supervisor and self-report instruments, such as the CCCI-R and MCI, can serve as important criterion-related validity. The intercultural sensitizer or standardized vignettes similarly can be used as additional means to assess MCC.

5. CONCLUSION

The purpose of this chapter was to review current approaches to assessing MCC, particularly as it relates to Asian American populations. We aimed to present a fair appraisal of these different assessment strategies, but we recognize that our own meta-assessment is biased by our own cultural worldviews. Having been raised, educated, and trained in the United States of America, we are heavily influenced by the prevailing Western social science perspective with its emphasis on internal validity. For example, we remain hesitant to fully endorse the use of the MCC standardized instruments until more rigorous research is conducted to validate the factor structure and utility of the instruments. At the same time, we have tried to strike a balance between issues of internal and external validity in multicultural research (S. Sue, 2000). A comprehensive assessment strategy, such as the portfolio model, therefore may be the best solution at this point in time to account for both the concrete and the more intangible and contextual elements of MCC.

We strongly encourage researchers to continue to examine issues of competency with specific racial groups. Although we attempted to address MCC as it relates to Asian American populations, the lack of research in this area made it difficult to assess competency with Asian Americans. Allison, et al.'s (1994) survey, however, does provide compelling evidence that there is a clear lack of competency working with Asian Americans. Similarly, studies of MCC with specific Asian American populations (e.g., Korean, Chinese, Indian, Pakistani, Thai, Vietnamese) is necessary, lest we also inadvertently essentialize group differences without consideration for within-group variability (Hare-Mustin & Maracek, 1988). There also is very little research at all on the multicultural competency of ethnic and racial minority psychologists, in this case Asian Americans. Tung (1981) as well as Chung

296   RICHARD M. LEE AND ADAM J. DARNELL

and Lu (1996) have presented poignant and compelling reasons why Asian American psychologists need to be fully conscious and aware of our own level of cultural competency, including issues of cultural countertransference and cross-cultural supervision. As practitioners and researchers pursue these lines of inquiry and research, we are confident that the theory and assessment of multicultural counseling competencies will bear fruitful findings pertinent to the psychological and social well-being of Asian Americans.

6. REFERENCES

Allison, K. W., Crawford, I., Echemendia, R., Robinson, L., & Knepp, D. (1994). Human diversity and professional competence. *American Psychologist, 49*, 792-796.

American Psychological Association (1987). *General guidelines for providers of psychological services.* Washington, DC: American Psychological Association.

American Psychological Association (1993). Guidelines for providers of psychological services to ethnic, linguistic, and culturally diverse populations. *American Psychologist, 48*, 45-48.

Arrendondo, P., Toporek, R., Brown, S. P., Jones, J., Locke, D., Sanchez, J., & Stadler, H. (1996). Operationalization of the multicultural counseling competencies. *Journal of Multicultural Counseling and Development, 24*, 42-78.

Atkinson, D. R., Casas, A., & Abreu, J. (1992). Mexican-American acculturation, counselor ethnicity and cultural sensitivity, and perceived counselor competence. *Journal of Counseling Psychology, 39*, 515-520.

Atkinson, D. R., Kim, B. S. K., & Caldwell, R. (1998). Ratings of helper roles by multicultural psychologists and Asian American students: Initial support for the three-dimensional model of multicultural counseling. *Journal of Counseling Psychology, 45*, 414-423.

Atkinson, D. R., Maruyama, M., & Matsui, S. (1978). Effects of counselor race and counseling approach on Asian Americans' perceptions of counselor credibility and utility. *Journal of Counseling Psychology, 25*, 76-83.

Atkinson, D. R., & Lowe, S. M. (1995). The role of ethnicity, cultural knowledge, and conventional techniques in counseling and psychotherapy. In J. G. Ponterotto, J. M. Casas, L. A. Suzuki, & C. M. Alexander (Eds.), *Handbook of multicultural counseling* (pp. 387-414). Thousand Oaks, CA: Sage.

Atkinson, D. R., & Matsushita, Y. J. (1991). Japanese-American acculturation, counseling style, counselor ethnicity, and perceived counselor credibility. *Journal of Counseling Psychology, 38*, 473-478.

Atkinson, D. R., & Wampold, B. E. (1982). A comparison of the Counselor Rating Form and the Counselor Effectiveness Rating Scale. *Counselor Education and Supervision, 22*, 25-36.

Atkinson, D. R., Wampold, B. E., Lowe, S. M., Matthews, L., & Ahn, H. (1998). Asian American preferences for counselor characteristics: Application of the Bradley-Terry-Luce model to paired comparison data. *The Counseling Psychologist, 26*, 101-123.

Barak, A., & LaCrosse, M. B. (1975). Multidimensional perception of counselor behavior. *Journal of Counseling Psychology, 22*, 25-36.

Bernal, M. E., & Castro, F. G. (1994). Are clinical psychologists prepared for service and research with ethnic minorities? A decade of progress. *American Psychologist, 49*, 797-805.

Bernal, M. E., & Padilla, A. M. (1982). Status of minority curriculum and training in clinical psychology. *American Psychologist, 37*, 780-787.

Betz, N. E., & Fitzgerald, L. F. (1993). Individuality and diversity: Theory and research in counseling psychology. *Annual Review of Psychology, 44*, 343-381.

Byington, K., Fischer, J., Walker, L., & Freedman, E. (1997). Evaluating the effectiveness of a multicultural counseling ethics and assessment training. *Journal of Applied Rehabilitation Counseling, 28*, 15-19.

Chung, H., & Lu, F. (1996). Ethnocultural factors in the development of an Asian American psychiatrist. *Cultural Diversity and Mental Health, 2*, 99-106.

Coleman, H. L. K. (1996). Portfolio assessment of multicultural counseling competence. *The Counseling Psychologist, 24*, 216-229.

THEORY AND METHOD OF MULTICULTURAL COUNSELING COMPETENCY ASSESSMENT

Coleman, H. L. K. (1998). General and multicultural counseling competency: apples and oranges? *Journal of Multicultural Counseling and Development, 26*, 147-156.

Constantine, M. G. (1997). Facilitating multicultural competency in counseling supervision: Operationalizing a practical framework. In D. B. Pope-Davis & H. L. K. Coleman (Eds.), *Multicultural Counseling Competencies: Assessment, Education and Training, and Supervision* (pp. 310-324). Thousand Oaks, CA: Sage.

Constantine, M. G., Ladany, N., Inman, A.G., & Ponterotto, J. G. (1996). Students' perceptions of multicultural training in counseling psychology programs. *Journal of Multicultural Counseling and Development, 24*, 241-253.

D'Andrea, M., & Daniels, J. (1991). Exploring the different levels of multicultural training in counselor education. *Journal of Counseling and Development, 70*, 78-85.

D'Andrea, M., Daniels, J., & Heck, R. (1991). Evaluating the impact of multicultural counseling training. *Journal of Counseling and Development, 70*, 143-148.

Gim, R. H., Atkinson, D., & Kim, S. J. (1991). Asian-American acculturation, counselor ethnicity, and cultural sensitivity, and ratings of counselors. *Journal of Counseling Psychology, 38*, 57-62.

Hare-Mustin, R. T., & Maracek, J. (1988). The meaning of difference: Gender theory, postmodernism, and psychology. *American Psychologist, 43*, 455-464.

Heppner, P., Kivlighan, D., & Wampold, B. (2000). *Research design in counseling* (2nd ed.). Boston: Brooks-Cole.

Hills, H. I., & Strozier, A. L. (1992). Multicultural training in APA-approved counseling psychology programs: A survey. *Professional Psychology: Research and Practice, 23*, 43-51.

Korman, M. (1973). *Levels and patterns of professional training in psychology.* Washington, DC: American Psychological Association.

Ladany, N., Inman, A. G., Constantine, M. G., & Hofheinz, E. W. (1997). Supervisee multicultural case conceptualization ability and self-reported multicultural competence as functions of supervisee racial identity and supervisor focus. *Journal of Counseling Psychology, 44*, 284-293.

LaFromboise, T. D., & Foster, S. L. (1992). Cross-cultural training: Scientist-practitioner model and methods. *The Counseling Psychologist, 20*, 472-489.

LaFromboise, T. D., Coleman, H. L. K., & Hernandez, A. (1991). Development and factor structure of the Cross-Cultural Counseling Inventory-Revised. *Professional Psychology: Research and Practice, 22*, 308-388.

Lee, R. G. (1999). *Orientals: Asian Americans in popular culture.* Philadelphia: Temple University Press.

Lee, R. M., Chalk, L., Conners, S. E., Kawasaki, N., Jannetti, A., LaRue, T., & Rodolfa, E. (1999). The status of multicultural counseling training at counseling center internship sites. *Journal of Multicultural Counseling and Development, 27*, 58-74.

Leong, F. T. L. (1986). Counseling and psychotherapy with Asian-Americans: Review of the literature. *Journal of Counseling Psychology, 33*, 196-203.

López, S. R., Grover, P., Holland, D., Johnson, M. J., Kain, C. D., Kanel, K., Mellins, C. A., & Rhyne, M. C. (1989). Development of culturally sensitive psychotherapists. *Professional Psychology: Research and Practice, 20*, 369-376.

Merta, R. J., Ponterotto, J. G., & Brown, R. D. (1992). Comparing the effectiveness of two directive styles in the academic counseling of foreign students. *Journal of Counseling Psychology, 39*, 214-218.

Murphy, M. C., Wright, B. V., & Bellamy, D. E. (1995). Multicultural training in university counseling center predoctoral internship programs: A survey. *Journal of Multicultural Counseling and Development, 23*, 170-180.

Neville, H. A., Heppner, M. J., Louie, C. E., Thompson, C. E., Brooks, L., & Baker, C. E. (1996). The impact of multicultural training on White racial identity attitudes and therapy competencies. *Professional Psychology: Research and Practice, 27*, 83-89.

Ottavi, T. M., Pope-Davis, D. B., & Dings, J. G. (1994). Relationship between White racial identity attitudes and self-reported multicultural counseling competencies. *Journal of Counseling Psychology, 41*, 149-154.

Pedersen, P. B. (1977). The triad model of cross-cultural counselor training. *Personnel and Guidance Journal, Oct*, 94-100.

Ponterotto, J. G. (1997). Multicultural counseling training: A competency model and national survey. In D. B. Pope-Davis & H. L. K. Coleman (Eds.), *Multicultural counseling competencies: Assessment, education and training, and supervision* (pp. 111-130). Thousand Oaks, CA: Sage.

Ponterotto, J. G., & Alexander, C. M. (1996). Assessing the multicultural competence of counselors and clinicians. In L. A. Suzuki, P. J. Meller, & J. G. Ponterotto (Eds.), *Handbook of multicultral assessment: Clinical, psychological, and educational applications* (pp. 651-672). San Francisco: Jossey-Bass.

Ponterotto, J. G., Alexander, C. M., & Grieger, I. (1995). A multicultural competency checklist for counseling training programs. *Journal of Multicultural Counseling and Development, 23*, 11-20.

Ponterotto, J. G., & Casas, J. M. (1991). *Handbook of racial/ethnic minority counseling research.* Springfield, IL: Thomas.

Ponterotto, J. G., Rieger, B. P., Barrett, A., & Sparks, R. (1994). Assessing multicultural counseling competence: A review of instrumentation. *Journal of Counseling and Development, 72*, 316-322.

Ponterotto, J. G., Rieger, B. P., Barrett, A., Harris, G., Sparks, R., Sanchez, C. M., & Magids, D. (1996). Development and initial validation of the Multicultural Counseling Awareness Scale. In G. R. Sodowsky & J. C. Impara (Eds.), *Multicultural assessment in counseling and clinical psychology* (pp. 247-282). Lincoln, NE: Buros Institute of Mental Measurement.

Ponterotto, J. G., Sanchez, C. M., & Magids, D. (1991, August). *Initial development of the Multicultural Counseling Awareness Scale.* Paper presented at the annual meeting of the American Psychological Association, San Francisco.

Pope-Davis, D. B., & Dings, J. G. (1994). An empirical comparison of two self-report multicultural counseling competency inventories. *Measurement and Evaluation in Counseling and Development, 27*, 93-102.

Pope-Davis, D. B., & Dings, J. G. (1995). The assessment of multicultural counseling competencies. In J. G. Ponterotto, J. M. Casas, L. A. Suzuki, & C. M. Alexander (Eds.), *Handbook of multicultural counseling* (pp. 287-311). Thousand Oaks, CA: Sage.

Pope-Davis, D. B., Reynolds, A. L., Dings, J. G., & Nielson, D. (1995). Examining multicultural counseling competencies of graduate students in psychology. *Professional Psychology: Research and Practice, 26*, 322-329.

Quintana, S. M., & Bernal, M. E. (1995). Ethnic minority training in counseling psychology: Comparisons with clinical psychology and proposed standards. *The Counseling Psychologist, 23*, 102-121.

Ramos-Sánchez, L., Atkinson, D. R., & Fraga, E. D. (1999). Mexican American's bilingual ability, counselor bilingualism cues, counselor ethnicity, and perceived counselor credibility. *Journal of Counseling Psychology, 46*, 125-131.

Rogers, M. R., & Ponterotto, J. G. (1997). Development of the Multicultural School Psychology Counseling Competency Scale. *Psychology in the Schools, 34*, 211-217.

Rogers, M. R., Ponterotto, J. G., Conoley, J. C., & Wiese, M. J. (1992). Multicultural training in school psychology: A national survey. *School Psychology Review, 21*, 603-616.

Said, E. (1979). *Orientalism.* New York: Random House.

Snowden, L. R., & Cheung, F. K. (1990). Use of inpatient mental health services by members of ethnic minority groups. *American Psychologist, 45*, 347-355.

Sodowsky, G. R. (1991). Effects of culturally consistent counseling tasks on American and International student observers' perception of counselor credibility: A preliminary investigation. *Journal of Counseling and Development, 69*, 253-256.

Sodowsky, G. R., Taffe, R. C., Gutkin, T. B., & Wise, S. L. (1994). Development of the Multicultural Counseling Inventory: A self-report measure of multicultural competencies. *Journal of Counseling Psychology, 41*, 137-148.

Speight, S. L., Thomas, A. J., Kennel, R. G., & Anderson, M. E. (1995). Operationalizing multicultural training in doctoral programs and internships. *Professional Psychology: Research and Practice, 26*, 401-406.

Suarez-Balcazar, Y., Durlak, J. A., & Smith, C. (1994). Multicultural training practices in community psychology programs. *American Journal of Community Psychology, 22*, 785-798.

Sue, D. W. (1991). A model for cultural diversity training. *Journal of Counseling and Development, 70*, 99-105.

Sue, D. W., Arrendondo, P., & McDavis, R. J. (1992). Multicultural counseling competencies and standards: A call to the profession. *Journal of Counseling and Development, 70*, 477-486.

THEORY AND METHOD OF MULTICULTURAL COUNSELING COMPETENCY ASSESSMENT

Sue, D. W., Bernier, Y., Durran, A., Feinberg, L., Pedersen, P. B., Smith, E. J., Vasquez-Nuttall, E. (1982). Position paper: Cross-cultural counseling competencies. *The Counseling Psychologist, 10*, 45-52.

Sue, S. (1988). Psychotherapeutic services for ethnic minorities: Two decades of research findings. *American Psychologist, 43*, 301-308.

Sue, S. (1998). In search of cultural competence in psychotherapy and counseling. *American Psychologist, 53*, 440-448.

Sue, S. (2000). Science, ethnicity, and bias: Where have we gone wrong? *American Psychologist, 54*, 1070-1077.

Sue, S., Fujino, D., Hu, L. T., Takeuchi, D., & Zane, N. W. S. (1991). Community mental health services for ethnic minority groups: A test of the cultural responsiveness hypothesis. *Journal of Clinical and Consulting Psychology, 59*, 533-540.

Sue, S., & Zane, N. (1989). The role of culture and cultural techniques in psychotherapy: A critique and reformulation. *American Psychologist, 42*, 37-45.

Takaki, R. (1989). *Strangers from a different shore: A history of Asian Americans*. Boston: Little, Brown.

Torres, S., Ottens, A. J., & Johnson, I. H. (1997). The multicultural infusion process: A research-based approach. *Counselor Education and Supervision, 37*, 6-18.

Tung, M. (1981). On being seen as a "Chinese therapist" by a Caucasian child. *American Journal of Orthopsychiatry, 51*, 654-661.

Uba, L. (1994). *Asian Americans: Personality patterns, identity, and mental health*. New York: Guilford.

Vázquez, L. A. (1997). A systematic multicultural curriculum model: The pedagogical process. In D. B. Pope-Davis & H. L. K. Coleman (Eds.), *Multicultural counseling competencies: Assessment, education and training, and supervision* (pp. 159-183). Thousand Oaks, CA: Sage.

JEAN LAU CHIN

CHAPTER 20

ASSESSMENT OF CULTURAL COMPETENCE IN MENTAL HEALTH SYSTEMS OF CARE FOR ASIAN AMERICANS

1. INTRODUCTION

There has been a growing emphasis on mental health services being culturally competent especially when working with diverse populations. How do we assess whether or not a system of care is culturally competent? How do we know when systems achieve cultural competency? When are these services adequate for an Asian American population? The focus of this chapter will address assessment of cultural competence within mental health systems of care as a quality of care issue and discuss guidelines for culturally competence when working with Asian American populations.

2. QUALITY OF CARE

With the rising cost of delivering services and the growth of managed care to contain costs within mental health, there has been a growing emphasis on the quality of care that is delivered. Professional associations, regulatory bodies, and funding sources are increasingly attempting to define what constitutes quality care. Guidelines or standards are the means through which professionals and service delivery systems are held accountable for the care they provide.

2.1 Guidelines Versus Standards

Guidelines are a set of practices and implicitly recognized principles of conduct which evolve over the history of every profession. They are aspirational in nature and suggest or recommend specific professional behavior. In contrast, standards of a profession are mandatory and may be accompanied by an enforcement mechanism (American Psychological Association, 1993). Ethics and values important to a profession are often included in guidelines and regulated through ethical codes. Standards tend to involve legislation, can be either clinical or administrative in nature, and are often monitored for compliance through regulatory bodies, accreditation, and licensure.

302 JEAN LAU CHIN

Increasingly, psychology as a profession has moved away from standards toward guidelines to define quality of care within the profession. The General Guidelines currently governing the behavior of psychologists is a set of aspirational statements that encourage continual improvement in quality of practice and service (Committee on Professional Standards, Board of Professional Affairs, 1987). These guidelines include an explicit statement that psychological services must be planned and implemented so that they are sensitive to factors such as age, gender, sexual orientation, culture and ethnicity that are related to life in a pluralistic society

Yet guidelines intended for the general population have been challenged for simply that. When Asian Americans make up only 3 to 5 percent within the general population and present with significant cultural differences, guidelines for the general population are not relevant for subgroup differences. Initially, cultural sensitivity or awareness of the importance of cultural differences was emphasized to provide services responsive to diverse populations. This shifted to an emphasis on the skills needed to provide these services (i.e., cultural competence). There is now an emphasis on cultural competence as a quality of care issue to hold providers accountable to providing responsive and culturally competent services.

2.2 Development of Clinical Practice Guidelines

For the reasons stated in the previous section, General Guidelines governing the profession of psychology have been supplemented by specialty clinical practice guidelines developed for clinical, industrial/organizational, and school psychologists, (American Psychological Association, 1981b), for forensic psychology (Committee on Professional Practice and Standards, 1994), child custody evaluations, and for providers of psychological services to ethnic, linguistic, and culturally diverse populations (Board of Ethnic Minority Affairs, 1990). Each of these specialty guidelines was developed because the General Guidelines did not address issues specific and unique to the specialty area.

The guidelines for services to ethnic, cultural, and linguistically diverse populations emphasize that psychological service providers need a sociocultural framework to consider diversity of values, interactional styles, and cultural expectations. They need knowledge and skills for multicultural assessment and intervention, should be cognizant of relevant research and practice as related to the population being served, and recognize ethnicity and culture as significant parameters in understanding psychological processes. To develop such a framework, providers would respect and attend to the influence of family, cultural, social, environmental factors on behavior.

In order to assess whether or not services conform to clinical practice guidelines, indicators and tools are needed to identify and measure quality of care. It is important to note that most indicators have focused on individual provider behavior as opposed to systems behaviors. Most tools have emphasized self-assessment. To develop a sociocultural framework relevant to Asian Americans, the indicators need to be relevant to the influence of cultural values, practices, and sociocultural

ASSESSMENT OF CULTURAL COMPETENCE IN MENTAL HEALTH SYSTEMS OF CARE FOR ASIAN AMERICANS

histories within an Asian American population and tools must be sensitive to identifying these differences.

2.3 Clinical Practice Versus Treatment Guidelines

Oftentimes, there has failed to be a distinction between clinical practice guidelines that govern the professional practice of providers, and treatment guidelines that govern the methods used by the profession. There has been an increasing trend toward the latter with an emphasis on empirical data over anecdotal and clinical evidence. Managed care organizations and payer sources now identify measurable outcomes and compare these outcomes to the bottom line value of dollars spent on services, and these outcomes are developed into quality of care indicators. Treatment guidelines are often available using empirical data to support the efficacy of psychotherapeutic procedures for a wide variety of specific disorders (Barlow, 1996); however, this is not the focus of this chapter.

3. PRINCIPLES OF CULTURAL COMPETENCE

Professional ethical guidelines and recent multicultural compete ncies for working with diverse populations (Arredondo et al., 1996) suggest that the delivery of culturally competent services is integral to the delivery of quality services. Principles of cultural competence are an important framework when developing indicators and tools to measure quality of care (i.e., to assess whether or not a system of care is culturally competent).

3.1 Assessment of Culture at All Levels of a System

Assessment of cultural competence can occur at many levels. The tools and processes used to diagnose and treat clients can be evaluated to ensure that they are respectful, appropriate, and informed of the client's culture, values, beliefs, and lifestyle. Skills of the provider can also be evaluated to ensure that they have the knowledge, skills, and framework when delivering care that is consistent with culturally competent principles. Finally, the system in which care is delivered can be evaluated to ensure that governing principles, policies, and practices that are culturally competent and valid for the populations being served.

Clinical practice guidelines and assessments of quality have typically focused on the client receiving care or the provider delivering the care. This initially focused on whether clinical tools such as psychological tests were translated for non-English speaking Asian Americans, or whether the provider diagnosing or treating Asian American clients knew about the Asian culture. This emphasis on cultural knowledge graduated to the provider competencies and skills necessary for working with culturally diverse populations (Chin, 2000). However, it is increasingly apparent that providers work within a system that has a culture of its own, and may

304   JEAN LAU CHIN

hold biases against different racial or ethnic populations that influence the delivery of care (Council on Ethical and Judicial Affairs, 1990).

3.2 Population Focus that is Inclusive of All Segments

Whereas Asian Americans make up a significant but relatively small percentage of the clients within the system, the system is likely to target its resources, skills, or services proportionate to their numbers (i.e., minimally). Governance and administrative protocols often define communities and boundaries based on geographic criteria as opposed to population criteria. Asian American communities often self-define by ethnicity and may cut across geographic boundaries; consequently, their numbers within geographically defined communities are often insufficient to impact allocation of resources to meet their needs.

Outcome data is important to evaluating quality, yet many data sets and survey methods do not identify ethnicity. When they do, they are inconsistently collected, both within and between datasets, making comparison and analysis impossible. Moreover, the relative size of the Asian American population makes representational sampling inadequate to capture the needs of the population.

A culturally competent system is inclusive of all segments of the population; it strives to ensure that a system is responsive to the "lowest common denominator" within its client population (e.g., Asian American population) rather than reaching the majority to get the "biggest bang for the buck."

3.3 Positive Integration of Difference and Diversity

System policies often give low priority to assessing culturally competence because it is costly. Often cultural competence is limited to inclusion of language in mission statements without operationalizing goals. The diversity of language and ethnic groups within the Asian American population often is a deterrent to systems responding to translation and interpreter needs.

Cultural competence presumes that difference and diversity between and within groups are valued and acknowledged; it presumes a positive integration of diversity, difference, and multiculturalism within a system of care. Universals and normative standards that reference "the average person" are avoided. Given the diversity within the Asian American population, failure to do so will mask differences that significantly influence access, utilization, and quality.

3.4 Value Added to Quality of Care

Clinical practice guidelines can be applied to a system of care, or organizational entity through which services are provided, as well as to individual providers. Guidelines can address administrative as well as clinical or practice dimensions of a service delivery system, i.e., how a system is organized, its policies and procedures for intake, triage, and patient flow through the system in addition to what a provider

ASSESSMENT OF CULTURAL COMPETENCE IN MENTAL HEALTH SYSTEMS OF CARE FOR ASIAN AMERICANS

does within a clinical session. These guidelines define quality of care within a system; cultural competence adds value to the quality of care within a system. To assess cultural competence within a system, quality indicators and tools derived from clinical practice guidelines identify and measure outcomes addressing several overarching criteria:

- The care is accessible for diverse segments of the population (i.e., Asian Americans can get the care they need).
- Utilization patterns among Asian American groups reflect the needs specific to those groups that are consistent with risk factors and prevalence rates.
- Quality of the care delivered to Asian Americans is good (i.e., patients were satisfied with improved health outcomes).
- There is added value when culturally competent services are delivered (Chin, 1999).

4. COMMUNITY HEALTH PSYCHOLOGY: A SYSTEMS PERSPECTIVE

A community health psychology model (De La Cancela, Chin, & Jenkins, 1998) provides a systems perspective through which to evaluate, assess, and audit a system as to whether or not it is culturally competent in meeting the needs of diverse individuals and communities. Community health psychology includes multiple bio-psycho-politico and social contexts in the formulation of our understanding of human behavior. Systems of health care must respond not only to the needs and health status of individuals, but also must be shaped by a wider perspective of the communities in which these individuals live. Hence, community health psychology expands the definition of psychology to be inclusive of health and community, expands the contexts from which information must be obtained, and expands the diversity of the lens through which we must view the problem. A key concept of the community health psychology perspective is a diversity orientation that is inclusive, systemic, culturally competent, and comprehensive in its approach. Intended outcomes are the improved health status of a population, empowerment for individuals and communities, and improved access to quality, culturally competent care (De La Cancela et al., 1998).

Using the community health psychology model, quality indicators can be defined to address the overarching criteria to assess whether or not a system is culturally competent. Questions are specific to Asian Americans, but can be modified for different stakeholders within a system (i.e., health plan, provider, care delivery system, consumer, or purchaser).

Regarding client access to culturally competent care:
1. Can all segments of the population get into the system? Do non-English speaking Asian Americans have more trouble getting into the system?

2. Are there barriers (e.g., language, cultural, economic) that prevent one group from having an easy access to the system? Are bilingual providers available for non-English speaking clients?
3. What is the understanding and integration of culturally based belief systems into intake, patient care, and patient flow procedures? Are patient information materials relevant to Asian practices and beliefs?
4. Does the gatekeeper function for triaging clients pose barriers to racial, cultural, and linguistic groups when they attempt to enter the system?

Regarding appropriate utilization and delivery of services:
1. Are linguistically, racially, culturally, and ethnically diverse groups appropriately utilizing the services offered by the system? Are Asian Americans using the services at least in proportion to their presence in the community?
2. Is it an integrated system of care that provides continuity of care consistent with client beliefs, values, and health care practices? How does the treatment consider beliefs about "talking cure" or ancestral spirits?
3. Does the system follow holistic principles in coordinating care with community, family, and spiritual support systems? What is the intake system in recognizing family names or referrals by family members?
4. Does it manage care in ways that offer comprehensive treatment, appropriate modalities and healing systems relevant to cultural practices, beliefs, and values? Is there a link between psychotherapy and other healers such as herbalists and acupuncturists?
5. Does the emphasis on cost containment result in limiting utilization to different segments of the population? Do outcome measures evaluate impact of administrative practices on utilization by Asian Americans?

Finally, regarding continuous quality improvement to promote community health:
1. Do the quality indicators address multiculturalism within the population? Are Asian American values and practices reflected?
2. Are outcomes identified to improve health status of diverse segments of the population? Do the outcomes address underutilization among Asian Americans or high rates of depression found among Asian college students?
3. Is it a community-based system that is responsive to the needs of diverse communities? How does it address high number of immigrants and refugees within the Asian American population?
4. Does the delivery of services use natural support systems within the community? Does it incorporate extended family systems in the treatment?
5. Does the delivery of care value and validate a collaborative and empowerment process? Does the system address perceived and actual dynamics of power common to the immigration experience or

ASSESSMENT OF CULTURAL COMPETENCE IN MENTAL HEALTH SYSTEMS OF CARE FOR ASIAN AMERICANS

experience of racism among Asian Americans?

6. Is it consumer driven to meet the needs of the community? Where in the system is feedback solicited from Asian Americans in the community? How can consumers register their voice to influence the delivery of services?

5. TOOLS FOR ASSESSING CULTURAL COMPETENCE

Empirical studies have demonstrated differences within Asian American populations on mental health concerns, access to care, and utilization of services. For example, primary mental health concerns among Asian Americans include sociodemographic variables of migration experience, and intergenerational conflict. The importance of ethnic specific services (Zane, Hatanaka, Park, & Akutsu, 1994), community-based approaches (Aponte & Morrow, 1995), and ethnic match in psychotherapy (Flaskerud & Liu, 1991) have been found to be significant for successful psychotherapy with Asian Americans. Asian Americans typically underutilize services (Sue, Fujino, Hu, Takeuchi, & Zane, 1991). These studies have led to recommendations for providing culturally competent services when working with Asian American clients.

Few tools however have been developed to assess cultural competence as a quality of care issue for working with Asian Americans (SAMHSA, CMHS, 1991). Several approaches have been used in developing tools to assess cultural competence within mental health systems: systems self-assessments, systems audits, and report cards.

5.1 Systems Self-Assessment

Systems self-assessments typically consist of self-assessment surveys for organizations to self-evaluate whether or not they have met aspirational goals based on cultural competence guidelines. These surveys, designed as questionnaires or checklists, are voluntary in nature, and internal tools not to meet external reporting requirements. They are intended as tools for agencies or provider organizations to establish baseline levels, assess growth, and promote systems change toward increased cultural competence.

Some self-assessment tools that have been developed include: the Children and Adolescent Service Systems Program (CASSP) model developed by Cross and associates out of Georgetown that identified policy, administrative, consumer, and provider as the four levels of a system which must be assessed for cultural competence (Cross, Bazron, Dennis, & Issacs, 1989); Cultural Competence Self-Assessment Questionnaire by Mason and colleagues for public sector and community agencies out of Oregon (Mason et al., 1995); and Program Self-Assessment Survey for Cultural Competence out of New Jersey (Weiss & Minsky, 1996).

308 JEAN LAU CHIN

5.2 Systems Audit

Systems audits, on the other hand, come from a compliance standpoint. They are external assessments, driven by regulatory or reporting requirements. While organizations often submit to them voluntarily, they often have the force of standards because they are used by organizations to gain competitive edge or to be eligible for reimbursement. Their growing use by payers and purchasers reflects a trend toward holding providers and care delivery systems accountable for quality care through value-based contracting. They are used by accreditation and regulatory bodies to assess an organization's compliance with externally defined clinical and administrative performance indicators. Systems audit tools are typically based on outcome measures, empirical data, and benchmark targets to be achieved. Outcome measures tend to be intermediary, for example, measuring how many members are screened for a disease as opposed to measuring the prevalence of a particular disease.

Some existing systems audits to measure clinical and systems outcomes in mental health include: Health Plan Employer Data and Information Set (HEDIS) developed by National Council on Quality Assurance (NCQA, 1997) to measure health plan compliance, Medicaid HEDIS by CMHS (1997) to measure organizations in the public sector, and Performance Measures for Managed Behavioral Healthcare Programs (PERMS) by American Managed Behavioral Health Association (AMHBA, 1998). All three tools collect information from medical records and administrative data. Each tool measures access and quality of care through utilization data.

All three have been criticized for their narrowness in identifying populations (SAMHSA, 1997) and their lack of responsiveness to ethnic minority populations. While none of these audit tools were developed to specifically assess cultural competence, all are relevant to culturally competent systems assessment. Because they measure an organization's compliance with overall quality of care standards and are used to determine an organization's accreditation status, it is important that they be expanded to include indicators of cultural competence.

While organizations such as National Council on Quality Assurance (NCQA), the organization that accredits managed care organizations, and the Joint Commission for the Accreditation of Clinics and Hospital Organizations (JACHO) that accredits provider organizations subscribe to principles of cultural competence in their preambles and principles, most have not emphasized assessment of cultural competence in their measures. HEDIS measures, for example, have only two indicators limited to the availability of services for clients whose primary language is not English (i.e., the number of bilingual/multilingual providers and staff available) while the PERMS collects no demographic information, making it impossible to identify utilization patterns among different racial/ethnic groups.

Yet, there is an emphasis on empirically validated therapies and data driven outcomes (i.e., a treatment guideline focus) by accrediting bodies, payers and purchasers who have used their funding leverage to set performance standards for the methods to be used when delivering care. There has been less emphasis on clinical practice guidelines (i.e., professional practice of providers to identify the

ASSESSMENT OF CULTURAL COMPETENCE IN MENTAL HEALTH SYSTEMS OF CARE FOR ASIAN AMERICANS

domains important to ensure that providers and systems are culturally competent when delivering services to diverse populations).

5.3 Consumer Report Cards

Not unlike systems audits, consumer report cards are external tools used to assess a system's competence and compliance. They too have been voluntary, but have the force of standards when the growing consumer movement creates a political climate that raises expectations for compliance and the inclusion of a consumer perspective in the assessment of service delivery systems, typically a most neglected aspect of systems assessment (Pope, 1996). Consumer empowerment, choice, and participation in health care decisions are becoming increasingly important aspirational goals for a quality service delivery system. Consumer report cards are growing increasingly popular among consumer groups to measure quality of care from the consumer perspective. Consumer advocacy groups are demanding that managed care organizations demonstrate their responsiveness as measured by annual patient satisfaction surveys. These report cards have not emphasized clinical outcome or improved health status.

Mental Health Statistics Improvement Program (MHSIP) developed by Center for Mental Health Services (CMHS) (MHSIP Task Force, 1996) has been a prototype consumer oriented report card to assess the quality and cost of mental health and substance abuse services. Domains and indicators of satisfaction and quality are defined from the consumer's perspective.

Given the data demonstrating disparities in health status among racial/ethnic groups, provision of care, prevalence rates, and response rates to different interventions across racial/ethnic groups, systems assessment must consider population differences in consumer needs if it is to be culturally competent. For example, while population specific differences (e.g., medication dosage) and population specific preferences (e.g., utilization of services) have been demonstrated among Asian Americans, measures on the MHSIP use universal and uniform standards to assess consumer satisfaction. Consequently, it is unresponsive to specific linguistic, cultural, and sociocultural needs within Asian American communities. Criteria from a consumer's perspective are: What do Asian American consumers want? How do the performance indicators and outcomes reflect Asian American consumer needs? Using the overarching criteria, consumers can ask in the report card:

1. Access: Can I get what I need? Do I have choice in choosing my provider?
2. Utilization: Are the services provided appropriate and relevant to what I need? Do I feel respected and empowered when I seek care?
3. Quality: Do I feel better? What are the risks of the treatment? How do I prevent relapse, or missed days of work?

310   JEAN LAU CHIN

5.4 National Surveys

National surveys represent a macro perspective using national or state datasets to identify utilization trends and quality outcomes. While these too are not designed specifically to assess cultural competence, they are important in their ability to identify trends, patterns, and outcomes among diverse populations.

The Medical Expenditure Panel Survey (MEPS), for example, is a nationally representative sample collected by the Agency for Health Care Policy and Research over multiple years to measure costs and identify utilization patterns. While not intended as a culturally competent tool, its use to measure utilization trends in the population at large suggests the importance for incorporating population differences into its design and measurement. Recently, MEPS has begun to present data on the differential utilization rates among racial/ethnic groups mirroring the demographic patterns found in the population. Unfortunately, it only presents data on Blacks and Hispanics. Its failure to include data on the Asian American population because of its small sample size reflect the inadequacies of most datasets to capture meaningful population differences within the Asian American population based on present methodology. The importance of including ethnic identifiers in these datasets and oversampling for the Asian American population is an important first step toward audit tools and surveys becoming culturally competent (Chin, 1999).

5.5 Audit Tools for Cultural Competence

Whereas the system audit tools and report card already discussed do not specifically assess cultural competence, there has been an attempt to develop audit tools that assess cultural competence within a system of care. The Center for Mental Health Services together with Western Interstate Commission for Higher Education (WICHE) mirrored the systems audit and developed a set of Cultural Competence Standards in managed mental health care for four underserved and underrepresented racial and ethnic groups (i.e., Black, Hispanic, Asian, and Native American). The project emphasized the concerns important to consumers (modeled after MHSIP report card) with the goal of recognizing the increasing diversity of the consumer population in the provision of mental health services. It defined a set of systems and clinical standards (e.g., cross-cultural communication is available at no additional cost, and access to services shall be available at the point of entry and throughout the course of services), and identified implementation guidelines, quality or performance indicators (e.g., number of bilingual professional staff) and benchmarks (i.e., % of limited English proficient individuals served). Outcomes relevant to racial and ethnic populations were identified under domains of access and availability, appropriateness (utilization), outcomes (quality), and priorities (satisfaction).

While the resulting product was called Cultural Competence Standards, they were not mandated; consequently, they constitute a set of voluntary guidelines of aspirational goals for states and managed care organizations to follow. The specificity of indicators and benchmarks for the outcomes to be achieved make it a

ASSESSMENT OF CULTURAL COMPETENCE IN MENTAL HEALTH SYSTEMS OF CARE FOR ASIAN AMERICANS

useful tool for assessing systems of care and health plans as to their level of cultural competence and responsiveness to racial and ethnic communities.

6. INDICATORS OF CULTURAL COMPETENCE

What are the indicators and benchmarks to assess the cultural competence of mental health systems of care? The following sections contain sample questions for assessing whether the systems and its practices are culturally competent. The questions can be used by systems and included in self-assessment surveys, system audit tools, report cards, or national surveys to define the domains relevant to providing culturally competent mental health services for Asian American populations. The questions reflect the principles of a community orientation, the integration of cultural values and beliefs into clinical practice and service delivery, and the incorporation of an integrated approach to care delivery as defined by the community health psychology model. The questions also build on the structure developed in the CMHS Cultural Competence Standards which distinguish systems and clinical standards, identifies implementation guidelines for auditing a system of care, and recommends performance indicators and outcomes. Lastly, questions should be framed differently depending on the sector through which the system of care is viewed (i.e., consumer, provider, or payer).

Systems competencies speak to the ways in which service delivery systems and health plans are organized in the provision of care or managing of benefits. They reflect the context in which services are provided, and the degree to which the system facilitates or poses barriers to care. System competencies must be assessed not only at the level of the care delivery system, but also at the levels of the payer, purchaser, and accrediting bodies. A population focus and community orientation is critical to identifying and assessing the competencies of a system.

1. Cultural Competence Planning: Does the planning of services incorporate those values and beliefs held to be important by diverse groups within the target population? For example, are differences in help seeking behaviors within the Asian American population accounted for?
2. Governance: Who is "at the table" to define and deliver care? Do they include professionals who reflect the interests of the diverse consumer groups being served? Are Asian Americans included?
3. Benefit Design: Does the benefit design include those used by diverse consumer groups? For example, is alternative medicine included? What is the eligibility for immigrants?
4. Prevention, Education, Outreach: How are population specific risk factors (e.g., high suicide rates among older Chinese women) identified and incorporated into outreach efforts and prevention targets? Do education materials identify risks and behaviors specific to diverse

312   JEAN LAU CHIN

groups (e.g., different transmission routes for HIV/AIDS among Asian Americans)?

5. Quality Monitoring and Improvement: What are the population-based criteria used in defining benchmarks for improving health status and utilization? Are there threshold criteria for defining when a system must address the needs of small population groups in its community (e.g., 3% or 2500)? How is client success defined? Are there culturally relevant outcomes to measure client success? Are there population groups who are more risk prone for certain diseases? How is this addressed within the system?

6. Are quality measures specific to population differences in utilization, health status, and outcomes? For example, how are population differences in response to medication dosage identified as benchmarks for provider compliance?

7. Decision support and MIS: Are ethnic identifiers collected on the characteristics of members and providers? How are these data used to promote health status and to eliminate disparities among different ethnic groups? For example, when sample sizes are insufficient, are Asian Americans over-sampled to provide meaningful data on utilization patterns?

8. Utilization: Is there higher out of network referral and utilization for specific groups because of a lack of flexibility in the system, or lack of availability of appropriate services? What is the utilization by consumers who are non-English speaking? What is the match between utilization of services and presenting complaint by population?

9. Human Resource Development: Is the workforce diverse and reflective of the consumer population? What are the benchmarks or quotas used to evaluate diversity within the workforce or provider network? For example, are there sufficient numbers of Asian American staff to serve Asian American clientele?

Clinical competencies, on the other hand, refer to the practice guidelines, clinical protocols, and provider skills in the actual provision of care.

1. Access and Service Authorization: How do non-English speaking clients access the system and the providers who speak their language? How are ethnic specific and bilingual providers recruited and retained in the network? How is the system responsive to an Asian American population whose concentrations may cut across geographic boundaries defined by catchment areas or network regions? Is there language capacity at all points of entry into system? What are the enabling services within the system to promote access to care?

2. Triage and Assessment: Do the intake worker, provider, benefits manager, utilization reviewer, and other workers incorporate diverse belief systems in the triage and authorization of benefits? For example, can a relative refer the family member to treatment or must the client call directly?

ASSESSMENT OF CULTURAL COMPETENCE IN MENTAL HEALTH SYSTEMS OF CARE FOR ASIAN AMERICANS

3. Care Planning: Is the care planning respectful of diverse patterns of childrearing and interpersonal relationships and family systems? For example, how is extended family incorporated into care planning? What is role given to children? Are they used as interpreters? Are allowance made for children in the waiting room?
4. Treatment Plan and Services: Is the treatment realistic to the life conditions of the client? Can consumers be matched with therapists of their culture if so desired? Are all ethnic therapists limited to serving only clients from their own culture?
5. Discharge Planning: Does the planning offer the least restrictive alternative? Are community-based alternatives such as community groups, civic associations, churches, extended family included where appropriate?
6. Case Management: Is extended family included where relevant?
7. Communication Styles and Linguistic support: Are appropriate interpreter services available to non-English speaking clients? Are bilingual professionals available in the network?

7. CONCLUSION

To assess cultural competence in mental health systems, we can use self-assessment or system audit tools. As a shift toward quality outcomes occurs, cultural competence should be considered integral to the definition of quality of care and included in accreditation tools, regulatory criteria, and national surveys. Quality indicators to identify, define, track, evaluate, and improve culturally competent practices and services are needed.

To date, language and interpreter services have been the primary criteria for defining cultural responsiveness and competence. This narrow definition must be expanded to include integration of culture into the delivery of care and ongoing training and staff development for working with diverse populations. Outcomes should respond to population differences in access to care and utilization of services and address population specific norms in symptom expression, thresholds of distress, clinical outcomes and treatment responsiveness.

Assessment of cultural competence should include all stakeholders (i.e., provider, care delivery system, purchaser, payer, and consumer) and the different perspectives they bring to the system of care. It is the composite of all stakeholders and perspectives that results in culturally competent systems of care.

8. REFERENCES

AMBHA (1998). *Performance Measures for Managed Behavioral Healthcare Programs* (PERMS) 2.0. Washington, DC: American Managed Behavioral Health Association.

American Psychological Association (1981b). Specialty guidelines for the delivery of services by clinical (counseling, industrial/organizational, and school) psychologists. *American Psychologist, 36,* 639-681.

314 JEAN LAU CHIN

American Psychological Association (1993). *Legal risk management.* Washington, DC: Author.

Aponte, J. F., & Morrow, C. A. (1995). Community approaches with ethnic groups. In J. F. Aponte, R. Y. Rivers, & J. Wohl (Eds.), *Psychological interventions and cultural diversity* (pp. 128-144). Boston: Allyn & Bacon.

Arredondo, P., Toperek, R., Brown, S. P., Jones, J., Locke, D. C., Sanchez, J., & Stadler, H. (1996). Operationalization of the multicultural counseling competencies. *Journal of Multicultural Counseling and Development, 24,* 42-78.

Barlow, D. (1996). Health care policy, psychotherapy research, and the future of psychotherapy. *American Psychologist, 51*(10), 1050-58.

Board of Ethnic Minority Affairs (1990). *Guidelines for providers of psychological services to ethnic, linguistic, and culturally diverse populations.* Washington, DC: Office of Ethnic Minority Affairs, American Psychological Association.

Chin, J. L. (1999). Issue Brief No. 5: Cultural competence and health care in Massachusetts: Where are we? Where should we be? *The Massachusetts Health Policy Forum.* MA: Heller School, Brandeis University.

Chin, J. L. (2000) Culturally competent health care. *Public Health Reports, 115,* 29-38.

Committee on Professional Practice and Standards (1994). Guidelines for child custody evaluations in divorce proceedings. *American Psychologist, 49*(7), 677-680.

Committee on Professional Standards, Board of Professional Affairs (1987). *General guidelines for providers of psychological services.* Washington, DC: American Psychological Association.

Council on Ethical and Judicial Affairs. (1990). Black-White Disparities in Health Care. *Journal of American Medical Association, 263,* 2344-2346.

Cross, T. L., Bazron, J., Dennis, K. W., & Issacs, M. R. (1989). *Toward a culturally competent system of care* (Vol. I). Washington, DC: Georgetown University, Children and Adolescent Service Systems Program Technical Assistance Center.

De La Cancela, V., Chin, J. L., & Jenkins, Y. M. (1998). *Community health psychology: Empowerment for diverse communities.* New York: Routledge.

Flaskerud, J., & Liu, P. Y. (1991). Effects of an Asian client-therapist language, ethnicity, and gender match on client outcomes. *Community Mental Health Journal, 17,* 31-42.

Mason, J. et al. (1995). *Cultural Competence Self-Assessment Questionnaire: A manual for users.* Portland, OR: Research and Training Center on Family Support and Children's Mental Health, Portland State University.

MHSIP Task Force (1996). *The final report of the Mental Health Statistics Improvement Program (MHSIP) Task Force on a Consumer-Oriented mental health report card.* Washington, DC: SAMHSA, Center for Mental Health Services.

NCQA (1997). *Health plan employer data and information set (HEDIS) 3.0: Travel copy* (vols. I and III). Washington, DC: National Committee on Quality Assurance.

Pope, K. S. (1992). Responsibilities in providing psychological test feedback to clients. *Psychological Assessment, 4*(3), 268-71.

SAMHSA, Center for Mental Health Services, The Western Interstate Commission for Higher Education (1998). *Cultural competence standards in managed care, mental health services for four underserved/underrepresented racial/ethnic groups.* Rockville, MD: SAMHSA, Center for Mental Health Services.

SAMHSA, Center for Mental Health Services (1997). *Mental health measures in Medicaid HEDIS.* Rockville, MD: SAMHSA, Center for Mental Health Services.

SAMHSA, Center for Mental Health Services (1997). *Mental Health standards of care literature review: Asian and Pacific Islander American populations.* Rockville, MD: SAMHSA, Center for Mental Health Services.

Sue, S., Fujino, D., Hu, L. T., Takeuchi, D., & Zane, N. W. S. (1991). Community mental health services for ethnic minority groups: A test of the cultural responsiveness hypothesis. *Journal of Consulting and Clinical Psychology, 59* (4), 533-540.

Weiss, C. I., & Minsky, S. (1996). *Program self-assessment survey for cultural competence: A manual.* New Jersey Division of Mental Health Services.

Zane, N. W. S., Hatanaka, H., Park, S., & Akutsu, P. (1994). Ethnic specific mental health services: Evaluation of the parallel approach for Asian American clients. *Journal of Community Psychology, 22,* 68-81.

SECTION V: CONCLUSIONS

21. Advances in the Scientific Study of Asian Americans
Stanley Sue

STANLEY SUE

CHAPTER 21

ADVANCES IN THE SCIENTIFIC STUDY OF ASIAN AMERICANS

1. INTRODUCTION

Three decades ago, researchers were lamenting the fact that little psychological research and knowledge were available concerning the Asian American population. The population was considered a model minority that had succeeded rather well in society. Both because of this image, which was in marked contrast to the well-publicized needs of other ethnic minority groups such as African American and Latinos, and because of their relatively small population in the United States, Asian Americans were not the target of much research attention. Over the past three decades, the situation has changed, albeit slowly. There is increasing recognition that the study of Asian Americans is important, not only for responding to the needs of this population but also for understanding more generally the nature of human beings. It should also be noted that while Asians constitute only 4 percent of the United States' population, they comprise 60 percent of the world's population. The advances in knowledge are apparent from the work of the researchers involved in this project. Their work has yielded new knowledge concerning Asian American well-being, the validity of research instruments and nosological systems, and appropriate research designs and methodological considerations.

2. WHAT DO WE KNOW?

Given the pervasive stereotype of Asian American well-being, one of the most important questions to address is their mental health status. What are the rates of psychopathology among Asian Americans? As noted by D. Chang (Chapter 2), the research evidence supports the notion that Asian Americans have rates of psychopathology that are similar to (and certainly not significantly lower than) those rates for other Americans. Her analysis suggests that Asian within group differences are important to consider—differences among various subgroups (e.g., Chinese, Filipinos, Koreans), immigration and acculturative stress, and social class. A similar conclusion was drawn by Suzuki, Mogami, and Kim (Chapter 11) in their review of the literature on cognitive and intellectual functioning of Asian Americans. In

317

contrast to the prevailing stereotype of Asian Americans as a homogenous group of smart and high-test scoring students, Suzuki and colleagues show that various pieces of evidence point to a great variability across Asian ethnic groups and to patterns of uneven verbal-quantitative performance profiles. The authors point to methodological and conceptual problems in cognitive assessment across different cultural groups, a theme that is apparent from the work of other contributors to this book.

We also know that culture as well as individual differences are major factors in human behavior. As noted by Leong and Tang (Chapter 18) in their review of career choices, researchers can focus on universal (across all human beings), group (e.g., cultural features), or individual (unique personal characteristics) factors that are responsible for career choices, personality patterns, or behaviors. Many of the contributors to the book provide insight into cultural, group, and individual influences that account for the behaviors of Asian Americans. For example, Kim and Wong (Chapter 13) note the importance of Asian cultural philosophies such as Confucianism that influence social roles and family relationships among Asian Americans. Similarly, Zane and Yeh (Chapter 9) draw attention to the importance of face in interpersonal relationships. Asians come from face cultures in which one's social integrity and appearance to others are important determinants of behavior. Zane and Yeh's research shows that loss of face is important to consider in the psychotherapeutic treatment of Asian Americans. If cultural characteristics are important in behaviors, is it possible that these characteristics predispose or inoculate one from specific forms of psychopathology? This is precisely the question posed by Okazaki (Chapter 8) in her investigations of interdependent self-construals, which is culturally more characteristic of Asians and independent self-construals, which is culturally more characteristic of Westerners. Her empirical research demonstrates that low independent self-construals and high interdependent self-construal were associated with elevated levels of depression and social anxiety for Asian Americans and White Americans.

Comparisons between groups such as Asians and Whites often point to interesting cultural differences but mask within group individual differences, sometimes resulting in stereotypic views of groups. In contrast to the focus on culture, Tsai and Chentsova-Dutton (Chapter 7), Roysircar and Maestas (Chapter 6), and Ying (Chapter 12) examine differences among Asians. Tsai and colleagues have found in their measure of cultural orientation that for immigrant Chinese "being Chinese" and "being American" were negatively correlated while for American born Chinese the two identity scales were largely independent. In other words, a bidimensional model of cultural orientation was applicable to American born Chinese while a unidimensional model was well suited for immigrant Chinese. The findings are enlightening because they shed insight into not only differences among Chinese Americans but also on the controversy over the model (i.e., bidimensional or unidimensional) used to account for acculturation effects. Similarly, Roysircar and Maestas argue that acculturation and effects of biculturalism affect immigrant and American born Asians differently. Immigrant Asians are more likely than American born Asians to be subjected to acculturative stress while bicultural stress is more likely to be experienced by American born (and later generation) Asians.

ADVANCES IN THE SCIENTIFIC STUDY OF ASIAN AMERICANS   319

Finally, Ying's chapter also point to the great variability among Chinese Americans in their conceptions of depression. Her studies have found that acculturated Chinese Americans hold similar conceptions of depression as White Americans, in which there are clearer body-mind and self-other differentiation. In contrast, less acculturated Chinese Americans tend to hold a more integrated conception of depression. These chapters clearly document the important issues that are often overlooked when ethnic comparisons are made without due consideration of within ethnic group differences.

3. HOW VALID ARE ASSESSMENT STRATEGIES AND THE DSM NOSOLOGICAL SYSTEM?

Much of our knowledge in psychological science is based on tests, measures, surveys, and classification schemes. One problem in assessment procedures and tools is that they often ignore one factor (e.g., cultural background) or lead to the confounding of one factor with another (e.g., mistakenly explaining behaviors on the basis of universal characteristics rather than culturally specific ones). Several contributors to this book discuss these particular problems. Kagawa-Singer and Chung (Chapter 4) find that assessment strategies often decontextualize human behavior from their social context. They need to be based on a more culturally informed model. Dana's work (Chapter 3) illustrates this point by critiquing the *Diagnostic and Statistical Manual of Mental Disorders, 4th edition* (DSM-IV) of the American Psychiatric Association (1994). DSM-IV is among the most widely used classification systems for diagnosing mental disorders. Dana attacks DSM-IV as an Anglo-American emic with assumptions concerning the origins, symptoms, and syndromes of psychopathologies that are not universally accepted. He proposes an alternative way of looking at psychopathology that is less culturally biased. Dana does note that the inclusion of Culture Bound Syndromes (CBSs) in DSM-IV is an attempt to recognize cultural influences. As noted in the DSM-IV (APA, 1994), CBS are locality-specific patterns of aberrant behavior and troubling experience that may or may not be linked to particular DSM-IV diagnostic categories. CBSs are generally limited to specific societies or cultures and are localized, folk, diagnostic categories that frame coherent meanings for certain repetitive, patterned, and troubling sets of experiences and observations. However, Lin and M. Lin (Chapter 5) argue that recognition of CBS implies that non-CBS disorders listed in DSM-IV are "culture-free," that is, universal. In other words, specifying that certain disorders are culture bound implies that the other major disorders listed in DSM-IV are applicable to all cultures. Lin and M. Lin believe that DSM-IV is culturally biased. They contrast Asian and Western views of disorders and the relationship between the mind and body to illustrate the pervasive effects of culture on the conceptions and manifestations of mental disorders.

320   STANLEY SUE

4. TOWARD CULTURALLY EFFECTIVE ASSESSMENTS OF ASIAN AMERICANS

In addition to questions over the validity of the diagnostic system, a number of contributors have pointed to validity issues and means to construct culturally valid measures and assessment tools. Sandoval (Chapter 17) discusses the importance of cultural factors in educational assessment and then provides procedures in cross-cultural assessment. Other researchers who have been involved in the assessment of Asians describe their experiences and draw implications for research and evaluation. By revealing the issues involved in constructing the Chinese Personality Assessment Inventory, Cheung (Chapter 10) notes those personality characteristics that appear to be universal and those that appear to be unique in human beings. Involved in the assessment of the mental health of Chinese Americans in Los Angeles, Kurasaki and Koike (Chapter 14) provide not only information on the prevalence of mental disorders but also insights into the sampling, design, translation, and instrumentation procedures that are necessary to study a small, predominantly immigrant population in the United States. Using examples from Cambodian American mental health, Uehara, Farwell, Yamashiro, and Smukler (Chapter 15) argue that qualitative research methods can often provide rich data that cannot be gained through quantitative methods. They demonstrate how qualitative methodologies and procedures such as the use of ethnography, grounded theory, and narrative analysis can yield important insights. Yeh and Yeh (Chapter 16) discuss a myriad of ways in which Asian cultural values influence the clinical presentation of Asian American children as well as special issues facing Asian American children and families that must be considered in conducting a culturally valid assessment. Finally, Lee and Darnell (Chapter 19) and Chin (Chapter 20) discuss ways in which cultural competency can be determined. However, the two chapters focus on different targets. Lee and Darnell examine cultural competency at the level of the provider or clinician. They indicate the problems in assessing the adequacy of providers in rendering treatment to ethnic minority clients. Chin is concerned with cultural competency not only at the provider level but also at the level of mental health systems and programs. Criteria to assess cultural competency include access to effective services, having bicultural/bilingual services, consumer surveys, utilization data, and so on.

In many ways, the authors in this book make a valuable contribution in informing us of who Asian Americans are, of inadequacies in our conceptions and assessment tools for human beings from different cultures, and means by which research designs and assessment instruments can be improved.

5. FUTURE DIRECTIONS

Research on ethnic minority groups has often been characterized as being descriptive, basic, and relatively unsophisticated because investigators have a difficult time finding validated assessment instruments, culturally appropriate research strategies, and suitable theories. This characterization is misleading. As is apparent from the work of the contributors to this book, the critiques, methods, and

ADVANCES IN THE SCIENTIFIC STUDY OF ASIAN AMERICANS

strategies are highly sophisticated. They inform us not only of the status of Asian Americans but also of the state of the mental health field. With respect to the latter point, in a profound manner the contributors point to limitations in the conceptualizations and research tools currently used in the field. Thus the value in their work goes well beyond Asian Americans; it has implications for the science and practice in the field as a whole.

What we need is to make more explicit how research on Asian Americans or non-mainstream groups has implications for the field as a whole. That is, while Asian Americans should be studied because of the lack knowledge of this population, we should also use studies to serve as a contrast to mainstream studies. Americans conduct the vast majority of assessment research studies. Most of the subjects of research are White Americans. Yet, Americans represent less than 5 percent of the world's population. Therefore, we would expect much of the research methods, assessment tools, theories, and practices to be most pertinent to this 5 percent of the world's population. By studying ethnic and non-American populations, much insight will be gained about cultural biases, universal and group-specific phenomenon, and valid assessment tools. Researchers have to more clearly identify the generality or specificity of findings and theories, depending on the cultural groups studied. In the future, it is important to address a number of mental health and assessment issues. How can valid assessment instruments be developed that have cross-cultural utility? Are mental disorders fundamentally the same, displaying differences only in symptoms, across cultures or can disorders be distinct in different cultures? How can effective treatment strategies be developed with different cultural groups? Do different competencies exist for different groups or does cultural competency reside in individuals (e.g., clinicians) independent of groups? Is cultural effectiveness a skill, or can manualized and scripted standard behaviors or procedures be considered culturally competent? We are beginning to address these questions as noted by the contributors.

With respect to Asian Americans, there continues to be a need to demonstrate the importance of culture and, simultaneously, the importance of individual differences. We have little knowledge about certain Asian American groups. For example, there is relatively little knowledge about the mental health and status of Pacific Islander Americans.

Advances in Asian American research can be described as a glass that is half empty or half full. Much more research is needed. For example, little is also known about issues involving Asian American drug abuse, family violence, youth gangs, and sexual orientation. On the other hand, as reflected in the work of the contributors to this book, an impressive array of facts, theories, methodological strategies, and critiques exists.

6. REFERENCES

American Psychiatric Association (1994). *Diagnostic and statistical manual of mental disorders* (4th ed.). Washington, DC: Author.

SUBJECT INDEX

A

Academic Achievement, 197
Acculturation, 9, 41, 56, 58, 77, 95, 267, 273, 275
  Acculturative Status, 42, 56, 177, 181, 243
  Acculturative Stress, 23, 24, 78, 83, 85, 87, 89, 317, 318
  Bicultural Stress, 85, 89
  Biculturalism, 85, 89, 110, 318
  Bidirectionality, 78, 79
  Career Choices, 275, 276
  Cultural Alienation, 89
  Cultural Conflict, 89
  Cultural Confusion, 89
  Ethnic Identity, 275
  Immigrant Status, 194
  Measurement, 78, 79, 84, 85
  Moderator Variables, 32, 84
  Multidimensionality, 86, 87
  Parental Influences, 243
  Parenting Practices, 193
  Self-Efficacy, 273
Acculturation Measures
  Acculturation Rating Scale for Mexican Americans (ARSMA), 79
  Acculturation Scale for Southeast Asians, 85
  Acculturation Scale for Vietnamese Adolescents, 79, 86
  Bicultural Acculturation Scale, 79
  Bidimensional Acculturation Scale for Hispanics, 79
  Children's Acculturation Scale, 85
  Cultural Awareness-Ethnic Loyalty Scale, 86
  Language Acculturation Scale for Mexican Americans, 86
  Minority-Majority Relations Scale, 86
  Suinn-Lew Asian Self-Identity Acculturation Scale (SL-ASIA), 100, 270
Acculturative Stress, 87, 90
Advocacy, 41, 42
Affective Moderation, 175, 177, 191, 198, 240

African Americans/Blacks, 14, 82, 287, 317
Anxiety Disorders, 16, 37
Asian Americans/Pacific Islanders
  Cambodian Americans, 32, 62, 84, 160, 212, 222, 223, 227, 228, 234, 320
  Census, 77, 205, 209, 251, 304
  Chinese Americans, 17, 18, 19, 21, 22, 23, 36, 38, 79, 81, 103, 167, 173, 176, 177, 179, 180, 181, 208, 209, 211, 214, 235, 318, 319, 320
  Filipino Americans, 23, 32, 36, 37, 81, 84, 127, 164, 165, 166, 167, 169, 176, 188, 236
  Generational Status, 207
  Hmong Americans, 18, 19, 36, 39, 95, 101, 102, 103, 160, 207, 212
  Immigration History, 19, 22, 77, 101, 155
  Japanese Americans, 19, 32, 37, 38, 79, 80, 83, 85, 90, 104, 207, 208
  Khmer Americans, 36, 222, 228
  Korean Americans, 19, 32, 37, 167
  Laotian Americans, 32, 36, 62, 160
  Mien Americans, 22, 36
  South Asians, 19, 24, 77, 79, 80, 81, 160, 285
  Southeast Asians, 19, 21, 24, 32, 37, 38, 160, 164, 165, 166, 167, 168, 169, 207, 223, 247
  Thai Americans, 295
  Vietnamese Americans, 32, 33, 36, 62, 79, 80, 84, 86, 127, 160, 164, 165, 168, 207, 234, 295
  Within-Group Variability, 18, 22, 58, 159, 160, 176, 180, 207, 233, 318
Asian Indians. *See* Asian Americans/Pacific Islanders, South Asians
Assertiveness, 238
Assessment, 319
  Actuarial Approach, 255
  Categorical Fallacy, 220
  Multimethod, 193
  Nonverbal Tests, 260, 261
  Qualitative Methods, 79, 85, 168, 221, 223, 230
  Quantitative Methods, 80, 168

323

SUBJECT INDEX

Response Sets, 124
Testing Accommodations, 258
Validity, 56, 220, 261, 320
Assimilation, 78, 275
Astronaut Parents. *See* Voluntary Family
Separation
Attachment, 245

B

Bilingualism, 168, 213, 238, 239, 258, 259, 306, 312, 313, 320
Biopsychosocial Model, 30, 39, 266
Buddhism, 49, 175, 176, 222, 230
Yuan, 175

C

Cambodian Americans. *See* Asian Americans/Pacific Islanders, Cambodian Americans
Cao Gio. See Health Beliefs, *Cao Gio*
Career Development Theories, 265
Cultural Accommodation Model, 266, 269, 274, 275, 277, 279
Cartesian Duality. *See* Mind-Body Dichotomy
Census. *See* Asian Americans/Pacific Islanders, Census
Chi. See Health Beliefs
Child Abuse, 246
Corporal Punishment, 246
Child Assessment Measures
Child Behavior Checklist (CBCL), 234, 235
Curriculum-Based Dynamic Assessment, 261
Junior Eysenck Personality Questionnaire, 235
Kinetic Family Drawings, 235
Offer Self-Image Questionnaire, 235
Peabody Picture Vocabulary Test, 260
Raven's Progressive Matrices, 260
Roberts Apperception Test for Children (RATC), 236
Thai Youth Checklist, 234
Thematic Apperception Test, 236
Childhood Disorders
Attention Deficit/Hyperactivity Disorder, 234

Autism, 241
Selective Mutism, 238
Chinese Americans. *See* Asian Americans/Pacific Islanders, Chinese Americans
Chinese Medicine. *See* Health Beliefs, Traditional Chinese Medicine
Chronic Fatigue Syndrome. *See* Somatoform Disorders, Chronic Fatigue Syndrome
Cognitive Abilities. *See* Standardized Tests *and* Intelligence Tests
Cognitive Errors
Anchoring Bias, 254
Availability Bias, 254
Confirmation Bias, 254
Prevention Strategies, 256, 257, 258
Representativeness Bias, 254
Collectivism, 30, 32, 33, 110, 125, 185, 270, 271, 277
Common Sense, 228, 230
Community Health Psychology, 305
Confucianism, 56, 174, 176, 190, 191, 196, 198, 242, 318
Construct Irrelevant Variance, 252, 253, 258, 261
Context, 284
Historical, 223
Sociocultural, 124, 223, 229
Coping Strategies
Collectivistic, 89
Individualist, 89
Cross-Cultural Studies
Australia, 34, 80, 111
China, 15, 16, 18, 20, 35, 38, 39, 113, 141, 142, 143, 144, 147, 152, 154, 155, 179, 195, 208, 211, 214, 240, 244, 246
England, 235
Hawai'i, 110, 112, 152, 153, 154, 240
Hong Kong, 15, 16, 18, 20, 22, 82, 110, 112, 113, 118, 141, 142, 143, 144, 145, 150, 151, 152, 153, 155, 169, 195, 208, 211, 240, 243, 244
Indonesia, 34, 49
Japan, 22, 34, 35, 38, 39, 110, 111, 113, 114, 115, 118, 161, 240, 244
Korea, 15, 16, 22, 34, 39, 69, 111, 244, 246
Singapore, 235
Sri Lanka, 34

SUBJECT INDEX

Taiwan, 15, 18, 22, 35, 69, 193, 194, 195, 208, 211, 244
Thailand, 234
Cultural Accommodation Model. *See* Career Development Theories, Cultural Accommodation Model
Cultural Competence, 42, 304
  Assessment, 62, 124, 136, 212, 222, 233, 237, 303, 313
  Audit Tools, 310
  Case Conceptualization, 124
  Center for Mental Health Services, 310
  Cultural Competence Planning, 311
  Cultural Competence Standards, 310, 311
  Curriculum, 283
  Diagnosis, 30, 40, 42, 62
  Indigenous Treatments, 55
  Multicultural Counseling Competency, 283, 284, 285, 286, 287, 288, 289, 290, 291, 292, 293, 294, 295
  Scale Development, 154
  Service Delivery, 53, 302, 303, 304, 305, 309, 310, 311. *See also* Quality of Care
  System Policies, 304
  Treatment, 181, 285, 305
  Western Interstate Commission for Higher Education, 310
Cultural Formulation, 31, 33, 38, 40, 67
Cultural Identity. *See* Ethnic Identity
Cultural Informants, 246
Cultural Orientation, 31, 40, 95, 96, 100, 101, 103, 104, 180, 318
  Activities, 96
  Birth Order, 104
  Feelings About One's Culture, 97
  Language, 96
  Models, 95, 97, 98, 100
  Social Affiliation, 96
  Treatment Implications, 103
  Well-Being, 98, 102
Cultural Orientation Measures. *See also* Acculturation Measures
  General Ethnicity Questionnaire, 101
Cultural Relativism, 51, 52, 53, 54, 55
Cultural Sensitivity, 293, 302
  Training, 256
Cultural Systems Approach, 48, 49, 55, 60, 61, 62
Culture

Operationalization, 57
Culture Bound Syndromes, 38, 39, 67, 68, 70, 319
  Amok, 68
  Hwa-Byung, 24, 32, 39, 70
  Kchall Koo, 222
  Koro, 24, 39, 68
  Koucharang, 223, 227
  Latah, 24, 39
  Neurasthenia, 18, 21, 23, 24, 32, 33, 37, 38, 53, 68, 69, 70, 174, 177, 214
  Peal Keutchreun, 223, 227
  Shenjing Shuairuo, 24, 68, 70
  Shenkui, 24, 39
  Shin-Byung, 24, 39
  Shink-Bu, 24
  Shinkeishitsu, 35, 36, 39
  Sudden Unexpected Nocturnal Dealth Syndrome (SUNDS), 39
  Taijin Kyofusho, 24, 39

D

Deference to Authority, 190, 195, 196, 198, 237, 238, 277
Depression. *See* Mood Disorders, Depression
Depression Measures
  Center for Epidemiologic Studies Depression Scale (CES-D), 36, 37, 176, 177, 179, 180, 181
  Zung Self-Rating Depression Scale, 208
Dermabrasion. *See* Health Beliefs, Dermabrasion
Diagnostic Measures
  Composite International Diagnostic Interview (UM-CIDI), 12, 17, 18, 19, 20, 23, 211, 215
  Diagnostic Interview Schedule, 10, 11, 12, 15, 16, 17, 19, 20, 211
  Diagnostic Interview Schedule (DIS), 211
  Self-Reporting Questionnaire (SRQ), 16
Diagnostic Systems
  Cultural Axis, 41
  Cultural Validity, 19, 208

326 SUBJECT INDEX

Diagnostic and Statistical Manual for
Mental Disorders, 3rd edition,
Revised (DSM-III-R), 12, 17, 18, 20
Diagnostic and Statistical Manual of
Mental Disorders, 1st edition
(DSM-I), 30
Diagnostic and Statistical Manual of
Mental Disorders, 3rd edition
(DSM-III), 10, 11, 12, 14, 15, 16,
17, 20, 30, 62
Diagnostic and Statistical Manual of
Mental Disorders, 4th edition
(DSM-IV), 21, 29, 30, 31, 34, 38,
39, 40, 41, 57, 62, 67, 208, 319
Group on Culture and Diagnosis, 67
International Classification of Diseases
(ICD-10), 18, 34, 38, 39
Not Otherwise Specified, 62, 69, 70
Response Bias, 20
Discrimination. *See* Prejudice

E

Eating Disorders, 53
Embarrassability, 240
Emic v. Etic, 20, 24, 40, 71
Imposed Etic, 142
Emotional Control. *See* Affective
Moderation
Empowerment, 305, 309
English as a Second Language, 125, 168,
253, 258. *See also* Bilingualism
Epidemiology
Chinese American Psychiatric
Epidemiological Study (CAPES),
17, 18, 19, 21, 22, 24, 35, 38, 39,
177, 205, 209, 210, 211, 214, 215,
216
Convenience Samples, 207
Cross-Cultural Comparisons, 16
Epidemiological Catchment Area, 10,
13, 14, 15, 16, 17, 20, 22, 23, 206,
207
Ethnic Differences, 14
Ethnocentric Bias, 56
Multi-Stage Probability Sampling, 209
National Comorbidity Study, 17, 18,
20, 22, 206, 207, 208
Prevalence Rates, 10, 12, 37, 207
Sampling, 320

Sampling Bias, 212
Sampling Cost, 206
Taiwan Psychiatric Epidemiological
Project, 15
Epiphenomena. *See* Emic v. Etic
Ethics, 31, 42, 283, 291, 301, 303
Ethnic Diversity. *See* Asian
Americans/Pacific Islanders, Within-
Group Variability
Ethnic Identity, 36, 42, 57, 58, 78, 79, 82,
84, 85, 87, 88, 89, 96, 133, 164, 267,
273, 275
Ethnic Matching, 33, 221
Ethnocentric Bias, 30, 31, 71
Ethos
Asian, 60, 151
European American, 49, 51, 54, 59
Etiology, 48
Explanatory Models, 19, 125, 179, 223
Extraversion-Introversion, 134

F

Face, 20, 32, 81, 124, 125, 126, 145, 147,
148, 151, 152, 237, 240, 255, 272, 318
Amae, 125, 134
Gaining Face, 126
Jen, 32, 134, 174
Losing Face, 126, 152, 318
Loss of Face Questionnaire, 126, 131,
133, 138
Personalisimo, 134
Saving Face, 239
Family Measures
Asian American Family Conflicts
Scale, 243
Family Adaptibility and Cohesion
Evaluation Scale (FACES), 188
Family Environment Scale (FES), 188
Family Relations
Father-Daughter Relationship, 196
Father-Son Relationship, 196
Mother-Daughter Relationship, 197
Mother-Son Relationship, 196
Filial Piety, 125, 152, 190, 191, 196, 198,
242
Criticism, 242

SUBJECT INDEX

G

Glass Ceilings. *See* Occupations, Occupational Discrimination
Graduate Record Exam. *See* Standardized Tests, Graduate Record Exam

H

Harmony. *See* Interpersonal Harmony
Health Beliefs, 32, 222, 306. *See also* Mind-Body Dichothomy
  Cao Gio, 247
  Chi (Qi), 59, 174, 181
  Dermabrasion, 247
  Syncretism, 222
  Traditional Chinese Medicine, 174, 181
Health Practices. *See* Health Beliefs
Help-Seeking, 34
Hispanics/Latinos, 37, 82, 84, 236, 251, 287, 317
Hmong Americans. *See* Asian Americans/Pacific Islanders, Hmong Americans
Human Rights, 41, 42

I

Idioms of Distress, 19, 20, 37, 38, 39, 48, 49, 54, 68, 70, 211, 212
  Heart Discomfort, 225
Indigeneous Psychology, 152
Individual Differences, 318
Individualism, 175, 185, 235, 277
Intelligence Conceptualizations
  Atama Ga Yoi, 169
  Chih Li, 169
Intelligence Tests. *See also* Standardized Tests
  Biligual Verbal Abilities Test (BVAT), 162
  Japanese Wechsler Intelligence Scale for Children-III, 162
  Stanford-Binet Intelligence Scale, 161
  Universal Nonverbal Intelligence Tests (UNIT), 161
  Wechsler Intelligence Scale for Children, Revised (WISC-R), 161

Woodcock-Johnson Tests of Cognitive Ability Revised, 162
Interpersonal Harmony, 126, 145, 151, 175, 238, 243
Interpreters, 260

J

Japanese Americans. *See* Asian Americans/Pacific Islanders, Japanese Americans

K

Khmer. *See* Asian Americans/Pacific Islanders, Khmer Americans
Korean Americans. *See* Asian Americans/Pacific Islanders, Korean Americans

L

Laotian Americans. *See* Asian Americans/Pacific Islanders, Laotian Americans
Locus of Control, 23, 134, 242, 271

M

Managed Care, 221, 251, 301, 303, 309
Measurable Outcomes, 303, 304
Mental Status, 233, 236
Mien. *See* Asian Americans/Pacific Islanders, Mien Americans
Mind-Body Dichotomy, 50, 68, 70, 174, 176, 177
Minnesota Multiphasic Personality Inventory (MMPI), 155
Minority Status, 21, 57, 58, 102, 103, 235, 283
Modesty, 175, 179, 189, 240, 243, 271, 279
Mood Disorders, 16
  Depression, 36, 70, 71, 173, 174, 176, 177, 180, 181, 208, 211, 319
Multicultural Counseling Competency Assessment
  Ethnic/Racial Groups, 295
  Idiographic, 287
  Norms, 293

328 SUBJECT INDEX

Pedagogical, 286
Portfolio Approach, 294, 295
Multicultural Counseling Competency
Measures
Cross-Cultural Counseling Inventory-
Revised (CCCI-R), 288, 289, 290,
293
Cross-Cultural Critical Incident
Quality Index (CCIQI), 289
Multicultural Awareness-Knowledge-
and-Skills Survey (MAKSS), 289
Multicultural Case Conceptualization
Ability (MCCA), 290
Multicultural Competency Checklist,
287
Multicultural Counseling Awareness
Scale-B (MCAS-B), 290
Multicultural Counseling Ethics and
Assessment Competency Scale
(MCEACS), 291
Multicultural Counseling Inventory
(MCI), 290, 293
Multicultural School Psychology
Counseling Competency Scale
(MSPCC), 288
Psychometrics, 292

N

National Institute of Mental Health, 211
National Multicultural Leadership
Summit, 284
National Research Center on Asian
American Mental Health, 1
Native Americans, 57
Nonverbal Communication, 238
Nosology, 67, 69, 70, 220, 317, 319
Asian, 58
Western, 61
Null Hypothesis, 30, 42

O

Obedience. *See* Deference to Authority
Occupational Measures
Career Maturity Inventory, 271
Minnesota Importance Questionnaire,
276
Ohio Work Values Inventory (OWVI),
270

Strong Interest Inventory, 270
Value Scale, 276
Occupations, 269
Career Maturity, 271
Career Self-Efficacy, 272
Family Influences, 273, 276
National Career Development Gallup
Survey, 270
Occupational Discrimination, 276
Occupational Segregation, 274, 276
Occupational Status, 272
Outcome Expectation, 272
Personality Variables, 270
Representation Index, 274
Underemployment, 271
Vocational Identity, 271

P

Pacific/Asian American Mental Health
Research Center, 15
Parachute Kids. *See* Voluntary Family
Separation
Parenting
Developmental Differences, 194
Developmental Outcomes, 197
Gender Differences, 195, 196
Parental Roles, 195, 198
Parenting Dimensions
Discipline, 187, 191
Family Obligation, 192
Guan, 192
Monitoring, 187, 191
Parental Control, 186, 187, 191, 193
Parental Warmth, 186, 187, 190, 193,
195, 197
Reasoning, 187
Parenting Measures
Child Rearing Practices Report
(CRPR), 187, 188
Parenting Styles
Authoritarian, 186
Authoritative, 186, 197
Personality Measures, 261
Chinese MMPI, 141, 142
Chinese Personality Assessment
Inventory (CPAI), 143, 144, 145,
147, 150, 151, 152, 154, 155, 320
Minnesota Multiphasic Personality
Inventory (MMPI), 130, 141, 142

SUBJECT INDEX

Population. *See* Census
Prejudice, 41, 52, 58, 80, 103, 104, 124,
   254, 255, 276
Psychotherapy
   Cultural Bias, 123, 124
   Process Variables, 134
   Self-Disclosure, 133
   Tripartite Integrative Framework, 266,
      267, 268
   Working Alliance, 125, 133

Q

Qi. See Health Beliefs
Qualitative Methods, 189, 190, 192, 211
Quality of Care, 301, 302, 305, 307. *See
   also* Cultural Competence:Service
   Delivery
   Benefit Design, 311
   Care Planning, 313
   Case Management, 313
   Center for Mental Health Services
      (CMHS), 309, 311
   Communication Styles, 313
   Discharge Planning, 313
   Governance, 311
   Human Resource Development, 312
   Joint Commission for the
      Accreditation of Clinics and
      Hospital Organizations, 308
   Monitoring, 312
   National Council on Quality Assurance
      (NCQA), 308
   Prevention, 311
   Service Authorization, 312
   Treatment Plans, 313
   Triage, 312
   Utilization Rates, 312
Quality of Care Assessment
   Children and Adolescent Service
      Systems Program (CASSP), 307
   Consumer Report Cards, 309
   Cultural Competence Self-Assessment
      Questionnaire, 307
   Health Plan Employer Data and
      Information Set (HEDIS), 308
   Medical Expenditure Panel Survey
      (MEPS), 310
   Mental Health Statistics Improvement
      Program (MHSIP), 309

National Surveys, 310
Performance Measures for Managed
   Behavioral Healthcare Programs
   (PERMS), 308
Systems Audit, 308
Systems Self-Assessment, 307

R

Racial Identity. *See* Ethnic Identity
Racism. *See* Prejudice
Refugees, 19, 21, 22, 24, 33, 36, 38, 80,
   82, 96, 101, 207, 222, 223, 272, 306
Relational Constructs, 134, 135
   Self-Other Integration, 174, 177
Relationship Orientation
   Nepotism, 151
   Ren Qing, 145, 147, 148, 151, 153

S

Scholastic Aptitude Test. *See*
   Standardized Tests, Scholastic
   Aptitude Test
Self-Consciousness Scale, 127, 128, 129
Self-Construal, 107
   Criticisms, 115
   Depression, 110, 111, 112
   Embarrassability, 110, 112
   Independent, 51, 108, 109, 185, 242,
      278, 318
   Interdependent, 51, 108, 109, 185, 242,
      278, 318
   Revised Self-Construal Scale, 111
   Social Anxiety, 110, 111, 112
   Well-Being, 108, 110, 112, 113, 114
Self-Construal Measures, 116
   Gundykunst et al., 111
   Implicit Measures, 117
   Implicit v. Explicit, 117
   Interdependence/Independence Scale
      (IIS), 111, 118
   Self-Construal Scale (SCS), 110, 111,
      112, 113, 116
   Takata, 110
   Twenty Statements Test, 118
Self-Esteem, 80, 110, 114, 134, 152, 175,
   185, 242, 246, 278
Self-Monitoring Scale, 127, 128, 129
Semantic Network Analysis, 224, 225

330 SUBJECT INDEX

Core Symbols, 225
Semantic Network Links, 225
Shame, 34, 56, 126, 133, 134, 238, 239, 240, 241, 246. *See also* Face
Social Desirability, 41, 127, 128, 130, 131, 235, 237, 292
Social Group Membership, 267
Social Reality, 213
Social Status, 127, 128, 151, 190, 196, 221, 272
Social Support, 36
Socioeconomic Status, 189
Sociological Models of Mental Illness
Etiological Approach, 52
Social Constructionist Model, 53
Social Response Model, 52
Sociological Psychology Model, 53
Sociosomatic Recticulum, 223
Somatization, 9, 14, 15, 16, 20, 32, 35, 36, 37, 60, 69, 70, 152, 153, 154, 174, 213, 255
Somatoform Disorders, 37, 68
Chronic Fatigue Syndrome, 21, 69
Standardized Tests, 252, 254
Achievement Tests, 160
Aptitude Tests, 160
Cultural Content, 253
Graduate Record Exam (GRE), 161
Language Proficiency, 162, 169, 253, 259
Reliability, 162, 163
Scholastic Aptitude Tests (SAT), 161
Standardization Samples, 161, 162
Validity, 162
Stereotypes, 276, 294, 317
Model Minority, 9, 159, 160, 169, 255, 273, 283, 284, 317
Stigma, 19, 34, 53, 70, 213
Substance Abuse Disorders, 16

Supervision, 257

T

Thai Americans. *See* Asian Americans/Pacific Islanders, Thai Americans
Therapeutic Alliance. *See* Psychotherapy, Working Alliance
Thought Disorders
Schizophrenia, 14, 16, 32, 35, 36, 52, 53
Transcultural Psychiatry, 67
Translation, 61, 259, 303
Back-Translation, 212
Conceptual Equivalence, 56, 61, 62, 124, 210, 212, 260
Level of Vocabulary, 213
Linguistic/Language Equivalence, 212
Measurement Equivalence, 189
Pilot Testing, 213
Test-Retest Reliability, 213
Triangulation, 256

V

Validity
Cultural, 267, 274, 320
External, 206, 293
Internal, 206, 293
Vietnamese Americans. *See* Asian Americans/Pacific Islanders, Vietnamese Americans
Voluntary Family Separation, 244, 245

W

Worldview, 49, 80, 123, 136, 284, 295

AUTHOR INDEX

A

Abe, J. S., 81, 129, 207
Abreu, J., 289
Achenbach, T. M., 234, 249
Adams, D. R., 160
Adler, S. R., 39
Advincula, A., 32
Agbayani-Siewert, P., 62
Ahn, H., 293
Ahuna, C., 81
Alarcon, O., 85
Alexander, C. M., 93, 287, 288, 296, 298
Allen, J., 42
Allison, K. W., 31, 286, 287, 295
Alpert, M., 125
Alvarado, C. G., 162
Ambady, N., 33, 164
American Educational Research
 Association, 261
American Psychiatric Association, 20, 25,
 29, 30, 67, 208, 211, 245, 319
American Psychological Association, 42,
 261, 283, 301, 302
Anderson, E. N., 190
Anderson, J., 32, 85, 86
Anderson, M. E., 286
Anderson, N. B., 58
Aneshensel, C. S., 64
Anker, M., 65
Antonovsky, A., 102, 221
Aranalde, M. A., 78
Armour-Thomas, E., 168, 169
Arnold, B., 79
Arrendondo, P., 283
Asai, M., 65
Ashmore, R. D., 116
Atkinson, D. R., 285, 289, 293
Averill, J., 48
Ayabe, H., 237
Azuma, H., 169, 199

B

Baker, C. E., 297
Baltes, P. B., 231
Baluch, S., 100
Bandura, A., 272
Bank, L., 193
Bankston, C. L., 165, 168
Barak, A., 281, 288
Barnes, D., 50, 63
Barrett, A., 283, 288, 289, 298
Barrett, R. J., 33
Bartlett, F. C., 257
Baumrind, D., 186
Beauvais, F., 98, 100, 130
Becker, W. C., 186
Bednarski, P., 25
Beiser, M., 22, 36, 61
Beit-Hallahmi, B., 100
Bellah, R. N., 51, 175
Bellamy, D. E., 286
Belsky, J., 193
Bempechat, J., 164, 165, 166
Bergin, A. E., 137
Berlin, J. A., 65
Bernal, G., 85
Bernal, H., 87, 89
Bernal, M. E., 283, 286
Berndt, T. J., 186, 195
Bernier, Y., 299
Berreman, G., 57
Berry, J. W., 78, 79, 82, 83, 87, 95, 98,
 100, 102, 142, 275
Berube, R. L., 234
Betancourt, H., 107, 121, 125
Betz, N. E., 272, 293
Birman, D., 96
Blackhall, L., 50, 63
Blair, S. L., 164, 165, 166, 167, 168
Blazer, D., 37
Block, J., 187
Bochner, S., 102
Boehnlein, J. K., 25
Bogue, D. J., 106

332 AUTHOR INDEX

Bond, M. H., 19, 110, 112, 121, 142, 150, 151, 152, 156, 157, 175, 182, 200, 201, 240, 248, 249
Bonstead-Bruns, M., 166
Bontempo, R., 121
Booth, A., 93
Borgen, F. H., 270, 280
Bornstein, M. H., 189
Boski, P., 97, 100
Boucher, J. D., 34
Bourne, E. J., 69
Bowlby, J., 245
Boyd, J. H., 25
Boyer, L. B., 44
Boyer, R., 105
Boyer, R. M., 44
Bracken, B. A., 161
Brandt, M. E., 34
Bravo, M., 61
Brennan, J., 25, 65
Brickman, P., 242
Briggs, S. R., 130
Brim, O. G., 231
Brislin, R., 117, 124
Brockner, J., 113
Brooks, L., 43, 265, 297
Brown, B. B., 167
Brown, D., 270, 271, 280
Brown, M., 265, 267, 268
Brown, R. D., 293
Brown, S., 272
Brown, S. D., 279
Brown, S. P., 314
Brown, W. J., 110
Bruce, M. L., 13
Bufka, L. F., 81
Bujaki, M., 78
Burgess, E., 106
Burgoon, M., 86
Burke, J. E., 65
Burnam, A., 25
Burnam, M. A., 85, 97
Buss, A. H., 127, 130
Butcher, J. N., 105, 142, 156, 157, 217
Byington, K., 289, 291

C

Cabacungan, L. F., 236
Cadavid-Hannon, E. B., 236

Cain, C., 223
Caldwell, R., 285
Calkins, D. R., 63
Callies, A., 21
Cameron, J. E., 110, 113
Canino, G. J., 26, 61, 217
Carielli, D., 100
Carlson, C. I., 193
Carroll, L., 47
Carter, R. T., 57, 263
Carter, W. B., 36, 37
Carver, C. S., 129
Casas, A., 289
Casas, J. M., 283, 293, 296, 298
Cassidy, J., 245
Castillo, R. J., 30, 39, 40, 56, 62
Castro, F. G., 82, 89, 286
Caudhill, W. A., 35
Cen, G., 199
Cervantes, R. C., 82, 89
Chaiyasit, W., 249
Chalk, L., 297
Chambon, A., 80
Chan, J. C., 104
Chan, S., 237, 238, 247
Chan, Y. Y., 19
Chang, D. F., 20
Chang, D.-S., 24
Chang, H., 175
Chang, L. Y., 15, 70, 208, 211, 234
Chang, S. C., 51
Chan-Ho, M.-W., 24, 216
Chao, R. K., 109, 141, 185, 186, 187, 188, 189, 192
Chapman, J. P., 254
Chapman, L. J., 254
Charmaz, K., 48, 49, 56
Chataway, C. J., 82
Chavira, V., 80, 89
Chen, C., 84, 163, 167, 187, 188, 194
Chen, C. L., 235
Chen, C.-N., 16, 208
Chen, H., 169, 199
Chen, H. C., 169
Chen, M., 164
Chen, M. J., 169
Chen, M. S., 43
Chen, M. S., Jr., 90
Chen, X., 193, 195, 197
Chen, Y., 113
Cheng, C.-H., 244

AUTHOR INDEX

Chen-Louie, T. T., 128
Chentosvoa, Y. E., 102
Cheung, F. K., 207, 284
Cheung, F. M., 19, 20, 33, 46, 68, 69,
141, 142, 143, 147, 150, 152, 153, 154,
173, 174, 217
Cheung, F. M. C., 240, 242
Cheung, P., 35
Cheung, P. C., 186
Cheung, S. T., 39
Cheung, T. S., 175
Chiang, L., 84
Chieh, L., 235
Chin, A. L. S., 201
Chin, J. L., 305, 310
Chiu, M. L., 188, 193
Chmielewski, P. M., 56
Cho, K. H., 72
Choe, J., 192, 243
Choi, J. O., 26, 72
Chou, E. L., 273, 275, 276, 277
Chu, C.-P., 236
Chun, C.-A., 46, 68, 69, 128
Chun, K. M., 19
Chung, H., 295
Chung, M., 189
Chung, R. C.-Y., 46, 48, 57, 59, 60, 61
Clarke, A. E., 64
Coates, D., 247
Cohen, D., 117
Cohen, J., 132
Cohen, M. L., 196
Cohler, B., 223
Cohn, E., 247
Cole, P. M., 43, 187
Coleman, H. L. K., 97, 285, 288, 294,
295, 297, 298, 299
Collins, R. C., 270
Comas-Diaz, L., 257
Conners, S. E., 297
Connor, J. W., 79, 80, 81, 84
Conoley, J. C., 199, 286
Constantine, M. G., 283, 286, 287, 290,
291
Constantinou, S. T., 96, 100, 103
Cook, W. L., 193
Coombs, M., 100
Cooper, A. M., 69, 71
Cooper, J. E., 65
Cooper, R. S., 48
Cortes, D. E., 61, 79, 82, 194

Costa, J. A., 25
Costa, P. T., Jr., 145, 147, 148, 151
Cox, C. I., 273
Cranach, M., 40
Crano, W. D., 86
Crawford, I., 31, 286
Crites, J. O., 271
Crocker, J., 113
Crosby, F., 110
Crosby, M., 110
Cross, S. E., 111, 307
Crouter, A. C., 93
Cuéllar, I., 40, 42, 43, 79, 84, 86, 99, 157
Cummins, J., 162
Curtis, R. C., 120

D

Dana, R. H., 29, 30, 31, 32, 40, 42, 43,
45, 46, 84, 93
Daniels, J., 286, 289, 292
Darling, N., 185, 186
Dasen, P. R., 90, 104
D'Avanzo, C. D., 222, 223, 228
Davidson, A. R., 41
Dawes, R. M., 255
Dawis, R. V., 277
Dawson, E. J., 86
Dawson, J. L. M., 136
Day, R., 65
De Anda, D., 89
De La Cancela, V., 305
DeBaryshe, B. D., 187
Delbanco, T. L., 63
Dembo, M. H., 163
Der-Karabetian, A., 97, 100
DeSipio, L., 103
Devins, G. M., 61
DeVos, G. A., 41, 57, 120, 182
Deyo, R. A., 86
Diaz-Guerrero, R., 41
Dickstein, S., 200
Diehl, A. K., 86
Diener, E., 108, 114, 121
Diener, M., 114
Dings, J. G., 288, 290, 292
Dinnel, D. L., 110
Dion, K. K., 23
Dion, K. L., 23
Dion, R., 61

334 AUTHOR INDEX

Dishion, T., 193
Dohrenwend, B. P, 22, 26
Dohrenwend, B. S., 22, 26
Doi, T., 59, 237
Dong, Q., 187
Dornbusch, S. M., 167, 186, 187, 188, 197
Dressler, W. W., 58, 87, 89
Dube, K. C.1, 25
Dube, R., 65
Dunbar, E., 154
Duran, R. P., 258
Durlak, J. A., 283
Durran, A., 299
Durvasula, R. S., 19, 141
Dyal, J. A., 89
Dyal, R. Y., 89

E

Eastman, K. L., 19
Eastman, L. E., 196
Eaton, M. J., 163
Eaton, W. W., 38
Ebata, A. T., 238
Ebata, K., 38
Echemendia, R., 31, 286
Edgerton, R., 25, 49, 53
Edwards, A. L., 127, 130, 131
Edwards, R. G., 61
Eisenberg, D. M., 54
Eisenberg, J. M., 65
Eisenberg, L., 54, 68
Elmen, J. D., 187
Enomoto, K., 68, 128, 141
Erkut, S., 85
Ernberg, G., 65
Ersak, M., 50, 63
Escarce, J. J., 65
Escobar, J. I., 25, 37, 85, 98, 105
Eshleman, S., 25, 216
Eysenck, S. B. G., 235

F

Fabrega, H., Jr., 31, 37, 44, 45, 48, 51, 53, 54, 55, 61, 67, 68, 70, 73
Facione, N. C., 55
Fan, F. M., 156
Fan, X., 164

Faust, D., 255
Fava, M., 71
Feinberg, L., 299
Feldman, S. S., 79, 80, 187, 188, 193
Fenigstein, A., 127, 129
Fenton, F. R., 35
Ferketich, S., 61
Fernandes, L. O., 56
Fernandez, M., 26, 217
Fernandez, T., 98
Fielding, R., 201
Fischer, J., 289
Fitzgerald, L. F., 293
Flannery, D. J., 197
Florio, L. P., 13
Folkman, S., 89, 221
Fong, J. Y., 92
Fong, S. L. M., 270, 276
Fontes, L. A., 249
Foster, C., 63
Foster, S. L., 286
Fouad, N. A., 263, 270, 272, 276
Fox, D., 166
Fraga, E. D., 289
Fraleigh, M. J., 188
Franco, J. N., 85
Frank, A. C., 269
Frank, J. D., 267
Freedman, E., 289
Freedman, M., 201
French, J. L., 255
Frensch, P. A., 197
Frey, M., 79, 82, 83, 85
Friedlander, M. L., 254
Friedman, R. J., 187
Frisby, C. L., 262, 263
Frye, B., 222, 223, 227, 228
Fu, V. R., 186, 187, 188, 193, 244
Fuertes, J. N., 160
Fugita, S. S., 18
Fujino, D., 284, 307
Fukuyama, M. A., 273
Fuligni, A. J., 160, 164, 166, 167, 188, 192
Furnham, A., 102
Furuto, S. M., 157
Fyffe, D., 32

AUTHOR INDEX

G

Gabrenya, W., Jr., 151, 152
Gabriel, S., 118
Gallin, B., 196
Galperin, C., 199
Gamba, R. J., 79
Gambrill, E., 257
Gan, Y. Q., 152, 153, 154, 156
Gao, G., 151
Garcia-Coll, C., 85
Gardner, H., 236
Gardner, J. W., 255
Gardner, W. L., 118
Garfield, S. L., 137, 254
Gaw, A. C., 36
Gay, E. G., 276
Ge, X., 48, 185, 187, 197
Geary, D. C., 150
Geertz, C., 48
Geisinger, K. F., 259, 262, 263
Genesee, F., 261
George, L., 25, 37, 214
Gersh, B. J., 65
Gerton, J., 97
Ghuman, P. A. S., 100
Gift, T., 25
Gilbert, M. J., 97
Gim, R. H. C., 273, 289
Giordano, J., 59, 137, 201, 249
Goffman, E., 126, 128, 133
Goldberg, N., 104
Golding, J. M., 105
Goldstein, M. J., 193
Gomez-Macqueo, E. L., 42
Gong-Guy, E., 22
Gonzalez, G., 40
Good, B. J., 20, 37, 39, 41, 45, 68, 70, 73,
  173, 182, 219, 220, 223, 224, 225, 226,
  227, 228, 230
Good, M., 219, 223, 224
Gordon, M. M., 97
Gordon, P., 36, 207
Gorman, J. C., 193
Goulde, M. S., 26
Graham, S. E., 164, 165, 166
Green, J., 223
Greenberger, E., 84, 187, 188, 194
Grenier, J. R., 257, 262, 263
Grieger, I., 287
Grover, P., 297

Guarnaccia, P. J., 21, 24, 41
Gudykunst, W. B., 49, 111, 116, 151
Guthrie, R., 43, 90
Gutkin, T. B., 284, 290
Gutkin, T. G., 161

H

Hackett, G., 272
Hagen, E. P., 161
Hale, R. L., 255
Hallowell, A. I., 56
Hamada, R., 21
Hammer, A. C., 270, 280
Hampson, S., 161
Han, J. H., 26, 72
Handler, L., 43
Hansen, J. C., 270
Hanson, M. J., 125, 248
Hao, L., 166
Harada, N., 110
Hare-Mustin, R. T., 295
Harless, W., 65
Harmon, L. W., 270
Harrell, S., 190
Harris, G., 298
Harris, L. C., 84
Harris, P., 35
Hartung, P. J., 277, 278
Harvey, M. E., 96, 100, 103
Hau, K. T., 186
Haverkamp, B. E., 270
Hayden, L. C., 193
Hayes, T. J., 273
Haynes, O. M., 199
Hazuda, H., 86
Healy, C. C., 272
Heck, R., 289, 292
Heelas, P., 48
Heiby, E., 65
Heine, S. J., 114, 175
Helzer, J. E., 26, 217
Hendel, D. D., 276
Heppner, M. J., 297
Heppner, P., 293
Heras, P., 246
Hernandez, A., 288
Hernandez, P., 221
Hess, D., 95
Hetts, J. J., 111, 117, 118

336 AUTHOR INDEX

Heyman, S., 119
Hills, H. I., 283
Hilsenroth, M., 43
Hinds, P. S., 65
Hinton, J., 49
Hinton, L., 19
Hirschfeld, R. M. A., 45
Hiruma, N., 110
Ho, D., 125, 126
Ho, D. Y. F., 125, 127, 134, 135, 191, 194, 195, 196, 246
Ho, R. M., 141
Hoagwood, K., 67, 69
Hoffman, L. W. H., 199
Hoffman, M. L., 199
Hofheinz, E. W., 290
Hofstede, G. H., 175
Hollan, D., 107
Holland, D., 297
Holland, J. L., 270
Holt, R., 175
Holzer, C. E., III, 13, 22
Hong, K.-H., 244
Honig, A. S., 189
Hopper, K., 53
Horowitz, L. M., 52, 53, 54, 125
Horridge, P. E., 100
Horwitz, A. V., 51, 52, 54, 56, 61, 232
Hough, R. L., 25, 85, 105
Hsia, C., 32
Hsia, J., 159, 160, 161, 164, 165, 168
Hsieh, S. J., 165
Hsu, F. L. K., 32, 120, 182
Hsu, J., 38
Hu, H. C., 125, 127, 128
Hu, L. T., 284, 307
Huang, J. S., 58, 176
Huang, L. N., 21, 237
Huang, M. G., 68
Huang, T. L., 244
Hughes, C. C., 21, 38, 67, 70, 72, 220, 221
Hughes, M., 25, 216
Hui, C. H., 41
Hutnik, N., 79, 81
Hwang, K. K., 97, 127, 128, 151, 152
Hwu, H.-G., 15, 70, 208, 211

I

Ickes, W., 129
Ingerman, C., 113
Inman, A. G., 283, 287, 290
Ino, S., 237
Inouye, A. R., 161, 170
Isajiw, W. W., 79
Ito, K., 59
Ivey, A. E., 263
Ivey, D., 272
Iwamasa, G. Y., 107
Izard, C. E., 249

J

Ja, D. Y., 59, 125, 196, 238
Jablensky, A., 25, 35, 65
Jaccard, J. J., 41
Jackson, J. S., 58
Jacob, T., 193
Jain, A., 193
Jannetti, A., 297
Jasso, R., 84
Jen, T., 244
Jenkins, J. H., 174, 305
Jensen, A. R., 161, 167
Jensen, M., 263
Jensen, P. S., 67, 69
Jepsen, D. A., 271
Jimenez, N. V., 164, 165, 166
Jitendra, A. K., 261
John, O. P., 10, 120, 255
Johnson, C. L., 50
Johnson, D. J., 166
Johnson, F. A., 50
Johnson, I. H., 286
Johnson, J. H., 22
Johnson, M. B., 162
Johnson, M. J., 297
Johnson-Powell, G., 73
Jones, E. E., 61
Jones, E. G., 61
Jones, J., 296, 314
Jung, M., 243
Junn, J., 104

K

Kagan, J., 240

AUTHOR INDEX

Kagawa-Singer, M., 48, 49, 50, 57, 58, 59, 60, 61, 63
Kahneman, D., 254
Kain, C. D., 297
Kamphaus, R. W., 262
Kanel, K., 297
Kao, G., 160
Kaplan, H. I., 68, 69
Kaptchuk, T. J., 174
Karno, M., 24, 85, 97
Karuza, J., Jr., 247
Kashima, Y., 104, 156
Kashiwagi, K., 169
Kato, K., 72, 111, 118
Katz, M. M., 20, 45
Kaufman, J. C., 169
Kaufman, J. S., 48
Kaufman, S., 49, 56
Kawanishi, Y., 62
Kawasaki, N., 297
Kay, M., 61
Keats, D. M., 106
Keefe, K., 141
Keefe, S. E., 97
Keitner, G., 200
Kelley, M. L., 189
Kellner, R., 71
Kendler, K. S., 25, 216
Kennard, B. D., 201
Kennedy, E., 165, 168
Kennel, R. G., 286
Kerner, J. F., 65
Kesselman, M., 125
Kessler, R. C., 17, 22, 38, 63, 205, 206, 208, 211, 216
Khoo, G., 81
Kidder, L., 247
Kiefer, C. W., 89
Kim, B. S. K., 285
Kim, E. J., 80
Kim, G., 192, 244
Kim, H. S., 72
Kim, K., 119, 206
Kim, M. S., 111, 116
Kim, S. C., 244
Kim, S. J., 289
Kim, S. Y., 187, 197
Kim, U., 78, 82, 87, 102, 156
Kim, Y. S., 26, 72
Kincaid, D. L., 272
King, C. R., 65

Kinzie, J. D., 21, 22, 36, 207
Kirk, B. A., 269, 271
Kirk, S. A., 49, 53, 56
Kirmayer, L. J., 44, 55, 69
Kitano, H. H., 10
Kitayama, S., 107, 109, 110, 114, 115, 116, 175, 182, 185, 278
Kivlighan, D., 293
Kleinknecht, E. E., 110
Kleinknecht, R. A., 110
Kleinman, A. M., 2, 19, 20, 31, 32, 36, 37, 39, 44, 45, 48, 50, 55, 56, 57, 62, 69, 70, 72, 73, 173, 182, 231, 249
Kleinman, J., 50, 56, 62, 70
Kluckhohn, C., 266, 267, 268
Knepp, D., 31, 286
Kochanska, G., 186
Koenig, B. A., 50, 63
Koizumi, K., 35
Kolody, B., 97
Koo, J., 33
Koplewicz, H. S., 234
Korchin, S. J., 61
Korman, M., 283
Korten, A., 65
Kramer, R. M., 120
Krishnan, A., 100
Kuhn, M. H., 118
Kunn, P., 43, 90
Kuo, H.-S., 206
Kuo, P. Y., 77, 79, 84, 85
Kuo, W. H., 22, 23, 36, 176, 207, 208
Kurasaki, K. S., 26, 27, 46, 205, 210, 217
Kurokawa, M., 114
Kurtines, W., 78, 98
Kurtz, R. M., 254
Kutchins, H., 49, 53, 56
Kwak, Y. S., 26, 72
Kwan, K.-L. K., 80, 85, 87
Kwan, V. S. Y., 110, 112, 152

L

LaCrosse, M. B., 288
Ladany, N., 283, 287, 290
LaFromboise, T. D., 97, 98, 263, 286, 288
Lai, C. S. Y., 110, 240
Lai, E. W. M., 79, 83, 87, 89
Lam, M., 192

AUTHOR INDEX

Lam, W. L., 188
Lamborn, S. D., 188
Landale, N., 93
Landerman, R., 37
Landrine, H., 107, 109
Lang, J. G., 85
Lang, O., 190, 191, 195, 196
Langenbucher, J. W., 30
Larkin, K. C., 272
LaRue, T., 297
Lasry, L., 98, 100
Lau, B. W., 69
Lau, J. K. C., 72
Lau, J. T.-F., 24, 216
Lau, S., 186, 188, 195
Lazarus, R., 48, 49, 89
Leaf, P. J., 13, 25, 206
Lebra, T., 49, 51, 60
Lee, A. Y., 118
Lee, C. K., 16, 69
Lee, F., 33
Lee, H. Y., 26
Lee, L. C., 26, 170, 249, 280
Lee, N., 24, 216
Lee, P. A., 58, 100, 102, 176, 180
Lee, R., 216
Lee, R. G., 284
Lee, R. M., 192, 243, 286, 291, 294
Lee, R. Y. P., 151
Lee, S., 20, 68
Lee, S. Y., 19
Lee, Y. H., 26, 72
Lee-Oh, J., 236
Lehman, D. R., 114, 175
Leiderman, P. H., 188
Leigh, J., 223
Lemelson, R. B., 52, 54, 55, 62
Lent, R. W., 272, 279
Leong, F. T. L., 154, 265, 266, 267, 268, 269, 270, 271, 273, 274, 275, 276, 277, 278, 279
Lese, K. P., 163
Leung, A. C. N., 244
Leung, K., 104, 150, 151, 152, 156, 187, 188, 189, 197
Leung, P. K., 25
Leung, S. A., 272, 273
Leung, T., 111, 116
Lew, A., 21, 237
Lew, S., 32
Lew, W. J., 186

Lewin, K., 268
Lewis, D. M., 277
Lewis-Fernandez, R., 31, 32
Li, B., 199
Li, D., 195
Li, X.-R., 234, 235
Lien, P., 104
Lim, R. F., 33
Lin, C. C., 186, 187, 188, 193
Lin, E. H. B., 36, 37, 57
Lin, J. C. H., 244, 248
Lin, K.-M., 21, 22, 33, 46, 70, 73
Lin, N., 36
Lin, T., 35, 38
Lindholm, K. J., 85, 276
Link, B., 26
Lipowski, Z. J., 36, 37
Littlewood, R., 68
Liu, J. Q., 65
Liu, M., 195
Liu, P. Y., 307
Liu, W. M., 160
Liu, W. T., 15, 27, 217
Lock, A., 48
Lock, M., 51, 59, 223
Locke, D., 296, 314
Lofquist, L. H., 277
Long, F. Y., 235
Lonner, W. J., 124, 136
López, S. R., 42, 107, 125, 221, 293
Louie, C. E., 297
Lowe, S. M., 285, 293
Lu, F., 296
Lukes, S., 50
Lung, C. T., 26, 217
Luo, X., 234
Lutz, C., 174, 175
Lynch, E. W., 125, 248
Lynn, R., 161

M

Maccoby, E. E., 186, 187
Madden, T., 192
Madsen, R., 51, 175
Maestas, M. V., 86, 87, 89
Magee, W. J., 38
Magids, D., 290, 298
Maital, S., 199
Maldonado, R., 79, 83, 99

AUTHOR INDEX

Malgady, R. G., 29, 30, 61, 79, 82, 194
Manaster, G. J., 104
Manese, J. E., 263
Mann, L., 106
Manson, S., 36, 73
Mao, L. M., 33
Maracek, J., 295
Marcos, L. R., 125
Marcus, M. B., 104
Marin, G., 79
Markus, H. R., 107, 109, 111, 114, 115, 116, 118, 175, 182, 185, 278
Marsella, A. J., 25, 35, 36, 50, 107, 108, 109, 182, 207, 208
Martin, J. A., 186, 187
Martinez, J. L., Jr., 79
Maruyama, M., 285
Mason, J., 307
Masuda, G. I., 244
Masuda, M., 22, 81, 83
Matsui, S., 285
Matsumoto, A. R., 164
Matsumoto, D., 109, 115, 116
Matsumoto, Y., 119
Matsuoka, J., 21, 154
Matsushita, Y. J., 285
Matthews, L., 293
Mau, W. C., 166
May, W. T., 29
McArthur, D. S., 236, 241
McBride-Chang, C., 201
McCallum, R. S., 161
McCrae, R. R., 145, 147, 148, 151
McDavis, R. J., 283
McGoldrick, M., 59, 137, 201, 249
McGonagle, K. A., 25, 216
McGraw, K. M., 113
McKinney, H., 10
McPartland, T., 118
Mechanic, D., 53, 56, 221
Meehl, P. E., 255
Mehta, S., 81
Meller, P. J., 44, 298
Mellins, C. A., 297
Mena, F. J., 83
Mendoza, R. H., 85
Meredith, G. M., 32, 83
Meredith, W. H., 243
Merta, R. J., 293
Messe, L. A., 79

Mezzich, J. E., 31, 41, 44, 67, 68, 69, 71, 73
Michels, R., 71
Michitsuji, S., 26
Miller, G. A., 56
Miller, I., 200
Miller, J. G., 107
Miller, L., 56
Miller, L. J., 162
Min, S. K., 26
Minde, T., 87
Minor, C. W., 270, 271, 280
Mishler, E. G., 223
Mizuta, I., 187
Moeschberger, M., 43, 90
Mok, D., 87
Mok, T. A., 80
Mokuau, N., 154
Mont-Reynaud, R., 79, 80, 187
Mookherjee, H. N., 25
Moore, L. J., 25
Moos, B. S., 188
Moos, R. H., 188
Morales, M. L., 41
Morishima, J. K., 125, 273
Morrissey, R. F., 234
Mounts, N. S., 187, 188
Mouw, T., 165, 168
Moy, S., 270, 277
Munet-Vilaro, F., 61
Munoz, R. F., 85
Munoz-Sandoval, A. F., 162
Munro, D., 106
Murase, K., 133
Murphy, M. C., 286
Murray, H. A., 266, 267, 268
Murthy, K., 81
Myers, H., 58
Myers, J. K., 25
Mylvaganam, G. A., 19

N

Nadelson, C., 25
Nakagawa, K., 166
Nakakuki, M., 237, 242, 243
Nakana, Y., 20, 25, 26, 38
Nakasaki, G., 72
Nathan, P. E., 30

340 AUTHOR INDEX

National Council on Measurement in
  Education, 261
National Institute of Mental Health, 205
Negy, C., 82, 86
Neider, J., 21
Nelson, C. B., 25, 216
Neugebaruer, D. D., 22
Neugebauer, R., 26
Nevill, D. D., 276
Neville, H. A., 289
Ng, M., 272
Ngo, V., 192, 244
Nguyen, H. H., 79, 86
Nguyen, N. A., 243
Nichols, D. S., 42
Nielson, D., 291
Nihonban WISC-III Kanko-Inakai, 162
Nisbett, R. E., 117
Nishida, T., 119
Nixon, J., 40
Norlock, F. E., 63
Norris, A. E., 85, 86
Nunnally, J., 130
Nuttall, E. V., 235
Nuttall, R. L., 235
Nyberg, B., 99

O

Oetting, E. R., 98, 100, 130
Oetzel, J. G., 111
Ogilvie, D. M., 116
Ogino, M., 199
Oh-Hwang, Y., 187
Ohnuki-Tierney, E., 59
Ohta, Y., 26, 38
Ohtsuka, T., 26
Okagaki, L., 197
Okamura, A., 246
Okano, K.-I., 240, 243
Okazaki, S., 30, 102, 110, 111, 112, 116,
  154, 155, 160, 161, 181, 207, 273
Olatawura, M., 25
Oldham, J. M., 44
Olesen, V. L., 64
Olmedo, E. L., 79, 86, 96, 98
Olson, D. H., 188
Ong Hing, B., 216
Ong, A., 192
Ong, P., 58

Opton, E., 48
Osipow, S. H., 272, 280
Osvold, L. L., 79, 82
Ots, T., 38, 62
Ottavi, T. M., 291
Ottens, A. J., 286
Owan, T. C., 45
Owen, S. V., 80
Ownbey, S. F., 100
Ozawa, K., 110

P

Padilla, A. M., 83, 85, 86, 90, 92, 96, 97,
  98, 104, 279, 286
Padilla, G., 56, 60
Padilla, J., 42
Painter, K., 199
Pak, A. W. P., 23
Pancheri, P., 142
Pang, K. Y. C., 32
Pangan, R. W., 62
Paniagua, F. A., 43, 157
Pannu, R., 85
Park, C., 221
Park, H. S., 165, 168
Park, R. E., 97
Park, S., 307
Parron, D. L., 31, 44, 45, 67, 68, 73
Pascual, L., 199
Pathak, D., 71
Patterson, G., 187, 193
Paul, B. D., 48, 255
Payton, C. R., 42
Pearce, J., 59, 137, 201, 249
Pearlin, I., 52
Pecheux, M.-G., 199
Pedersen, P. B., 286, 299
Pelham, B. W., 111, 117, 118
Pelletier, L. G., 61
Peng, K., 117
Peng, S. S., 159, 160, 161, 164, 165, 166,
  168
Perry, S., 69, 71
Phelan, J. C., 63, 64
Phillips, L., 61
Phillips, S. D., 254
Phinney, J. S., 80, 81, 82, 83, 89, 96, 100,
  186, 189, 192
Pilkonis, P. A., 240

AUTHOR INDEX

Pittinsky, T. L., 164
Plake, B. S., 79, 80, 86
Plog, S., 25
Ponterotto, J. G., 44, 93, 100, 263, 283, 286, 287, 288, 289, 290, 291, 293, 296, 298
Pope-Davis, D. B., 288, 290, 292, 297, 298, 299
Price, R. K., 25
Prince, R., 70

Q

Qian, Z., 164, 165, 166, 167, 168
Qu, G. Y., 26, 217
Quintana, D., 100
Quintana, S. M., 283, 286

R

Rabinowitz, V. C., 247
Radford, M., 26
Radloff, L., 176, 177, 180
Rahn, C., 199
Ramos-Sánchez, L., 289
Ramsey, E., 187
Rao, N., 201
Rasmussen, S., 200
Redding, S. G., 272
Ree, H., 26
Reglin, G. L., 160
Reiger, D. A., 10, 26, 205, 206, 207
Reynolds, C. R., 262, 291
Reznick, J. S., 240
Rhee, S., 24, 72
Rhodes, C., 104
Rhyne, M. C., 297
Riba, M. B., 44
Ricco, R., 32
Rickard-Figueroa, K., 32
Rieger, B. P., 298
Riley, C., 25
Rin, H., 35, 68
Ritter, P. L., 188
Robbins, J. M., 44
Robbins, S. B., 163
Roberts, D. F., 188
Roberts, G. E., 236, 241
Robins, L. N., 10, 26, 205, 206, 207
Robinson, L., 31, 161, 286

Rodolfa, E., 297
Rodriguez, N., 58
Rogers, M. R., 286, 288
Rogler, L. H., 21, 24, 53, 61, 69, 79, 82, 85, 194, 220, 230
Rohena-Diaz, E., 261
Roid, G. H., 162
Rooney, R. A., 272
Rosenbaum, J., 71
Rosenberg, M., 48
Rosenthal, D. A., 33, 79, 80, 96, 186, 187, 188, 193
Rossell, J., 89
Rotherman-Borus, M. J., 80, 83
Rowe, D. C., 197
Rubin, K. H., 199
Ruef, M. L., 162
Ruiz, Y., 97, 100
Rumbaut, R. G., 36, 77, 80, 84
Rushton, J. P., 163, 167
Russell, C. S., 188
Russell, J. A., 175
Ruzek, S. B., 64

S

Sadock, B. J., 68
Said, E., 284
Sakuma, M., 111
Sameroff, S., 200
Sanchez, C. M., 290
Sanchez, J., 296, 314
Sandelowski, M., 219
Sandoval, J., 252, 254, 258, 262
Sanjek, R., 58
Santana, F., 25
Santiago, E. S., 89
Sarason, I. G., 22
Sartorius, N., 25, 53, 69, 90, 104
Sato, T., 110, 113
Sattler, J. M., 161, 236, 257
Sayegh, L., 98, 100
Schaefer, E. S., 186
Scheier, M. F., 127, 129
Scheueneman, J. D., 262, 263
Schiller, M., 200
Schooler, C., 35
Schulman, K. A., 58
Schwebel, A. I., 25
Schweder, R. A., 69

AUTHOR INDEX

Scopetta, M. A., 78
Scott, R., 235
Scriven, M., 255
Sedlacek, W. E., 160
Seifer, R., 200
Seike, M., 111
Serafica, F. C., 25, 274, 275, 276, 278
Sharkey, W. F., 110, 111, 240
Shaver, P. R., 245
Shay, J., 223
Shea, B. M., 13, 25
Shek, D. T. L., 194, 195
Shen, H., 26, 46, 97, 217
Shih, M., 164
Shon, S. P., 59, 125, 196, 238
Siegel, J. M., 22
Siegfried, J., 219, 228, 229, 230
Silva, E., 25
Simons, R. C., 21, 38, 72
Singelis, T. M., 110, 111, 112, 113, 116, 152, 240, 242, 243
Sistrunk, S., 65
Skinner, M., 193
Slaughter-Defoe, D. T., 166
Smith, C., 283
Smith, D., 25
Smith, E. J., 299
Smith, E. M. J., 89
Smith, P. L., 272, 276
Smith, R., 51
Smith, S. K., 107
Snidman, N., 240
Snowden, 14, 19, 56, 207, 284
Snowden, L. R., 19, 22
Snyder, M., 127, 130
Sodowsky, G. R., 77, 79, 80, 81, 82, 83, 85, 86, 87, 89, 284, 285, 290, 298
Song, W. Z., 141, 142, 150, 156
Sorenson, S. B., 85, 97
Sparks, R., 283, 288, 289, 298
Speight, J. D., 277
Speight, S. L., 286
Spielberger, C. D., 156
Spiro, M., 48, 49
Sprenkle, D. H., 188
Stadler, H., 296, 314
Steinberg, L., 167, 185, 186, 187, 188
Stern, M. P., 86
Sternbach, R., 48
Stewart, S. L., 192, 199
Stollak, G. E., 79

Stonequist, E. V., 97
Strongman, K. T., 108
Strozier, A. L., 283
Su, L.-Y., 234
Suarez-Balcazar, Y., 283, 286
Sue, D., 20, 154, 237
Sue, D. W., 10, 20, 141, 207, 237, 238, 269, 271, 283
Sue, L., 10
Sue, S., 10, 18, 19, 23, 24, 30, 33, 38, 46, 68, 102, 107, 141, 154, 155, 161, 206, 207, 210, 212, 271, 273, 284, 293, 295
Suh, E. M., 108, 121
Suinn, R. M., 32, 81
Sulieman, R., 100
Sullivan, W. M., 51, 175
Sun, H. F., 152
Sun, Y., 166
Super, D. E., 276
Suryani, L. K., 65
Suwanlert, S., 249
Suzuki, L. A., 44, 93, 161, 272, 296, 298
Svy, D., 223, 227
Swanson, J. W., 13, 25
Swartz, M., 37
Swidler, A., 51, 175
Szapocznik, J., 78, 98

T

Taffe, R. C., 284, 290
Takada, K., 38
Takahashi, R., 25
Takaki, R., 283
Takanishi, R., 166
Takata, T., 110, 112, 116
Takeuchi, D. T., 10, 18, 19, 22, 23, 35, 37, 46, 62, 206, 207, 209, 217, 284, 307
Takeuchi, M., 235
Tally, S. R., 187
Tanaka-Matsumi, J., 32
Tang, J., 272
Tang, M., 272, 273, 274, 276
Tata, S. P., 270, 276
Taylor, K. M., 185, 272
Teleghani, C. K., 65
Telles, C. A., 85
Thakker, J., 108
Thich, N. H., 175

AUTHOR INDEX

Thoits, P., 221
Thomas, A. J., 286
Thompson, C. E., 297
Thompson, L. L., 113
Thorndike, R. L., 161
Thorndike, R. M., 124
Timbers, D. M., 25
Time, 185
Ting-Toomey, S., 49, 79, 81, 119, 151, 181
Tipton, S. M., 51, 175
Toda, S., 199
Tokuno, K. A., 238
Toperek, R., 314
Toporek, R., 296
Tori, C. D., 165
Torres, S., 286
Tou, L. A., 270
Townes, B. D., 234
Tozuma, L., 22
Tran, T. V., 22
Triandis, H. C., 41, 108, 113, 134, 185
Tropp, L. R., 85
Trull, T. J., 150
Tryon, W. W., 61
Tsai, J. L., 58, 95, 97, 98, 100, 101, 102, 176, 180
Tsai, R., 243
Tsai, Y.-M., 22, 23, 36
Tseng, H. M., 189
Tseng, V., 188, 192
Tseng, W. S., 38, 55, 182
Tung, M., 174, 181, 295
Turner, R. G., 129
Tursky, B., 48
Tversky, A., 254
Tyler, F. B., 96
Tyler, T. R., 120

U

U.S. Bureau of the Census, 77, 100, 173, 251
Uba, L., 58, 126, 195, 196, 207, 238, 284
Uchino, J., 38
Upshur, J. A., 261
Urcuyo, L., 125

V

van de Vijver, F., 42
Varley, C. K., 234
Vasquez-Nuttall, E., 299
Vaughn, C. A., 41
Vázquez, L. A., 286
Vazsonyi, A. T., 197
Vega, W. A., 97
Venuti, P., 199
Vernon, P. E., 161
Veroff, J., 104
Verran, J., 61
Vigil, P., 32
Vignoe, D., 234
Vyt, A., 199

W

Wagatsuma, Y., 85, 276
Walker, L., 289
Walsh, J. A., 42, 280
Wampold, B. E., 289, 293
Wan, G., 234, 243
Wang, A., 243
Wang, C. H., 15, 208
Wang, C. H. C., 186, 189
Wang, G. C. S., 19
Wang, L., 199
Wang, X., 26
Wang, Y., 46, 217
Wang, Y. W. V., 84
Ward, B. E., 194
Ward, C., 154
Ward, T., 108
Wartofsky, L., 224
Waxler, N. E., 53
Weiss, B., 249
Weiss, C. I., 307
Weiss, D. J., 276
Weissman, M. M., 13, 25
Weisz, J. R., 234
Wellenkamp, J., 49
Wellesz, E., 50
Wells, K. M., 105
Welsh, G. S., 130
Wen, J. K., 65
Werth, E. B., 199
Westermeyer, J., 21, 35
Wewers, M. E., 43, 90

344 AUTHOR INDEX

Whang, P. A., 167
Wibulswasdi, P., 65
Wiese, M. J., 286
Williams, D., 58
Williams, H. L., 243
Williams, S., 65
Williamson, L., 80
Wilson, L. G., 35
Wilson, R. W., 240
Windle, M., 193
Wing, J., 40
Wintrob, R. M., 38
Wise, S. L., 284, 290
Wittchen, H. U., 25, 38, 216
Wittig, M. A., 42
Wolf, M., 191, 194, 195, 196, 197
Wong, J., 24, 216
Wong, K. C., 68
Wong, N. Y. C., 117
Wong, Y., 95
Wong-Kerberg, L., 246
Wong-Rieger, D., 100
Woodcock, R. W., 162
Woods, D. J., 82, 86
World Health Organization, 52, 214
Wright, B., 164, 165, 166, 199, 286
Wu, D. Y. H., 174, 182, 190, 194
Wu, S., 272
Wunsch-Hitzig, R., 26
Wyer, R. S. J., 119
Wynne, L. C., 25

X

Xia, Z. Y., 15, 26, 217
Xie, D., 150
Xie, Y., 165, 168
Xu, C. L., 26, 217
Xu, D., 38

Y

Yamada, A. M., 110
Yamaguchi, S., 156

Yamamoto, J., 21, 24, 26, 72
Yan, H., 26
Yan, Y., 58
Yang, D. C., 235
Yang, K.-S., 152, 175, 242, 243
Yang, M.-C. U., 127, 128, 196
Yang, Z., 234
Yao, E. L., 32
Yee, B. W. K., 21, 237
Yee, C. M., 56
Yeh, E. K., 182, 211
Yik, M. S. M., 142, 150, 175
Ying, Y.-W., 23, 58, 95, 97, 100, 102,
    176, 177, 179, 180, 181
Yoon, E., 19
Young, A., 69
Young, D., 35
Young, K., 45, 133
Young, M., 78
Yu, E., 15
Yu, E. S. H., 26, 217
Yu, L. C., 272
Yuhua, C., 38
Yum, J. O., 272

Z

Zak, I., 98
Zane, N. W. S., 25, 26, 32, 33, 45, 81, 83,
    128, 129, 133, 170, 181, 207, 249, 280,
    284, 293, 307
Zhang, A. Y., 14, 19, 22, 207
Zhang, J. P., 156
Zhang, J. X., 156
Zhang, M. Y., 15, 26, 217
Zhao, S., 25, 216
Zheng, Y. P., 35, 72
Zheng, Y.-P., 18, 19, 21, 23
Zhou, M., 165, 168
Zimbardo, P. G., 240